Understanding Patient Safety

Second Edition

Robert M. Wachter, MD

Professor and Associate Chairman
Department of Medicine
Marc and Lynne Benioff Endowed Chair
Chief of the Division of Hospital Medicine
University of California, San Francisco
Chief of the Medical Service
UCSF Medical Center
San Francisco, California

McGraw Hill Medical

New York   Chicago   San Francisco   Lisbon   London   Madrid   Mexico City
Milan   New Delhi   San Juan   Seoul   Singapore   Sydney   Toronto

Understanding Patient Safety, Second Edition

1 2 3 4 5 6 7 8 9 0 CTP/CTP 17 16 15 14 13 12

ISBN 978-0-07-176578-7
MHID 0-07-176578-6

This book was set in Times New Roman PS by Thomson Digital.
The editors were James F. Shanahan and Kim J. Davis.
The production supervisor was Sherri Souffrance.
Project management was provided by Gaurav Srivastava of Thomson Digital.
China Translation & Printing, Ltd. was the printer and binder.

Library of Congress Cataloging-in-Publication Data

Wachter, Robert M.
  Understanding patient safety / Robert M. Wachter. —2nd ed.
   p. ; cm.
  Includes bibliographical references and index.
  ISBN-13: 978-0-07-176578-7 (pbk. : alk. paper)
  ISBN-10: 0-07-176578-6 (pbk. : alk. paper)
   I. Title.
  [DNLM: 1. Medical Errors—prevention & control. 2. Safety Management—
methods. WB 100]
  610.28'9—dc23
                                                    2011042733

Contents

Chapter 16

Workforce Issues 281

Chapter 17

Education and Training Issues 303

Chapter 18

The Malpractice System 321

SECTION IV: APPENDICES

Preface

In late 1999, the Institute of Medicine published *To Err is Human: Building a Safer Health Care System*.[1] Although the IOM has published more than 600 reports since *To Err*, none have been nearly as influential. The reason: extrapolating from data from the Harvard Medical Practice Study,[2,3] performed a decade earlier, the authors estimated that 44,000 to 98,000 Americans die each year from medical errors. More shockingly, they translated these numbers into the now-famous "jumbo jet units," pointing out that this death toll would be the equivalent of a jumbo jet crashing each and every day in the United States.

Although some critiqued the jumbo jet analogy as hyperbolic, I like it for several reasons. First, it provides a vivid and tangible icon for the magnitude of the problem (obviously, if extended to the rest of the world, the toll would be many times higher). Second, if in fact a jumbo jet were to crash every day, who among us would even consider flying electively? Third, and most importantly, consider for a moment what our society would do—and spend—to fix the problem if there were an aviation disaster every day. The answer, of course, is that there would be no limit to what we would do to fix *that* problem. Yet prior to the IOM Report, we were doing next to nothing to make patients safer.

This is not to imply that the millions of committed, hardworking, and well-trained doctors, nurses, pharmacists, therapists, and healthcare administrators *wanted* to harm people from medical mistakes. They did not—to the degree that Albert Wu has labeled providers who commit an error that causes terrible harm "second victims."[4] Yet we now understand that the problem of medical errors is not fundamentally one of "bad apples" (though there are some), but rather one of competent providers working in a chaotic system that has not prioritized safety. As Kaveh Shojania and I wrote in our book, *Internal Bleeding*:

> Decades of research, mostly from outside healthcare, has confirmed our own medical experience: Most errors are made by good but fallible people working in dysfunctional systems, which means that making care safer depends on buttressing the system to prevent or catch the inevitable lapses of mortals. This logical approach is common in other complex, high-tech industries, but it has been woefully ignored in medicine. Instead, we have steadfastly clung to the view that an error is a moral failure by an individual, a posture that has

left patients feeling angry and ready to blame, and providers feeling guilty and demoralized. Most importantly, it hasn't done a damn thing to make healthcare safer.[5]

Try for a moment to think of systems in healthcare that were truly "hardwired" for safety prior to 1999. Can you come up with any? I can think of just one: the double-checking done by nurses before releasing a unit of blood to prevent ABO transfusion errors. Now think about other error-prone areas: preventing harmful drug interactions or giving patients medicines to which they are allergic; ensuring that patients' preferences regarding resuscitation are respected; guaranteeing that the correct limbs are operated on; making sure primary care doctors have the necessary information after a hospitalization; diagnosing patients with chest pain in the emergency department correctly—none of these were organized in ways that ensured safety.

Interestingly, many of the answers were there for the taking—from industries as diverse as take-out restaurants to nuclear power plants, from commercial aviation to automobile manufacturing—and there are now dozens of examples of successes in applying techniques drawn from other fields to healthcare safety and quality (Table P–1).[6] Why does healthcare depend so much on the experiences of other industries to guide its improvement efforts? In part, it is because other industries have long recognized the diverse expertise that must be tapped to produce the best possible product at the lowest cost. In healthcare, the absence of any incentive (until recently) to focus on quality and safety, our burgeoning biomedical knowledge base, our siloed approach to training, and, frankly, professional hubris have caused us to look inward, not outward, for answers. The fact that we are now routinely seeking insights from aviation, manufacturing, education, and other industries, and embracing paradigms from engineering, sociology, psychology, and management, may prove to be the most enduring benefit of the patient safety movement.

All of this makes the field of patient safety at once vexing and exciting. To keep patients safe will take a uniquely interdisciplinary effort, one in which doctors, nurses, pharmacists, and administrators forge new types of relationships. It will demand that we look to other industries for good ideas, while recognizing that caring for patients is different enough from other human endeavors that thoughtful adaptation is critical. It will require that we tamp down our traditionally rigid hierarchies, without forgetting the importance of leadership or compromising crucial lines of authority. It will take additional resources, although investments in safety may well pay off in new efficiencies, lower provider turnover, and fewer expensive complications. It will require a thoughtful embrace of this new notion of systems

Table P-1   **EXAMPLES OF PATIENT SAFETY PRACTICES DRAWN AT LEAST IN PART FROM NON-HEALTHCARE INDUSTRIES**

Strategy (Described in Chapter X)	Nonhealthcare Example	Study Demonstrating Value in Healthcare	Impetus for Wider Implementation in Healthcare
Improved ratios of providers to "customers" (Chapter 16)	Teacher-to-student ratios (such as in class-size initiatives)	Needleman et al. (2011)	Legislation in many states mandating minimum nurse-to-patient ratios, other pressure
Decrease provider fatigue (Chapter 16)	Consecutive work-hour limitations for pilots, truck drivers	Landrigan et al. (2004)	Accreditation Council for Graduate Medical Education (ACGME) regulations limiting resident duty hours
Improve teamwork and communication (Chapter 15)	Crew resource management (CRM) in aviation	Neily et al. (2010)	Some hospitals now requiring team training for individuals who work in risky areas such as labor and delivery or surgery
Use of simulators (Chapter 17)	Simulator use in aviation and the military	Bruppacher et al. (2010)	Medical simulation now required for credentialing for certain procedures; technology improving and costs falling
Executive Walk Rounds (Chapter 22)	"Management by Walking Around" in business	Thomas et al. (2005)	Executive Walk Rounds not required, but remain a popular practice
Bar coding (Chapter 13)	Use of bar coding in manufacturing, retail, and food sales	Poon et al. (2010)	U.S. Food and Drug Administration now requires bar codes on most prescription medications; bar coding or its equivalent may ultimately be required in many identification processes

Reproduced and updated with permission from Wachter RM. Playing well with others: "translocational research" in patient safety. *AHRQ WebM&M* (serial online); September 2005. Available at: http://webmm.ahrq.gov/perspective.aspx?perspectiveID=9.

Bruppacher HR, Alam SK, LeBlanc VR, et al. Simulation-based training improves physicians' performance in patient care in high-stakes clinical setting of cardiac surgery. *Anesthesiology* 2010;112:985–992.

Landrigan CP, Rothschild JM, Cronin JW, et al. Effect of reducing interns' work hours on serious medical errors in intensive care units. *N Engl J Med* 2004;351:1838–1848.

Needleman J, Buerhaus P, Pankratz VS, et al. Nurse staffing and inpatient hospital mortality. *N Engl J Med* 2011;364:1037–1045.

Neily J, Mills PD, Young-Xu Y, et al. Association between implementation of a medical team training program and surgical mortality. *JAMA* 2010;304:1693–1700.

Poon EG, Keohane CA, Yoon CS, et al. Effect of bar-code technology on the safety of medication administration. *N Engl J Med* 2010;362:1698–1707.

Thomas EJ, Sexton JB, Neilands TB, et al. The effect of executive walk rounds on nurse safety climate attitudes: a randomized trial of clinical units. *BMC Health Serv Res* 2005;5:28.

thinking, while recognizing the absolute importance of the well-trained and committed caregiver. Again, from *Internal Bleeding*:

> Although there is much we can learn from industries that have long embraced the systems approach,... medical care is much more complex and customized than flying an Airbus: At 3 A.M., the critically ill patient needs superb and compassionate doctors and nurses more than she needs a better checklist. We take seriously the awesome privileges and responsibilities that society grants us as physicians, and don't believe for a second that individual excellence and professional passion will become expendable even after our trapeze swings over netting called a "safer system." In the end, medical errors are a hard enough nut to crack that we need excellent doctors *and* safer systems.[5]

I wrote the first edition of *Understanding Patient Safety* in 2007. In preparing this new volume four years later, I was astounded by the deepening understanding of some very fundamental issues in safety, and by how remarkably dynamic this field has proven to be. Some of the recent epiphanies and trends, all of which will be discussed in detail, include:

> *Information technology (Chapter 13)*: In the early days of the safety movement, many people saw information technology (IT) as the holy grail. Our naïveté—about the value of IT and its ease of implementation—has been replaced by a much more realistic appreciation of the challenges of implementing healthcare IT systems and leveraging them to prevent harm. Several installations of massive and expensive IT systems have failed (including one at my own hospital), and the adoption curve for IT has remained sluggish. The U.S. federal government is providing more than $20 billion to support the diffusion of computerized systems that meet certain standards ("meaningful use"), which is finally leading to a significant uptick in implementations.[7] With more systems going online, we are beginning to gain a better appreciation of the true value of IT in patient safety, as well as how to mitigate some of the unanticipated consequences and potential harms.[8]

> *Measurement of safety, errors, and harm (Chapters 1 and 14)*: In the early years of the safety field, the target was errors, and we focused on measuring, and decreasing, error rates. This paradigm has largely given way to a new focus on measuring and attacking "harm" or "adverse events." The Global Trigger Tool[9]—an instrument that supports a focused chart review looking for harm—has become increasingly popular, particularly as the limitations of other methods (incident reports, the AHRQ

Patient Safety Indicators) have become clearer.[10] One influential and disheartening study found no significant improvement in harm measures in North Carolina hospitals between 2003 and 2008, driving additional pressure for improvement.[11]

The checklist (Chapter 15): The remarkable success of checklist-based interventions in preventing central line–associated bloodstream infections[12] and surgical complications,[13,14] coupled with articles and books by respected safety leaders,[15–17] have given the "lowly checklist" a newly exalted status in the patient safety field. The same leaders, however, caution that checklists are not a magic bullet, and that they can fail when introduced without sufficient attention to questions of culture and leadership.[18,19]

Safety targets: The safety field's embrace of healthcare-associated infections as a key target was driven by the fact that such infections are more easily measured and, in some cases, prevented than many other kinds of harm. This prioritization is natural but risks paying inadequate attention to other crucial targets that are less easily measured and fixed. One of my pet peeves is the short shrift we've given to diagnostic errors (Chapter 6), a state of affairs that has begun to change only in recent years.[20]

Policy issues in patient safety: In the early years of the safety field, much of the pressure to improve came from accreditors such as the Joint Commission and from the media, local and regional collaborations, and nongovernmental organizations such as the Institute for Healthcare Improvement.[21] We are finally witnessing the emergence of a true business case for safety, driven by public and governmental reporting systems,[22] along with fines for serious cases of harm and "no pay for errors" policies.[23] Increasingly, concerns about the cost of healthcare are being coupled with concerns about patient safety—leading to payment penalties tied to substandard performance in areas such as readmissions, healthcare-associated infections, and others.[24] In other words, we have entered an era in which the business case for patient safety has become sufficiently robust that many boards and CEOs now consider it a mission-critical endeavor.

Balancing "no blame" and accountability: As I mentioned earlier, the focus of the early years of the safety field was on improving systems of care and creating a "no blame" culture. This focus was not only scientifically correct (based on what we know about errors in other industries) but also politically astute. Particularly for U.S. physicians—long conditioned to hearing the term "error" and, in a kind of Rorschach test, thinking "medical malpractice"—the systems approach generated goodwill and buy-in.

But perhaps the greatest change in my own thinking between writing the first and second editions of this book is an increased appreciation of the need to balance a "no blame" approach (for the innocent slips and mistakes for which it is appropriate) with an accountability approach (including blame and penalties as needed) for caregivers who are habitually careless, disruptive, unmotivated, or fail to heed reasonable quality and safety rules.[25] Getting this balance right is one of the most central questions we face in patient safety over the next decade.

This is just a short list designed to hint at some of the major changes that have influenced, even rocked, the still-young field of patient safety in the past few years. Another measure of the field's evolution is the fact that this second edition is about 30% longer than the first and has more than twice as many references. In other words, if you're looking for a stable, settled field, look elsewhere.

This book aims to teach the key principles of patient safety to a diverse audience: physicians, nurses, pharmacists, other healthcare providers, quality and safety professionals, risk managers, hospital administrators, and others. It is suitable for all levels of readers: from the senior physician trying to learn this new way of approaching his or her work, to the medical or nursing student, to the risk manager or hospital board member seeking to get more involved in institutional safety efforts. The fact that the same book can speak to all of these groups (whereas few clinical textbooks could) is another mark of the interdisciplinary nature of this field. Although many of the examples and references are from the United States (mostly because they are more familiar to me), my travels and studies (including the time I spent in England as a Fulbright Scholar in 2011) have convinced me that most of the issues are the same internationally, and that all countries can learn much from each other. I have made every effort, therefore, to make the book relevant to a geographically diverse audience, and have included key references and tools from outside the United States.

The book is divided into three main sections. In the introduction, I'll describe the epidemiology of error, distinguish safety from quality, discuss the key mental models that inform our modern understanding of the safety field, and summarize the policy environment for patient safety. In Section II, I'll review different error types, taking advantage of real cases to describe various kinds of mistakes and safety hazards, introduce new terminology, and discuss what we know about how errors happen and how they can be prevented. Although many prevention strategies will be touched on in Section II, more general issues regarding various strategies (from both individual institutional and broader policy perspectives) will be reviewed in Section III. After a concluding chapter, the Appendix includes a wide array of resources, from helpful Web sites to a patient safety glossary. To keep the book a manageable size, my goal is to be more useful and engaging than comprehensive—readers wishing to dig deeper will find relevant references throughout the text.

Some of the material for this book is derived or adapted from other works that I have edited or written. Specifically, some of the case presentations will be drawn from *Internal Bleeding: The Truth Behind America's Terrifying Epidemic of Medical Mistakes*,[5] the "Quality Grand Rounds" series in the *Annals of Internal Medicine* (Appendix I),[26] and AHRQ WebM&M.[27] Many of the case presentations came from cases we used for the QGR series, and I am grateful to the patients, families, and caregivers who allowed us to use their stories (often agreeing to be interviewed). Of course, all patient and provider names have been changed to protect privacy.

I am also indebted to my partner in many of these efforts, Dr. Kaveh Shojania, now of the University of Toronto, for his remarkable contributions to the safety field and for reviewing an earlier draft of this book and authoring the glossary. Thanks too to my other partners on Quality Grand Rounds (Dr. Sanjay Saint and Amy Markowitz), AHRQ WebM&M and AHRQ Patient Safety Network[28] (Drs. Brad Sharpe, Niraj Sehgal, Russ Cucina, John Young, and Sumant Ranji [a special tip of the hat to Sumant, who is the primary author of the superb AHRQ PSNet Patient Safety Primers, which proved to be a rich source of information for this edition]; Professors Mary Blegen, Brian Alldredge, and Joe Guglielmo; and Lorri Zipperer and Erin Hartman), and to the sponsoring organizations (Rugged Land, publisher of *Internal Bleeding*; the California HealthCare Foundation and the *Annals of Internal Medicine* for Quality Grand Rounds; and the U.S. Agency for Healthcare Research and Quality for AHRQ WebM&M and PSNet).

I wrote this second edition during my sabbatical at Imperial College London, and owe a special thanks to my British colleagues, particularly Professor Charles Vincent, to the US–UK Fulbright Commission for sponsoring my time in the United Kingdom, and to Brad Sharpe and Maria Novelero and the rest of the UCSF Division of Hospital Medicine for holding down the proverbial fort during my absence. Additional thanks to Bryan Haughom, who coauthored the original version of Chapter 7, to my colleagues on the American Board of Internal Medicine, to my administrative assistant Mary Whitney, and to Jim Shanahan of McGraw-Hill, who conceived of this book and has nurtured it every step of the way. This book would not have been possible without the contributions of all these extraordinary people and organizations. Katie Hafner, with whom I share my life, is a joy, an inspiration, and one hell of a great writer and editor. Katie, I dedicate this book to you, and us.

Finally, although this is not primarily a book written for patients, it is a book written *about* patients. As patient safety becomes professionalized (with "patient safety officers"), it will inevitably become jargon-heavy—"We need a

root cause analysis!" "What did the Failure Mode Effects Analysis show?"—
and this evolution will make it easy to take our eyes off the ball. We now know
that tens of thousands of people in the United States and many times that
number around the world die each year because of preventable medical errors.
Moreover, every day millions of people check into hospitals or clinics worried
that they'll be killed in the process of receiving chemotherapy, undergoing
surgery, or delivering a baby. Our efforts must be focused on preventing these
errors, and the associated anxiety that patients feel when they receive medical
care in an unsafe, chaotic environment.

Some have argued that medical errors are the dark side of medical
progress, an inevitable consequence of the ever-increasing complexity of
modern medicine. Perhaps a few errors fit this description, but most do
not. I can easily envision a system in which patients benefit from all the
modern miracles available to us, and do so in reliable organizations that
take advantage of all the necessary tools and systems to "get it right" the
vast majority of the time. Looking back at the remarkable progress that has
been made in the 12 years since the publication of the Institute of Medicine
report on medical errors, I am confident that we can create such a system.
My hope is that this book makes a small contribution toward achieving
that goal.

REFERENCES

1. Kohn L, Corrigan J, Donaldson M, eds. *To Err is Human: Building a Safer Health System*. Committee on Quality of Health Care in America, Institute of Medicine. Washington, DC: National Academy Press; 2000.
2. Brennan TA, Leape LL, Laird NM, et al. Incidence of adverse events and negligence in hospitalized patients. Results of the Harvard Medical Practice Study I. *N Engl J Med* 1991;324:370–376.
3. Leape LL, Brennan TA, Laird N, et al. The nature of adverse events and negligence in hospitalized patients. Results of the Harvard Medical Practice Study II. *N Engl J Med* 1991;324:377–384.
4. Wu AW. Medical error: the second victim. *West J Med* 2000;172:358–359.
5. Wachter RM, Shojania KG. *Internal Bleeding: The Truth Behind America's Terrifying Epidemic of Medical Mistakes*. New York, NY: Rugged Land; 2004.
6. Wachter RM. Playing well with others: "translocational research" in patient safety. *AHRQ WebM&M* (serial online); September 2005. Available at: http://webmm.ahrq.gov/perspective.aspx?perspectiveID=9.
7. Blumenthal D. Launching HITECH. *N Engl J Med* 2010;362:382–385.
8. Sittig DF, Singh H. Defining health information technology–related errors. New developments since *To Err is Human. Arch Intern Med* 2011;171:1281–1284.

9. IHI Global Trigger Tool for Measuring Adverse Events. Available at: http://www.ihi.org/knowledge/Pages/Tools/IHIGlobalTriggerToolforMeasuringAEs.aspx.

10. Shojania KG. The elephant of patient safety: what you see depends on how you look. *Jt Comm J Qual Patient Saf* 2010;36:399–401.

11. Landrigan CP, Parry GJ, Bones CB, et al. Temporal trends in rates of patient harm resulting from medical care. *N Engl J Med* 2010;363:2124–2134.

12. Pronovost P, Needham D, Berenholtz S, et al. An intervention to decrease catheter-related bloodstream infections in the ICU. *N Engl J Med* 2006;355:2725–2732.

13. Haynes AB, Weiser TG, Berry WR, et al.; for the Safe Surgery Saves Lives Study Group. A surgical safety checklist to reduce morbidity and mortality in a global population. *N Engl J Med* 2009;360:491–499.

14. de Vries EN, Prins HA, Crolla RM, et al.; SURPASS Collaborative Group. Effect of a comprehensive surgical safety system on patient outcomes. *N Engl J Med* 2010;363:1928–1937.

15. Gawande A. The checklist. *The New Yorker*. December 10, 2007;83:86–95.

16. Gawande A. *The Checklist Manifesto: How to Get Things Right.* New York, NY: Metropolitan Books; 2009.

17. Pronovost P, Vohr E. *Safe Patients, Smart Hospitals: How One Doctor's Checklist can Help Us Change Health Care from the Inside Out.* New York, NY: Hudson Street Press; 2010.

18. Bosk CL, Dixon-Woods M, Goeschel CA, et al. Reality check for checklists. *Lancet* 2009;374:444–445.

19. Dixon-Woods M, Bosk CL, Aveling EL, et al. Explaining Michigan: developing an ex post theory of a quality improvement program. *Milbank Q* 2011;89:167–205.

20. Wachter RM. Why diagnostic errors don't get any respect—and what can be done about them. *Health Aff (Millwood)* 2010;29:1605–1610.

21. Wachter RM. Patient safety at ten: unmistakable progress, troubling gaps. *Health Aff (Millwood)* 2010;29:165–173.

22. Rosenthal J. Advancing patient safety through state reporting systems. *AHRQ WebM&M* (serial online); June 2007. Available at: http://webmm.ahrq.gov/perspective.aspx?perspectiveID=43.

23. Wachter RM, Foster NE, Dudley RA. Medicare's decision to withhold payment for hospital errors: the devil is in the details. *Jt Comm J Qual Patient Saf* 2008;34:116–123.

24. Nelson B. Value-based purchasing raises the stakes. *The Hospitalist.* May 2011. Available at: http://www.the-hospitalist.org/details/article/1056049/Value-Based_Purchasing_Raises_the_Stakes.html.

25. Wachter RM, Pronovost PJ. Balancing "no blame" with accountability in patient safety. *N Engl J Med* 2009;361:1401–1406.

26. Wachter RM, Shojania KG, Saint S, et al. Learning from our mistakes: quality grand rounds, a new case-based series on medical errors and patient safety. *Ann Intern Med* 2002;136:850–852.

27. Available at: http://webmm.ahrq.gov.

28. Available at: http://psnet.ahrq.gov.

AN INTRODUCTION TO PATIENT SAFETY AND MEDICAL ERRORS

THE NATURE AND FREQUENCY OF MEDICAL ERRORS AND ADVERSE EVENTS

1

ADVERSE EVENTS, PREVENTABLE ADVERSE EVENTS, AND ERRORS

Although Hippocrates said "first, do no harm" over 2000 years ago and many hospitals have long hosted conferences to discuss errors (Morbidity and Mortality, or "M&M," conferences), until recently medical errors were considered an inevitable by-product of modern medicine or the unfortunate detritus of bad providers. This began to change in late 1999, with the Institute of Medicine's (IOM) publication of *To Err is Human: Building a Safer Health System.*[1] This report, which estimated that 44,000 to 98,000 Americans die each year from medical mistakes, generated tremendous public and media attention, and set the stage for unprecedented efforts to improve patient safety. Of course, these seminal works built on a rich tapestry of inquiry and leadership in the field of patient safety (Appendix III), familiar to a small group of devotees but generally unknown to mainstream providers, administrators, policymakers, and patients.

The IOM death estimate, which was drawn from thousands of chart reviews in New York,[2,3] Colorado, and Utah[4] in the late 1980s and early 1990s, was followed by studies that showed huge numbers of medication errors, communication problems in intensive care units (ICUs), gaps in the discharge process, retained sponges in the operating room—in short, everywhere one looked there was evidence of major problems in patient safety. Moreover, accompanying this information in the professional literature were scores of dramatic reports in the lay media: errors involving the wrong patient going to a procedure or the wrong limb being operated on, chemotherapy overdoses, botched transplants, patients released from the emergency department (ED)

3

only to die later from myocardial infarction or aortic dissection, and more (Table 1-1).

The patient safety literature contains many overlapping terms to describe safety-related issues. Although the terms sometimes confuse more than clarify, two key distinctions underlie most of the terminology and allow one to keep it relatively straight. First, because patients commonly experience adverse outcomes, it is important to distinguish adverse outcomes as a result of medical care from morbidity and mortality that patients suffer as a consequence of their underlying medical conditions. The former are known as *adverse events* or *harm* (the two terms are generally used interchangeably) and have been defined by the Institute for Healthcare Improvement as:

> Unintended physical injury resulting from or contributed to by medical care (including the absence of indicated medical treatment) that requires additional monitoring, treatment, or hospitalization, or that results in death.[5]

Second, because patients may experience harm from their medical care in the absence of any errors (i.e., from accepted complications of surgery or medication side effects), the patient safety literature separates *preventable adverse events* from *nonpreventable* ones. Figure 1-1 shows a Venn diagram depicting these various terms.

Now, where do *errors* or *mistakes* fit in? The safety literature commonly defines an error as "an act of commission (doing something wrong) or omission (failing to do the right thing) leading to an undesirable outcome or significant potential for such an outcome."[6] Note that many errors do not result in adverse events (Figure 1-1)—we generally characterize the more serious ones as "near misses" or "close calls." Note too that some errors involve care that falls below a professional standard of care—these are called *negligence* and may create legal liability or a duty to compensate the patient in some systems (Chapter 18). Finally, although most preventable adverse events involve errors, not all of them do (see "The Challenges of Measuring Errors and Safety," below).

In the early days of the patient safety movement, most of the focus was on measuring and decreasing the incidence of errors. Increasingly, safety experts prefer to highlight preventable adverse events or preventable harm—rather than errors—as the main target of the field. Framing this issue in the language of the Donabedian process–outcome–structure triad (Chapter 3),[7] one might think about harm as the "outcome" and errors as the "process." Advocates of this new approach see several advantages to it. First, focusing on adverse events removes the implication that a specific provider was responsible for the harm, which may generate defensiveness by caregivers or an inordinate focus by the organization on dealing with the individual rather than the system

Table 1-1	SELECTED MEDICAL ERRORS THAT GARNERED EXTENSIVE MEDIA ATTENTION IN THE UNITED STATES*		
Error	**Institution**	**Year**	**Impact**
An 18-year-old woman, Libby Zion, daughter of a prominent reporter, dies of a medical mistake, partly due to lax resident supervision	Cornell's New York Hospital	1984	Public discussion regarding resident training, supervision, and work hours. Led to New York law regarding supervision and work hours, ultimately culminating in ACGME duty hour regulations (Chapter 16)
Betsy Lehman, a *Boston Globe* healthcare reporter, dies of a chemotherapy overdose	Harvard's Dana-Farber Cancer Institute	1994	New focus on medication errors, role of ambiguity in prescriptions and possible role of computerized prescribing and decision support (Chapters 4 and 13)
Willie King, a 51-year-old diabetic, has the wrong leg amputated	University Community Hospital, Tampa, Florida	1995	New focus on wrong-site surgery, ultimately leading to Joint Commission's Universal Protocol, and later the surgical checklist, to prevent these errors (Chapter 5)
18-month-old Josie King dies of dehydration	Johns Hopkins Hospital	2001	Josie's parents form an alliance with Johns Hopkins' leadership (leading to the Josie King Foundation and catalyzing Hopkins' safety initiatives), demonstrating the power of institutional and patient collaboration
Jesica Santillan, a 17-year-old girl from Mexico, dies after receiving a heart–lung transplant of the wrong blood type	Duke University Medical Center	2003	New focus on errors in transplantation, and on enforcing strict, high reliability protocols for communication of crucial data (Chapters 2 and 8)
The twin newborns of actor Dennis Quaid are nearly killed by a large heparin overdose	Cedars-Sinai Medical Center	2007	Renewed focus on medication errors and the potential value of bar coding to prevent prescribing errors (Chapters 4 and 13)

ACGME, Accreditation Council for Graduate Medical Education.
*Other countries have had similar errors that also helped catalyze the safety field. For example, in the United Kingdom the 2001 publication of a national inquiry into a childhood deaths after surgery at the Bristol Royal Infirmary was a defining event for the patient safety movement. See Walshe K, Offen N. A very public failure: lessons for quality improvement in healthcare organizations from the Bristol Royal Infirmary. *Qual Saf Health Care* 2001;10:250–256.

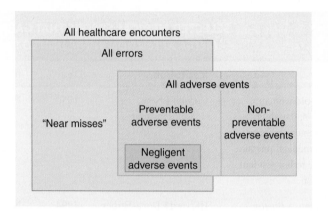

Figure 1-1 ■ Venn diagram depicting patient safety terminology.

(Chapter 2).[8–10] Moreover, patients, quite naturally, care more about what happened to them than whether their doctor or nurse made a mistake.

Although these advocates make a strong argument (and I find myself in their camp with increasing frequency), it is worth appreciating the fear on the part of other experts that the terms "preventable adverse events" or "preventable harm" seem a bit too careful, perhaps even politically correct, lacking the visceral punch of "error" or "mistake" that helped launch the safety field. One can be sure that this vigorous debate—which has been with us since the early days of the field[11,12]—will continue. For now, it is clear that patient safety's center of gravity has shifted toward adverse events/harm as the focus of measurements and interventions.

These distinctions are important to understand as one tries to wade through the safety literature or interpret individual cases. To help illustrate the point, let's consider three scenarios involving a patient placed appropriately on warfarin for chronic atrial fibrillation who develops a gastrointestinal (GI) bleed. If the bleeding began while the patient's international normalized ratio (INR) was therapeutic, he would be said to be the victim of an adverse event (often called a *side effect* when caused by a medication), but not a preventable adverse event or a medical error. Such cases should prompt us to reevaluate the benefit-to-risk ratio of the intervention (in this patient and others like him) and to try to improve the science (i.e., identify a strategy with a comparable benefit but lower risk), but not to infer that there was a mistake in the patient's care or that the harm was preventable.

If, on the other hand, the patient had bled in the setting of a supratherapeutic INR, but there was no overt error on the part of the physician (she was following standard guidelines for warfarin dosing and monitoring), the patient would be said to have suffered a *preventable adverse event*, but the case would still not be characterized as having been caused by an error. Here too, the focus should be on reassessing the benefit-to-risk ratio in this and similar patients and on improving the science, although it is worth considering systems changes (such as more frequent monitoring) that might have made a difference in this case and ones like it.

Finally, it would be a preventable adverse event *and an error* if the INR was supratherapeutic because the physician prescribed a new medication without checking for possible drug interactions. As we'll see, before focusing too narrowly on the failures of the individual caregiver (unless such carelessness was habitual or willful), the more productive stance will likely be to consider systems changes (a computerized order entry system with robust decision support,[13] or a dedicated anticoagulation clinic[14]) that might prevent such errors and harm in the future. Ideally, of course, warfarin would be replaced by a medication that delivered the same therapeutic benefit but lacked its drug interactions and monitoring requirements.[15]

Before leaving the area of patient safety terminology, I should add that some safety experts bristle at the distinction between preventable and nonpreventable adverse events, reminding us that certain types of harm previously thought unpreventable are now known to be preventable with better systems. Some even contend that labeling such events "nonpreventable" is defeatist and self-fulfilling. Probably the strongest support for this argument comes from the story of central line–associated bloodstream infections, which were once felt to be inevitable consequences of modern medicine but are now known to be largely preventable with the consistent application of a "bundle" of safety practices[16] (Chapter 10). Although this point of view has considerable merit, the distinction between preventability and nonpreventability permeates the literature, and blurring it risks a public perception that all adverse events result from errors, which they do not. As one point of reference, studies of cases of harm in hospitalized patients generally find about half to have been preventable.[9,10]

This debate is likely to continue because measurement is so fundamental to our efforts to improve safety. Robust and reliable measurement is the cornerstone for conducting sound research about patient safety practices, prioritizing areas of focus for study and implementation, holding individuals and institutions accountable for performance, and assessing how we are faring in our efforts to improve safety.[8] So, although matters of terminology and measurement might seem arcane and of only marginal relevance to patients, caregivers, administrators, and policymakers, they are really quite central to the field.

THE CHALLENGES OF MEASURING ERRORS AND SAFETY

At Douglastown Hospital, the patient safety officer has become concerned about the frequency of medication errors. One patient received a 10-fold overdose of insulin when the order "please give

10U regular insulin" was interpreted as "100 regular insulin." Another patient received a cephalosporin antibiotic for pneumonia, despite being allergic to this class of drugs. A third suffered a GI bleed when an overdose of warfarin led to over-anticoagulation.

In response to these incidents, the hospital is considering whether to invest in a $50 million computerized provider order entry system. The Chief Financial Officer, knowing that this expense will mean that the hospital will have to forego its planned purchase of a new 256-slice computed tomography scanner and the construction of two new operating rooms (investments with near-guaranteed positive returns on investment), asks the safety officer, "How will we know that we've made a difference?"

The CFO's question seems relatively straightforward, but is much harder to answer than you might think. Let's consider various ways of measuring errors.

The most common method is through self-reports of errors by providers, usually referred to as *incident reports*. These reports have traditionally been completed by pencil and paper; they are increasingly being inputted through a computerized system. Incident reports (see also Chapter 14) might seem to be a reliable way of tracking errors, but there are several problems with using them to measure the frequency of errors.[17] First, although nurses tend to report errors through incident reporting systems, few doctors do,[18] either not reporting at all or reporting through informal channels (such as, in teaching programs, telling the chief residents). Secondly, as most reporting systems are voluntary, the frequency of reports will be influenced by many factors other than the number of errors. Let's say the institution has improved its safety culture (Chapter 15), such that reporting of errors is now strongly encouraged by local leaders and incident reports result in tangible action. Under these circumstances, an increase in incident reports might well reflect the same number of, or even fewer, errors being reported more assiduously. This conundrum distinguishes measuring patient safety from measuring the quality of care, which is less dependent on voluntary reporting and thus can be done more reliably (Chapter 3).

Another method of measuring safety is through a series of *patient safety indicators* gleaned from large administrative datasets. The most widely used indicator set is the Agency for Healthcare Research and Quality's (AHRQ) Patient Safety Indicators (PSIs), which consists of 25 outcomes or processes that are plausibly related to safety[19] (Appendix V). Although AHRQ cautions that these indicators should only be used as clues for problems (because their source is administrative rather than clinical data, they produce results that may be inaccurate or do not correlate very well to actual safety[20–22]), some commercial vendors do just that, and the media disseminate these (often sensational) findings widely.

Given the problem in using incident reports and administrative data to measure the frequency of errors or harm, are there other ways? One could *review charts* for evidence of errors. This, in fact, is what the Harvard Medical Practice Study investigators did as they searched for "preventable adverse events."[2–4] Unfortunately, chart review is expensive and labor intensive (this burden may be eased somewhat by electronic medical record systems, particularly if they capture data in organized ways rather than as free text; Chapter 13), poor charting may be on the same gene as the propensity to commit errors (thus penalizing institutions and providers who document well), the medicolegal climate almost certainly induces some "buffing of the chart" after an error, and chart review is simply not a very reliable way to determine whether an error has occurred.[23] The latter problem is partly due to the inevitability of hindsight bias, in which knowledge of the final outcome influences the reviewer's determination regarding whether a given act was an error, a problem that also besets many malpractice investigations.[24]

Over the past several years, the use of *trigger tools* has emerged as a favored method to measure the incidence of adverse events in many healthcare settings. The most popular of these is the *Global Trigger Tool*, developed by the Institute for Healthcare Improvement. The premise behind trigger tools is that some errors in care will engender a response that can be tracked—in essence, a clue that an adverse event (and perhaps an error) may have occurred.[25] For example, the patient with a warfarin overdose may be given a dose of Vitamin K or fresh frozen plasma to counteract the excess anticoagulant, or a patient who has received too much morphine may be treated with an opiate antagonist such as naloxone. Or, a patient insufficiently observed on the medical ward may need to be transferred urgently to the ICU, another event captured by the Global Trigger Tool.

Although trigger tools are neither perfectly sensitive nor specific, they have reasonably good interrater reliability[26] and often identify cases of medical errors that incident reporting or administrative data-based systems miss. Because many triggers do not represent errors or even true harm, they are best used as a screen, followed by more detailed chart review. The use of the Global Trigger Tool currently involves significant labor costs (largely for the follow-up chart reviews), but some of this effort may eventually be automated. Selected triggers from the Global Trigger Tool are shown in Table 1-2.

Several recent studies have utilized the IHI Global Trigger Tool to assess the state of patient safety. The results are sobering. Landrigan and colleagues tracked the rates of adverse events of nine hospitals in North Carolina from 2003 to 2008, and found no significant improvement in harm rates during these years, despite major efforts to improve safety.[9] A study by the U.S. Office of the Inspector General (OIG) of the Department of Health and Human Services found that one in eight Medicare patients experienced

Table 1-2   SELECTED TRIGGERS FROM THE INSTITUTE FOR HEALTHCARE IMPROVEMENT'S (IHI) GLOBAL TRIGGER TOOL

Care module triggers
   Any code or arrest
   Abrupt drop of >25% in hematocrit
   Patient fall
   Readmission within 30 days
   Transfer to higher level of care

Surgical module triggers
   Return to surgery
   Intubation/reintubation in postanesthesia care unit
   Intra- or postoperative death
   Postoperative troponin level >1.5 ng/mL

Medication module triggers
   PTT >100 s
   INR >6
   Rising BUN or creatinine >2 times baseline
   Vitamin K administration
   Narcan (Naloxone) use
   Abrupt medication stop

Intensive care module triggers
   Pneumonia onset
   Readmission to intensive care
   Intubation/reintubation

Perinatal module
   Third- or fourth-degree lacerations

ED module
   Readmission to ED within 48 h
   Time in ED >6 h

BUN, blood urea nitrogen; ED, emergency department; PTT, partial thromboplastin time.
Reproduced with permission from Griffin FA, Resar RK. *IHI Global Trigger Tool for Measuring Adverse Events.* Cambridge, MA: Institute for Healthcare Improvement; 2009. (Available at: www.IHI.org.)

a significant adverse event during their hospitalization.[10] Finally, Classen and colleagues found that approximately one in three hospitalized patients experienced an adverse event of some kind.[8] This study, which compared the test characteristics of the Global Trigger Tool with that of voluntary incident reports and the AHRQ Patient Safety Indicators, found that the former was far more sensitive and specific (Table 1-3). Table 1-4 highlights some of the

Table 1-3	**SENSITIVITY AND SPECIFICITY OF THREE METHODS OF MEASURING ADVERSE EVENTS**	
Method	**Sensitivity (%)**	**Specificity (%)**
Global Trigger Tool	94.9	100
AHRQ Patient Safety Indicators	5.8	98.5
Voluntary Error Reporting	0	100

From Classen DC, Resar R, Griffin F, et al. 'Global Trigger Tool' shows that adverse events in hospitals may be ten times greater than previously measured. *Health Aff (Millwood)* 2011;30:581–589.

Table 1-4	**ADVANTAGES AND DISADVANTAGES OF VARIOUS STRATEGIES FOR MEASURING SAFETY AND HARM**	
Measurement Strategies	**Advantages**	**Disadvantages**
Retrospective Chart Review (by itself or after use of a trigger tool)	Considered the "gold standard," contains rich detailed clinical information	Costly, labor-intensive, data quality variable due to incomplete clinical information, retrospective review only. Efficiency improved by focusing chart reviews on cases identified by a reliable trigger tool
Voluntary Incident Reporting Systems	Useful for internal quality improvement and case-finding, highlights adverse events that providers perceive as important	Capture small fraction of adverse events, retrospective review only based on provider self-reports, no standardization or uniformity of adverse events reported
Automated Surveillance	Can be used retrospectively or prospectively, helpful in screening patients who may be at high risk for adverse events using standardized protocols	Need electronic data to run automated surveillance, high proportion of "triggered" cases are false positives
Administrative/Claims Data (e.g., AHRQ Patient Safety Indicators)	Low-cost, readily available data, useful for tracking events over time across large populations, can identify "potential" adverse events	Lack detailed clinical data, concerns over variability and inaccuracy of *ICD-9-CM* codes across and within systems, may detect high proportion of false positives

Adapted with permission from Rosen AK. Are we getting any better at measuring patient safety. *AHRQ WebM&M* [serial online], November 2010. Available at: http://webmm.ahrq.gov/perspective.aspx?perspectiveID=94.

advantages and disadvantages of the most common methods of measuring errors and adverse events.[27]

There are two other assessment methods that bear mention. Several years ago, there was considerable enthusiasm for using *hospital standardized mortality ratios* (HSMR), a method pioneered by Professor Brian Jarman of Imperial College London. The attractiveness of using risk-adjusted over-all mortality can be inferred through its nickname in many U.S. hospitals: the "Big Dot." In other words, a single risk-adjusted mortality statistic is an intuitively appealing "roll-up" measure that seems to capture many aspects of safety and quality and can be followed over time. In part because of this natural appeal to policymakers, in the UK this measure has become a major focus of quality and safety efforts, and the finding of outlier HSMR results has triggered several hospital investigations.[28] However, Lilford and Pronovost, in highlighting the HSMR's methodologic problems (poor signal-to-noise ratio, uncertain case-mix adjustment, poor reliability, etc.), have called its use a "bad idea that won't go away,"[29] and I am convinced by their arguments. Moreover, a 2010 study found that four different popular methods of measuring hospital mortality came to wildly different conclusions about hospital quality.[30]

A recent trend has been to *ask patients themselves to identify instances of harm or errors*. This too is an appealing idea, in that it grows out of a broader movement to engage patients in their own safety and respect their roles as active participants in care. Early studies demonstrated that patients are able to identify some errors missed by other assessment methods.[31,32] That said, the overall util-ity of this strategy, including whether placing patients in this position compro-mises their sense of trust in their caregivers, is yet to be fully defined. Chapter 21 delves more deeply into the role of patients in preserving their own safety.

As we've seen, there are many ways to try to measure the number of errors and cases of harm. The key point is that the frequency will vary markedly depending on the method used,[33] and a robust institutional or external program to assess the state of patient safety and learn from errors and adverse events will need to integrate several of these methods (Chapters 20 and 22). Kaveh Shojania calls this the "elephant of patient safety," in that what you see depends on what part of the animal you're looking at.[34]

THE FREQUENCY AND IMPACT OF ERRORS

In part because of different definitions and assessment methods, various stud-ies have shown differing rates of adverse events. Overall, while early studies[2–4] identified adverse events in approximately 1 in 10 admissions, recent ones, using the Global Trigger Tool, have found rates ranging from 1 in 8 (the OIG study[10]) to 1 in 3 (Classen et al.[8]). Whether this change represents a true increase in harm or more sensitive measures is unknown. (Interestingly, over-all hospital mortality rates have fallen markedly in recent years, further high-lighting the "elephant" of patient safety measurement.) In any case, given the substantial efforts that have gone into improving safety over the past decade, the adverse events figures are sobering, and should cause us to redouble our efforts and be sure that we are on the correct path.

Of course, not all adverse events are created equal: we are more con-cerned about adverse events that result in death or disability than those that lead to an extra day in the hospital or a delay in a radiograph or a medication. (The caveat here, as always, is that some near misses—cases in which there was no harm at all—illustrate important systems problems and have tremen-dous learning value for organizations.[35]) Many safety studies use the National Coordinating Council for Medication Error Reporting and Prevention's Index for Categorizing Errors (*NCC MERP Index*), which grades errors on a scale of A to I (Figure 1-2). Most published studies focus on cases in which errors reached patients and caused harm: labeled "E" (temporary harm that requires intervention) through "I" (death). Most healthcare systems that use trigger tools or similar methods to analyze their own adverse events do the same.

Overall, although about two-thirds of adverse events cause little or no patient harm, about one-third do—ranging from minor harm (such as a pro-longed hospitalization) to permanent disability (Figure 1-3). This risk is not evenly distributed—some unfortunate patients have a far higher chance of suf-fering a significant adverse event, and these patients often experience multiple events.[36] For example, it has been estimated that the average patient in the ICU has 1.7 errors in his or her care per ICU day[37] and the average hospital-ized medical patient experiences one medication error per day![38] Patients on multiple medications or on particularly risky medications (e.g., anticoagu-lants, opiates, insulin, and sedatives)[39,40] are more likely to be harmed, as are older patients (Figure 1-3).

The financial impact of medical errors and adverse events is enormous. The IOM report estimated that the overall national (U.S.) cost for preventable adverse events (in the late 1990s) was between 17 billion and 29 billion dol-lars;[1] this estimate was essentially stable in a 2011 study.[41] Including "nonpre-ventable" adverse events would double these figures. As these numbers come exclusively from hospital-based studies, adding in the impact of adverse events in ambulatory clinics,[42] nursing homes and assisted living facilities,[43] and other settings would drive them still higher.

When viewed this way, it becomes difficult to argue that we cannot afford to fix the problem of medical errors. But—particularly in fee-for-service pay-ment systems (like most of the United States)—part of the problem is that both providers and institutions are generally compensated (often quite handsomely) for unsafe care, providing little financial incentive to make the requisite

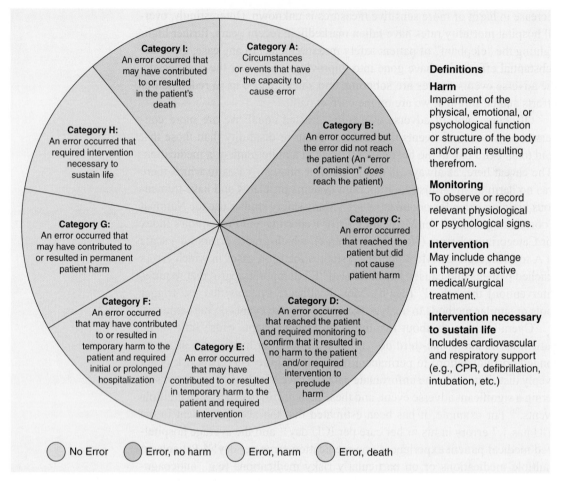

Definitions

Harm
Impairment of the physical, emotional, or psychological function or structure of the body and/or pain resulting therefrom.

Monitoring
To observe or record relevant physiological or psychological signs.

Intervention
May include change in therapy or active medical/surgical treatment.

Intervention necessary to sustain life
Includes cardiovascular and respiratory support (e.g., CPR, defibrillation, intubation, etc.)

Figure 1-2 ▪ The NCC MERP Index for categorizing errors. (Reprinted with permission from the National Coordinating Council for Medication Error Reporting and Prevention, © 2001. Available at: http://www.nccmerp.org/pdf/indexBW2001-06-12.pdf.)

investments in safer systems. Even in countries and organizational structures that *do* lose money from errors and harm (e.g., capitated systems such as Kaiser Permanente or the Veterans Affairs system in the United States, or the United Kingdom's National Health Service), doing the accounting to determine the "return on investment" from spending on safety is tricky.[44] Many recent policy initiatives are designed to increase the cost of errors and harm to systems, in an effort to promote investment in safety.

All of that said, one should not get too distracted by the numbers and dollars. The largest impact of medical errors and adverse events is on patients and their

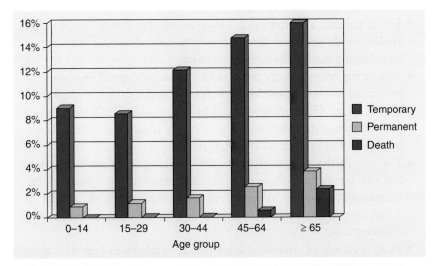

Figure 1-3 ■ Proportion of patients experiencing an adverse event who suffer temporary (<1 year) disability, permanent disability, or death; by age group. Note that not only does the severity of harm go up with age, but so does the chance of an adverse event (in this Australian study it was approximately 10% per admission in younger patients, up to nearly 25% per admission in patients over 65). (Reproduced with permission from Weingart SN, Wilson RM, Gibberd RW, et al. Epidemiology of medical error. *BMJ* 2000;320: 774–777; Wilson RM, Runciman WB, Gibberd RW, et al. The quality in Australian health care study. *Med J Aust* 1995;163:458–471.)

loved ones, and the toll is best measured in anxiety, harm, and deaths. Moreover, in so many cases, providers are "second victims" of unsafe systems that let them down when they most needed the support.[45] For all of these reasons, the moral and ethical case for patient safety remains the most powerful motivator of all.

KEY POINTS

- The modern patient safety movement began with the publication of the Institute of Medicine's report on medical errors, *To Err is Human: Building a Safer Health System,* in late 1999.
- Adverse events (also known as harms) are injuries resulting from medical care, as opposed to adverse outcomes arising from underlying disease. Not all adverse events are preventable—those that are usually involve errors. In many cases, preventability relies on system changes that reduce the likelihood of the adverse events in question.

- Errors are acts of commission (doing something wrong) or omission (failing to do the right thing) leading to an undesirable outcome or significant potential for such an outcome.
- Measuring errors is very tricky. Many systems depend on voluntary reports by providers (incident reports), which detect only a small fraction of errors. Other methods, such as patient safety indicators drawn from administrative datasets, may be overly sensitive and thus should be augmented by detailed chart review.
- The use of the Global Trigger Tool—seeking clues about a possible adverse event, followed by detailed chart review—has become increasingly popular in recent years, in keeping with a shift in focus from errors to adverse events as targets for measurement and interventions.
- From a variety of studies, at least 1 in 10 (perhaps as high as 1 in 3) hospital admissions is marred by an adverse event, and about half of these are preventable. About one-third of these adverse events cause true patient harm.

REFERENCES

1. Kohn L, Corrigan J, Donaldson M, eds. *To Err is Human: Building a Safer Health System*. Washington, DC: Committee on Quality of Health Care in America, Institute of Medicine: National Academy Press; 2000.
2. Brennan TA, Leape LL, Laird NM, et al. Incidence of adverse events and negligence in hospitalized patients. Results of the Harvard Medical Practice Study I. *N Engl J Med* 1991;324:370–376.
3. Leape LL, Brennan TA, Laird N, et al. The nature of adverse events and negligence in hospitalized patients. Results of the Harvard Medical Practice Study II. *N Engl J Med* 1991;324:377–384.
4. Thomas EJ, Studdert DM, Burstin HR, et al. Incidence and types of adverse events and negligent care in Utah and Colorado. *Med Care* 2000;38:261–271.
5. Available at: http://www.IHI.org
6. Available at: http://webmm.ahrq.gov/glossary.aspx
7. Donabedian A. The quality of care. How can it be assessed? *JAMA* 1988;260: 1743–1748.
8. Classen DC, Resar R, Griffin F, et al. 'Global Trigger Tool' shows that adverse events in hospitals may be ten times greater than previously measured. *Health Aff (Millwood)* 2011;30:581–589.
9. Landrigan CP, Parry GJ, Bones CB, et al. Temporal trends in rates of patient harm resulting from medical care. *N Engl J Med* 2010;363:2124–2134.

10. Levinson DR. *Adverse Events in Hospitals: National Incidence Among Medicare Beneficiaries.* Washington, DC: US Department of Health and Human Services, Office of the Inspector General; November 2010. Report No. OEI-06-09-00090.

11. Layde PM, Maas LA, Teret SP, et al. Patient safety efforts should focus on medical injuries. *JAMA* 2002;287:1993–1997.

12. McNutt RA, Abrams R, Aron DC, et al. Patient safety efforts should focus on medical errors. *JAMA* 2002;287:1997–2001.

13. Classen DC, Phansalkar S, Bates DW. Critical drug–drug interactions for use in electronic health records systems with computerized physician order entry: review of leading approaches. *J Patient Saf* 2011;7:61–65.

14. Franco AC, Maxwell P, Green K, Barthol C. Anticoagulation patient safety goal compliance at a university health system: methods for achieving the goal. *Hosp Pharm* 2009;44:776–780, 784.

15. Connolly SJ, Ezekowitz MD, Yusuf S, et al. Dabigatran versus warfarin in patients with atrial fibrillation. *N Engl J Med* 2009;361:1139–1151 [Erratum, *N Engl J Med* 2010;363:1877.]

16. Pronovost P, Needham D, Berenholtz S, et al. An intervention to decrease catheter-related bloodstream infections in the ICU. *N Engl J Med* 2006;355:2725–2732.

17. Shojania KG. The frustrating case of incident-reporting systems. *Qual Saf Health Care* 2008;17:400–402.

18. Wild D, Bradley EH. The gap between nurses and residents in a community hospital's error reporting system. *Jt Comm J Qual Patient Saf* 2005;31:13–20.

19. Available at: http://www.qualityindicators.ahrq.gov/.

20. Isaac T, Jha AK. Are Patient Safety Indicators related to widely used measures of hospital quality? *J Gen Intern Med* 2008;23:1373–1378.

21. Romano PS, Mull HJ, Rivard PE, et al. Validity of selected AHRQ Patient Safety Indicators based on VA National Surgical Quality Improvement program data. *Health Serv Res* 2009;44:182–204.

22. White RH, Sadeghi B, Tancredi D, et al. How valid is the ICD-9-CM based AHRQ Patient Safety Indicator for postoperative venous thromboembolism? *Med Care* 2009;47:1237–1243.

23. Thomas EJ, Lipsitz SR, Studdert DM, et al. The reliability of medical record review for estimating adverse event rates. *Ann Intern Med* 2002;136:812–816.

24. Caplan RA, Posner KL, Cheney FW. Effect of outcome on physician judgments of appropriateness of care. *JAMA* 1991;265:1957–1960.

25. Classen DC, Lloyd RC, Provost L, et al. Development and evaluation of the Institute for Healthcare Improvement global trigger tool. *J Patient Saf* 2008;4:169–177.

26. Sharek PJ, Parry G, Goldmann D, et al. Performance characteristics of a methodology to quantify adverse events over time in hospitalized patients. *Health Serv Res* 2011;46:654–678.

27. Rosen AK. Are we getting any better at measuring patient safety. *AHRQ WebM&M* [serial online], November 2010. Available at: http://webmm.ahrq.gov/perspective.aspx?perspectiveID=94.

28. Bottle A, Jarman B, Aylin P. Strengths and weaknesses of hospital standardised mortality ratios. *BMJ* 2011;342:c7116.

29. Lilford R, Pronovost P. Using hospital mortality rates to judge hospital performance: a bad idea that just won't go away. *BMJ* 2010;340:955–957.

30. Shahian DM, Wolf RE, Iezzoni LI, et al. Variability in the measurement of hospital-wide mortality rates. *N Engl J Med* 2010;363:2530–2539.

31. Weissman JS, Schneider EC, Weingart SN, et al. Comparing patient-reported hospital adverse events with medical record review: do patients know something that hospitals do not? *Ann Intern Med* 2008;149:100–108.

32. Zhu J, Stuver SO, Epstein AM, et al. Can we rely on patients' reports of adverse events? *Med Care* 2011;49:948–955.

33. Levtzion-Korach O, Frankel A, Alcalai H, et al. Integrating incident data from five reporting systems to assess patient safety: making sense of the elephant. *Jt Comm J Qual Patient Saf* 2010;36:402–410.

34. Shojania KG. The elephant of patient safety: what you see depends on how you look. *Jt Comm J Qual Patient Saf* 2010;36:399–401, AP1–AP3.

35. Wu AW, ed. *The Value of Close Calls in Improving Patient Safety*. Oakbrook Terrace, IL: Joint Commission Resources; 2011.

36. Weingart SN, Wilson RM, Gibberd RW, et al. Epidemiology of medical error. *BMJ* 2000;320:774–777.

37. Donchin Y, Gopher D, Olin M, et al. A look into the nature and causes of human errors in the intensive care unit. *Crit Care Med* 1995;23:294–300.

38. Aspden P, Wolcott J, Bootman JL, et al., eds. *Preventing Medication Errors: Quality Chasm Series. Committee on Identifying and Preventing Medication Errors*. Washington, DC: National Academy Press; 2007.

39. Kanjanarat P, Winterstein AG, Johns TE, et al. Nature of preventable adverse drug events in hospitals: a literature review. *Am J Health Syst Pharm* 2003;60:1750–1759.

40. Bates DW, Boyle D, Vander Vliet M, et al. Relationship between medication errors and adverse drug events. *J Gen Intern Med* 1995;10:199–205.

41. Van Den Bos J, Rustagi K, Gray T, et al. The $17.1 billion problem: the annual cost of measurable medical errors. *Health Aff (Millwood)* 2011;30:596–603.

42. Sarkar U, Wachter RM, Schroeder SA, et al. Refocusing the lens: patient safety in ambulatory chronic disease care. *Jt Comm J Qual Patient Saf* 2009;35:377–383.

43. Young HM, Gray SL, McCormick WC, et al. Types, prevalence, and potential clinical significance of medication administration errors in assisted living. *J Am Geriatr Soc* 2008;56:1199–1205.

44. Weeks WB, Bagian JP. Making the business case for patient safety. *Jt Comm J Qual Saf* 2003;29:51–54.

45. Wu AW. Medical error: the second victim. *West J Med* 2000;172:358–359.

| ADDITIONAL READINGS

Advances in Patient Safety: New Directions and Alternative Approaches. Rockville, MD: Agency for Healthcare Research and Quality; July 2008. AHRQ Publication Nos. 080034 (1–4).

Hilfiker D. Facing our mistakes. *N Engl J Med* 1984;310:118–122.

Millman EA, Pronovost PJ, Makary MA, et al. Patient-assisted incident reporting: including the patient in patient safety. *J Patient Saf* 2011;7:106–108.

Murff HJ, FitzHenry F, Matheny ME, et al. Automated identification of postoperative complications within an electronic medical record using natural language processing.
JAMA 2011;306:848–855.

Pronovost PJ, Colantuoni E. Measuring preventable harm: helping science keep pace with
policy. *JAMA* 2009; 301:1273–1275.

Pronovost PJ, Lilford R. Analysis and commentary: a road map for improving the performance of performance measures. *Health Aff (Millwood)* 2011;30:569–573.

Rosenthal MM, Sutcliffe KM, eds. *Medical Error: What Do We Know? What Do We Do?*
San Francisco, CA: Jossey-Bass; 2002.

Spath PL, ed. *Error Reduction in Health Care: A Systems Approach to Improving Patient
Safety*. 2nd ed. San Francisco, CA: Jossey-Bass; 2011.

Thomas EJ, Studdert DM, Newhouse JP, et al. Costs of medical injuries in Utah and Colorado. *Inquiry* 1999;36:255–264.

Vincent C. *Patient Safety*, 2nd ed. London: Elsevier; 2010.

Vincent C. Understanding and responding to adverse events. *N Engl J Med* 2003;348:
1051–1056.

BASIC PRINCIPLES OF PATIENT SAFETY | 2

THE MODERN APPROACH TO PATIENT SAFETY: SYSTEMS THINKING AND THE SWISS CHEESE MODEL

The traditional approach to medical errors has been to blame the provider who delivers care directly to the patient, acting at what is sometimes called the "sharp end" of care: the doctor performing the transplant operation or diagnosing the patient's chest pain, the nurse hanging the intravenous medication bag, or the pharmacist preparing the chemotherapy. Over the last decade, we have recognized that this approach overlooks the fact that most errors are committed by hardworking, well-trained individuals, and such errors are unlikely to be prevented by admonishing people to be more careful, or by shaming, firing, or suing them.

The modern patient safety movement replaces "the blame and shame game" with an approach known as *systems thinking.* This paradigm acknowledges the human condition—namely, that humans err—and concludes that safety depends on creating systems that anticipate errors and either prevent or catch them before they cause harm. Such an approach has been the cornerstone of safety improvements in other high-risk industries but has been ignored in medicine until the past decade.

British psychologist James Reason's "*Swiss cheese model*" of organizational accidents has been widely embraced as a mental model for system safety[1,2] (Figure 2-1). This model, drawn from innumerable accident investigations in fields such as commercial aviation and nuclear power, emphasizes that in complex organizations, a single "sharp-end" (the person in the control booth in the nuclear plant, the surgeon making the incision) error is rarely enough to cause harm. Instead, such errors must penetrate multiple incomplete layers of protection ("layers of Swiss cheese") to cause a devastating result. Reason's model highlights the need to focus less on the (futile) goal of trying to perfect human behavior and more on aiming to shrink the holes in

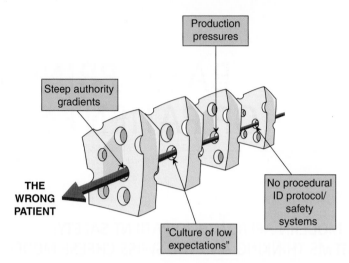

Figure 2-1 ▪ James Reason's Swiss cheese model of organizational accidents. The analysis is of "The Wrong Patient" case in Chapter 15. (Reproduced with permission from Reason JT. *Human Error*. New York, NY: Cambridge University Press, 1990. Copyright © 1990 Cambridge University Press.)

the Swiss cheese (sometimes referred to as *latent errors*) and create multiple overlapping layers of protection to decrease the probability that the holes will ever align and let an error slip through.

The Swiss cheese model emphasizes that analyses of medical errors need to focus on their "root causes"—not just the smoking gun, sharp-end error, but all the underlying conditions that made an error possible (or, in some situations, inevitable) (Chapter 14). A number of investigators have developed schema for categorizing the root causes of errors; the most widely used, by Charles Vincent, is shown in Table 2-1.[3,4] The schema explicitly forces the error reviewer to ask whether there should have been a checklist or read back, whether the resident was too fatigued to think clearly, or whether the young nurse was too intimidated to speak up when she suspected an error.

ERRORS AT THE SHARP END: SLIPS VERSUS MISTAKES

Even though we now understand that the root cause of hundreds of thousands of errors each year lies at the "blunt end," the proximate cause *is* often an act committed (or neglected, or performed incorrectly) by a caregiver. Even as we embrace the systems approach as the most useful paradigm, it would be wrong not to tackle these human errors as well. After all, even a room filled with flammable gas will not explode unless someone strikes a match.

Table 2-1	CHARLES VINCENT'S FRAMEWORK FOR CATEGORIZING THE ROOT CAUSES OF ERRORS	
Framework	Contributory Factors	Examples of Problems That Contribute to Errors
Institutional	Regulatory context Medicolegal environment	Insufficient priority given by regulators to safety issues; legal pressures against open discussion, preventing the opportunity to learn from adverse events
Organization and management	Financial resources and constraints Policy standards and goals Safety culture and priorities	Lack of awareness of safety issues on the part of senior management; policies leading to inadequate staffing levels
Work environment	Staffing levels and mix of skills Patterns in workload and shifts Design, availability, and maintenance of equipment Administrative and managerial support	Heavy workloads, leading to fatigue; limited access to essential equipment; inadequate administrative support, leading to reduced time with patients
Team	Verbal communication Written communication Supervision and willingness to seek help Team leadership	Poor supervision of junior staff; poor communication among different professions; unwillingness of junior staff to seek assistance
Individual staff member	Knowledge and skills Motivation and attitude Physical and mental health	Lack of knowledge or experience; long-term fatigue and stress
Task	Availability and use of protocols Availability and accuracy of test results	Unavailability of test results or delay in obtaining them; lack of clear protocols and guidelines
Patient	Complexity and seriousness of condition Language and communication Personality and social factors	Distress; language barriers between patients and caregivers

Reproduced with permission from Vincent C. Understanding and responding to adverse events. *N Engl J Med* 2003;348:1051–1056; Vincent C, Taylor-Adams S, Stanhope N. Framework for analyzing risk and safety in clinical medicine. *BMJ* 1998; 316:1154–1157.

In thinking about human errors, it is useful to differentiate between "slips" and "mistakes", and to do this, one must appreciate the difference between *conscious* behavior and *automatic* behavior. Conscious behavior is what we do when we "pay attention" to a task, and it is especially important when we are doing something new, like learning to play the piano or program our DVD player. On the other hand, automatic behaviors are the things we do almost unconsciously—they may have required a lot of thought initially, but after a while we do them virtually "in our sleep." Humans prefer automatic behaviors because they take less energy, have predictable outcomes, and allow us to "multitask"—do other things at the same time. Some of these other tasks are also automatic behaviors, like driving a car while drinking coffee or talking on the phone, but some require conscious thought. These latter moments—when a doctor tries to write a "routine" prescription while also pondering his approach to a challenging patient—are particularly risky, both for making errors in the routine, automatic process ("slips") or in the conscious process ("mistakes").

Now that we've distinguished the two types of tasks, let's turn to slips versus mistakes. *Slips* are inadvertent, unconscious lapses in the performance of some automatic task: you absently drive to work on Sunday morning because your automatic behavior kicks in and dictates your actions. Slips occur most often when we put an activity on "autopilot" so we can manage new sensory inputs, think through a problem, or deal with emotional upset, fatigue, or stress (a pretty good summing up of most healthcare environments). *Mistakes*, on the other hand, result from incorrect choices. Rather than blundering into them while we are distracted, we usually make mistakes because of insufficient knowledge, lack of experience or training, inadequate information (or inability to interpret available information properly), or applying the wrong set of rules or algorithms to a decision (we'll delve into this area more deeply when we discuss diagnostic errors in Chapter 6).

When measured on an "errors per action" yardstick, conscious behaviors are more prone to mistakes than automatic behaviors are prone to slips. However, slips probably represent the greater overall threat to patient safety because so much of what healthcare providers do is automatic. Doctors and nurses are most likely to slip while doing something they have done correctly a thousand times: asking patients if they are allergic to any medications before writing a prescription, remembering to verify a patient's identity before sending her off to a procedure, or loading a syringe with heparin (and not insulin) before flushing an IV line (the latter two cases are described in Chapters 15 and 4, respectively).

The complexity of healthcare work adds to the risks. Like pilots, soldiers, and others trained to work in high-risk occupations, doctors and nurses are programmed to do many specific tasks, under pressure, with a high degree of accuracy. But unlike most other professions, medical jobs typically combine three very different types of tasks: lots of conscious behaviors (complex decisions, judgment calls), many "customer" interactions, and innumerable automatic behaviors. Physician training, in particular, has traditionally emphasized the highly cognitive aspects with a small focus on the human interactions. But, until very recently, it has completely ignored the importance, and risky nature, of automatic behaviors.

With all of this in mind, how then should we respond to the inevitability of slips? Our typical response would be to reprimand (if not fire) a nurse for giving the wrong medication, admonishing her to "be more careful next time!" Even if the nurse did, she is just as likely to commit a different error while automatically carrying out a different task in a different setting. As James Reason reminds us, "Errors are largely unintentional. It is very difficult for management to control what people did not intend to do in the first place."[2] And it is not just managers whose instinct is to blame the provider at the sharp end—we providers blame ourselves! When we make a slip—a stupid error in something that we usually do perfectly "in our sleep"—we feel embarrassed. We chastise ourselves harder than any supervisor could, and swear we'll never make a careless mistake like that again.[5] Realistically, though, such promises are almost impossible to keep.

Whatever the strategy employed to prevent slips (and they will be discussed throughout the book), a clear lesson is that boring, repetitive tasks can be dangerous and are often performed better by machines. In medicine, these tasks include monitoring a patient's oxygen level during a long surgery, suturing large wounds, holding surgical retractors steady for a long time, and scanning mountains of data for significant patterns. As anesthesiologist Alan Merry and legal scholar and novelist Alexander McCall Smith have observed:

> people have no need to apologize for their failure to achieve machine-like standards in those activities for which machines are better suited. They are good at other things—original thought, for one, empathy and compassion for another. . . It is true that people are distractible—but in fact this provides a major survival advantage for them. A machine (unless expressly designed to detect such an event) will continue with its repetitive task while the house burns down around it, whereas most humans will notice that something unexpected is going on and will change their activity. . .[6]

COMPLEXITY THEORY AND COMPLEX ADAPTIVE SYSTEMS

The decisions made and actions taken by individual doctors and nurses occur in the context of the structure, policies, and culture of their organizations and healthcare systems. We will explore these issues later in this book because appreciating this context is often the key to improving safety. For now, as we think about mental models relevant to safety, it is worth introducing the topic of complexity theory.[7]

You'll recall that I referred to complexity earlier when discussing many of the decisions that frontline caregivers need to make every day. But another type of complexity—that of the entire ecosystem of care—is also at play when we consider patient safety. This area goes under the broad heading of *complexity theory,* a branch of management thinking that holds that large organizations don't operate like predictable and static machines, in which Inputs A and B predictably lead to Result C. Rather, they operate as *complex adaptive systems*, with elements of unpredictability, codependancy, and nonlinearity that must be appreciated as we try to make them work better.[8]

Complexity theory divides decisions and problems into three general categories: simple, complicated, and complex.[9] *Simple* problems are ones in which the inputs and outputs are known; they can be managed by following a recipe or a set of rules. Baking a cake is a simple problem; so is choosing the right antibiotics to treat pyelonephritis. *Complicated* decisions involve substantial uncertainties: the solutions may not be known, but they are potentially knowable. An example is designing a rocket ship to fly to the moon—if you were working for NASA in 1962 and heard President Kennedy declare this as a national goal, you probably believed it was not going to be easy but, with enough brainpower and resources, it could be done. Finally, *complex* decisions are likened to raising a child. Although we may have a general sense of what works, the actual formula for success is, alas, unknowable (or certainly seems so most days!).

Understanding these differences is vital because we need to match our approaches to the types of problems at hand. A checklist may be a wonderful solution for a simple problem, but a distraction for a complex one. Enacting a series of rules and policies may seem like progress, but may actually set us back if it stifles innovation and collegial exchange among frontline workers. Sometimes the best approach to a complex problem is to try something that seems sensible, measure the results (making sure workers feel able to speak truthfully and staying attuned to unanticipated consequences), and repeat this cycle many times.

But, as organizational expert Paul Plesk points out, our recognition of the complexity of healthcare systems is not a call for chaos. "A somewhat surprising finding from research on complex adaptive systems," he writes, "is that relatively simple rules can lead to complex, emergent, innovative system behavior."[8] Atul Gawande expands on this point in *The Checklist Manifesto*.[9] A good checklist, by specifying a few behaviors and encouraging cross-talk among frontline caregivers, can lead to remarkable improvements that go well beyond adherence to the items on the list (Chapter 15).

Table 2-2 presents a distillation of some of the key lessons from studies of complex adaptive systems. We'll return to these issues several times over

Table 2-2 **SOME KEY PRINCIPLES AND ASSUMPTIONS DRAWN FROM COMPLEXITY THEORY AND THE STUDY OF COMPLEX ADAPTIVE SYSTEMS**

- Relationships between parts are more important than the parts themselves.
- Neither the system nor its external environment is, or ever will be, constant—emergence and natural creativity are the norm. Equilibrium is actually an unhealthy state.
- Individuals within a system are independent and creative decision makers and highly interdependent.
- Uncertainty and paradox are inherent within the system.
- Problems cannot be solved like a machine can solve something, but they can nevertheless be "moved forward" if you understand the patterns that are creating them.
- Effective solutions can emerge from minimum specifications or simple rules rather than overspecification.
- Small changes can have big effects (nonlinearity).
- Behavior exhibits patterns (that can be termed "attractors").
- Change is more easily adopted when it taps into attractor patterns.

Reproduced with permission from Tamarack—An Institute for Community Engagement. Complexity—A Conversation with Brenda Zimmerman. Available at: http://tamarackcommunity.ca/ssi8.html.

the course of the book, such as when we discuss culture and High Reliability Organizations (Chapter 15) and consider how to build strong institutional patient safety programs (Chapter 22).

GENERAL PRINCIPLES OF PATIENT SAFETY IMPROVEMENT STRATEGIES

Drawing on these mental models, the modern patient safety field emphasizes the need to shore up systems to prevent or catch errors rather than to create "goof-proof" individual providers. For example, errors in routine behaviors ("slips") can best be prevented by *building in redundancies and cross checks*, in the form of checklists, read backs ("let me read your order back to you"), and other standardized safety procedures (e.g., signing the surgical site prior to an operation, asking patients their name before medication administration). It also emphasizes the need for *standardization and simplification*. For example, standardizing the process of taking a patient to the magnetic resonance imaging scanner makes it far easier to "bake in" the correct safety procedures.

Recently, there has been increased emphasis on decreasing errors at the person–machine interface through the use of *forcing functions*—engineering solutions that decrease the probability of human error. The classic example outside medicine was the 1980s-era modifications to automobile braking systems that rendered it impossible to place a car in reverse when the driver's foot is off the brake. In healthcare, forcing functions include changing the gas nozzles and connectors so that anesthesiologists cannot mistakenly hook up the wrong gas to a patient. Given the ever-increasing complexity of modern medicine, building in such forcing functions (in intravenous pumps, cardiac defibrillators, mechanical ventilators, and computerized order entry systems) will be crucial to safety (Chapter 7).

In addition to systems enhancements, there has been a growing recognition of the importance of improving communication and teamwork. Commercial pilots all participate in "*crew resource management*" courses in which they train for emergencies with other crew, learning to encourage open dialogue, communicate clearly using standard language, and utilize checklists, debriefings, and other systemic approaches. The evidence that such training enhances patient safety is increasingly persuasive.[10] The term "*culture of safety*" is used as shorthand for an environment in which teamwork, clear communication, and openness about errors (both to other healthcare professionals and to patients) are operative (Chapter 15).

Another key patient safety principle is to *learn from one's mistakes*. This may take multiple forms. Safe systems have a culture in which errors are openly discussed, often in morbidity and mortality (M&M) conferences. There is a new push to make sure that such discussions include members of the appropriate disciplines (such as nursing and hospital administration, not just physicians), point out errors rather than gloss over them in the name of avoiding a punitive atmosphere, and emphasize systems thinking and solutions.[11,12] In addition to open discussions at conferences, safe organizations build in mechanisms to hear about errors from frontline staff, often via incident reporting systems or unit-based safety teams,[12,13] and to perform detailed ("root cause") analyses[14] of major errors ("sentinel events") in an effort to define all the "layers of Swiss cheese" that need attention (Chapter 14). They also recognize the realities of complex adaptive systems: overmanaging workers through boatloads of top-down, prescriptive rules and directives may be more unsafe than tolerating some degree of flexibility and experimentation on the frontlines.

Finally, there is increasing appreciation of the importance of a *well-trained, well-staffed, and well-rested workforce* in delivering safe care. There is now evidence linking low nurse-to-patient ratios, long resident work hours, and lack of board certification to poor patient outcomes (Chapter 16).[15–19] Such research is catalyzing a more holistic view of patient safety, recognizing that the implementation of "safer systems" will not create safe patient care if the providers are overextended, poorly trained, or undersupervised. Nor is "systems thinking" an excuse to allow caregivers or their leaders to remain unaccountable for being unwilling to follow appropriate and well-vetted safety rules (Chapter 19).[20]

This long list of potential approaches to improving safety (each of which will be discussed in greater detail later) highlights one of the great challenges in the field: in the absence of comparative evidence, and in light of the high cost of some of the interventions (e.g., improved staffing, computerized order entry, simulation, teamwork training), even organizations committed to safety can become bewildered as they consider which approach to emphasize.[21] Institutions quite naturally focus on the practices that are measured, publicly reported, and compensated. As the next chapter will show, such a prioritization scheme will tend to elevate quality improvement strategies over those focused on patient safety because the results of the former are easier to measure. Thankfully, many of the approaches to improving quality, such as computerization and standardization, will also yield safety benefits. On the other hand, because improving culture is both difficult and hard to measure, it risks being shuffled to the bottom of the deck, notwithstanding its importance to patient safety. Pronovost, Miller, and I have suggested a measurement scheme for patient safety that takes these considerations into account (Table 2-3).[22]

Table 2-3 **A PROPOSED METHOD FOR MEASURING PROGRESS IN PATIENT SAFETY**

Measures that can be feasibly captured as rates

1. How often are patients harmed? (e.g., rates of healthcare-associated infections, postoperative venous thromboembolism, or medication errors)
2. How often do clinicians provide appropriate interventions? (e.g., measures of processes that have been strongly linked to safety outcomes: higher nurse-to-patient ratios, pharmacist presence on hospital units, functioning computerized provider order entry)

Measures that generally cannot be presented as rates

1. Have clinicians learned from mistakes? (evidence that incident reports or root cause analyses led to meaningful changes, such as new policies or procedures)
2. How successful are clinicians and healthcare systems in creating a culture of safety? (has the system administered a validated safety culture survey to the staff, and demonstrated improvement on it?)

KEY POINTS

- The modern approach to patient safety hinges on "systems thinking"—a recognition that most errors are made by competent, careful, and caring providers, and preventing these errors often involves embedding providers in a system that anticipates glitches and catches them before they do harm.
- James Reason's "Swiss cheese model" is the dominant paradigm for understanding the relationship between active ("sharp end") errors and latent ("blunt end") errors; it is important to resist the temptation to focus solely on the former and neglect the latter.
- A variety of strategies should be employed to create safer systems, including simplification, standardization, building in redundancies, improving teamwork and communication, and learning from past mistakes.
- There is a growing appreciation of the complexity of healthcare delivery organizations, which are vivid examples of complex adaptive systems. Such systems rarely respond in linear, predictable ways to prescriptive policies. This means that efforts to improve safety must combine rules and standards with messier activities that account for the importance of culture, innovation, and iterative learning.

REFERENCES

1. Reason JT. *Human Error*. New York, NY: Cambridge University Press; 1990.
2. Reason JT. *Managing the Risks of Organizational Accidents*. Aldershot, Hampshire, England: Ashgate; 1997.
3. Vincent C. Understanding and responding to adverse events. *N Engl J Med* 2003; 348:1051–1056.
4. Vincent C, Taylor-Adams S, Stanhope N. Framework for analyzing risk and safety in clinical medicine. *BMJ* 1998;316:1154–1157.
5. Waterman AD, Garbutt J, Hazel E, et al. The emotional impact of medical errors on practicing physicians in the United States and Canada. *Jt Comm J Qual Patient Saf* 2007;33:467–476.
6. Merry A, Smith AM. *Errors, Medicine, and the Law*. Cambridge, England: Cambridge University Press; 2001.
7. Plsek P, Greenhalgh T. The challenge of complexity in health care. *BMJ* 2001; 323:625–628.

8. Plesk P. Redesigning health care with insights from the science of complex adaptive systems. Appendix B in: Committee on Quality Health Care in America, Institute of Medicine. *Crossing the Quality Chasm: A New Health System for the 21st Century.* National Academy Press; 2001: 309–322.

9. Gawande A. *The Checklist Manifesto: How To Get Things Right.* New York: Metropolitan Books; 2009.

10. Neily J, Mills PD, Young-Xu Y, et al. Association between implementation of a medical team training program and surgical mortality. *JAMA* 2010;304:1693–1700.

11. Pierluissi E, Fischer MA, Campbell AR, et al. Discussion of medical errors in morbidity and mortality conferences. *JAMA* 2003;290:2838–2842.

12. Berenholtz SM, Hartsell TL, Pronovost PJ. Learning from defects to enhance morbidity and mortality conferences. *Am J Med Qual* 2009;24:192–195.

13. Pronovost P, Weast B, Rosenstein B. Implementing and validating a comprehensive unit-based safety program. *J Patient Saf* 2005;1:33–40.

14. Wu AW, Lipshutz AKM, Pronovost PJ. Effectiveness and efficiency of root cause analysis in medicine. *JAMA* 2008;299:685–687.

15. Needleman J, Buerhaus P, Pankratz VS, et al. Nurse staffing and inpatient hospital mortality. *N Engl J Med* 2011;364:1037–1045.

16. Landrigan CP, Rothschild JM, Cronin JW, et al. Effect of reducing interns' work hours on serious medical errors in intensive care units. *N Engl J Med* 2004;351: 1838–1848.

17. Brennan TA, Horwitz RI, Duffy FD, et al. The role of physician specialty board certification status in the quality movement. *JAMA* 2004;292:1038–1043.

18. Hugonnet S, Chevrolet JC, Pittet D. The effect of workload on infection risk in critically ill patients. *Crit Care Med* 2007;35:76–81.

19. Ong M, Bostrom A, Vidyarthi A, et al. House staff team workload and organization effects on patient outcomes in an academic general internal medicine inpatient service. *Arch Intern Med* 2007;167:47–52.

20. Wachter RM, Pronovost PJ. Balancing "no blame" with accountability in patient safety. *N Engl J Med* 2009;361:1401–1406.

21. Wachter RM. Patient safety at ten: unmistakable progress, troubling gaps. *Health Aff (Millwood)* 2010;29:165–173.

22. Pronovost PJ, Miller MR, Wachter RM. Tracking progress in patient safety: an elusive target. *JAMA* 2006;296:696–699.

| ADDITIONAL READINGS

Berwick DM. The science of improvement. *JAMA* 2008;299:1182–1184.

Dixon-Woods M, Bosk CL, Aveling EL, et al. Explaining Michigan: developing an ex post theory of a quality improvement program. *Milbank Q* 2011;89:167–205.

Garvin DA, Edmondson AC, Gino F. Is yours a learning organization? *Harv Bus Rev* 2008;86:109–116.

Helmreich RL. On error management: lessons from aviation. *BMJ* 2000;320:781–785.

32 I I AN INTRODUCTION TO PATIENT SAFETY AND MEDICAL ERRORS

Leape LL. Error in medicine. *JAMA* 1994;272:1851–1857.

Pronovost PJ, Faden RR. Setting priorities for patient safety: ethics, accountability, and public engagement. *JAMA* 2009;302:890–891.

Rogers J, Gaba DM. Have we gone too far in translating ideas from aviation to patient safety? *BMJ* 2011;342:c7309–c7310.

Wachter RM, Shojania KG. *Internal Bleeding: The Truth Behind America's Terrifying Epidemic of Medical Mistakes*. New York, NY: Rugged Land; 2004.

Weick KE, Sutcliffe KM. *Managing the Unexpected: Assuring High Performance in an Age of Complexity*. 2nd ed. San Francisco, CA: John Wiley & Sons; 2007.

Woods DD, Dekker S, Cook R, et al. *Behind Human Error*. 2nd ed. Burlington, VT: Ashgate; 2010.

SAFETY, QUALITY, AND VALUE | 3

WHAT IS QUALITY?

Quality of care has been defined by the Institute of Medicine (IOM) as "the degree to which health services for individuals and populations increase the likelihood of desired health outcomes and are consistent with current professional knowledge." In its seminal 2001 report, *Crossing the Quality Chasm,* the IOM advanced six aims for a quality healthcare system (Table 3-1): patient safety, patient-centeredness, effectiveness, efficiency, timeliness, and equity.[1] Note that this framework depicts safety as one of these six components, in essence making it a subset of quality. Note also that, though many clinicians tend to think of quality as being synonymous with the delivery of evidence-based care, the IOM's definition is much broader and includes matters that are of particular importance to patients (patient-centeredness and timeliness) and to society (equity).

Although the IOM makes clear that quality is more than the provision of care supported by science, evidence-based medicine *does* provide the foundation for much of quality measurement and improvement. For many decades, the particular practice style of a senior clinician or a prestigious medical center determined the standard of care (this tradition is now sometimes called "eminence-based medicine," with more than a hint of derision). Without discounting the value of experience and mature clinical judgment, the modern paradigm for identifying optimal practice has changed, driven by the explosion in clinical research over the past two generations (the number of randomized clinical trials has grown from less than 500 per year in 1970 to 20,000 per year in 2010). This research has helped define "best practices" in many areas of medicine, ranging from preventive strategies for a 64-year-old woman with diabetes to the treatment of the patient with acute myocardial infarction and cardiogenic shock.

Table 3-1   **THE IOM'S SIX AIMS FOR A QUALITY HEALTHCARE SYSTEM**
■ Healthcare must be safe
■ Healthcare must be effective
■ Healthcare must be patient-centered
■ Healthcare must be timely
■ Healthcare must be efficient
■ Healthcare must be equitable

Reproduced with permission from Committee on Quality of Health Care in America, Institute of
  Medicine. *Crossing the Quality Chasm: A New Health System for the 21st Century.* Washington, DC:
  National Academy Press, 2001.

Health services researcher Avedis Donabedian's taxonomy is widely used for measuring the quality of care. "*Donabedian's Triad*" divides quality measures into *structure* (how is care organized), *process* (what was done), and *outcomes* (what happened to the patient).[2] When used to assess the quality of care, each element of the Triad has important advantages and disadvantages[3] (Table 3-2). In recent years, as clinical research has established the link between certain processes and improved outcomes, process measures have often been used as proxies for quality. Examples include measuring whether hospitalized patients with pneumonia received influenza and pneumococcal vaccinations, and measuring glycosylated hemoglobin (hemoglobin A1c) at appropriate intervals in outpatients with diabetes.

There is a nuance in the last sentence that is worth highlighting. If the latter measure was of whether the physician *checked* the hemoglobin A1c (or the blood pressure or cholesterol; the point would be the same) at appropriate intervals, that would be a classic process measure. On the other hand, if the measure was of the *actual value* of the hemoglobin A1c (i.e., fraction of patients with hemoglobin A1c below 7%), that would be an outcome—more specifically, an *intermediate outcome,* as it is really a proxy for outcomes we care about, such as mortality, kidney function, or retinopathy.[4] Although such intermediate outcomes may seem like attractive hybrids between process measures and true outcomes, care is warranted as intermediate outcomes may, like true outcome measures (see below), require case-mix adjustment to fairly assess the quality of care. More importantly, the medical literature is replete with cautionary reports on the results of interventions that produced beneficial effects on plausible intermediate outcomes (such as suppression of premature ventricular contractions or raising levels of HDL cholesterol) but no effect—or even harm—on the main outcomes of interest.[5–7]

Table 3-2 **ADVANTAGES AND DISADVANTAGES OF USING STRUCTURE, PROCESS, AND OUTCOME (THE "DONABEDIAN TRIAD") TO MEASURE THE QUALITY OF CARE**

Measure	Simple Definition	Advantages	Disadvantages
Structure	How was care organized?	May be highly relevant in a complex health system	May fail to capture the quality of care by individual physicians Difficult to determine the "gold standard"
Process	What was done?	More easily measured and acted upon than outcomes May not require case-mix adjustment May directly reflect quality (if carefully chosen) No time lag—can be measured when care is provided	A proxy for outcomes All may not agree on "gold standard" processes May promote "cookbook" medicine, especially if physicians and health systems try to "game" their performance
Outcome	What happened to the patient?	What we really care about	May take years to occur May not reflect quality of care Requires case-mix and other adjustment to prevent "apples-to-oranges" comparisons

Reproduced with permission from Shojania KG, Showstack J, Wachter RM. Assessing hospital quality: a review for clinicians. *Eff Clin Pract* 2001;4:82–90.

When the science of case-mix adjustment is suitably advanced (e.g., in cardiac bypass surgery[8]), measures of outcomes such as mortality rates are often used. The caveat is crucial: if case-mix adjustment is not done well, the surgeon or hospital that accepts (or is referred) the sickest patients may appear to be worse than the lesser surgeon or institution that takes only easy cases.

Finally, when the processes are quite complex and the science of case-mix adjustment is immature, structural measures are often used as proxies for quality. As with process measures, using structural measures in this way assumes that good research has linked such elements to overall quality. Examples here include the presence of intensivists in critical care units, a dedicated stroke service, nurse-to-patient ratios, and computerized provider order entry (CPOE).

It is worth highlighting another special kind of outcome measure. As we've seen, the IOM appropriately considers the patient's experience to be one of the key dimensions of quality. Accordingly, assessments of such experience—generally collected through patient surveys—have become important quality measures, both because they reflect an outcome that we intrinsically care about, and because patients may identify quality problems missed by other methods.[9,10] In Medicare's new *"value-based purchasing"* program, rolling out in 2012–2014, 70% of the weight is placed on clinical measures such as care processes (e.g., administration of aspirin and beta-blockers to patients with myocardial infarction) and outcomes (30-day readmission rates, case-mix adjusted mortality rates), and fully 30% is given to the results of patient experience surveys.[11]

Harvard Business School professor Michael Porter has argued that we should focus our attention on outcome measures, as they are what really matters to patients.[12] Although I agree in theory, as the Chapter 1 discussion of using hospital mortality rates as quality/safety measures made clear (and at the risk of being obvious), good process measures are more helpful and valid than bad outcome measures.[13]

Moreover, even good outcome measures don't obviate the need for process and structural measurement. Let's say we find that our readmission rates for heart failure patients or our mortality rates for stroke admissions are higher than we would like. The next step, of course, is to examine our processes and structures and compare them to those of our peers or to known best-practice benchmarks. This is what we mean when we say that one of the downsides of outcome measures is that they are not directly actionable.[3] In the end, it is clear that a thoughtful mix of all elements of the Donabedian Triad—process, structure, and outcome—is important to any sound program of quality measurement and improvement.

THE EPIDEMIOLOGY OF QUALITY PROBLEMS

In a series of pioneering studies, Wennberg and colleagues demonstrated large and clinically indefensible variations in care from one city to another for the same problem or procedure.[14] Other studies have demonstrated large variations in the quality of care for patients based on race, income, and gender (*healthcare disparities*).[15] Together, these studies hint at a fundamental flaw in modern medical practice: we see such profound variations in common processes and procedures, as well as in the outcomes of comparable patient groups, that we can only conclude that care is often inconsistent with evidence.

Stimulated by these early studies on disparities and variations, researchers have more directly measured the frequency with which doctors and healthcare organizations provide care that comports with best evidence. McGlynn and colleagues studied more than 400 evidence-based measures of quality, and found that practice was consistent with the evidence *only 54% of the time.*[16] Adherence to evidence-based processes generally correlates with ultimate clinical outcomes,[17] although, soberingly, some studies have found a weaker relationship than one would anticipate.[18,19] Nevertheless, these large differences between best and actual practice have caused patients, providers, and policymakers to seek methods to drive and support quality improvement (QI) activities.

CATALYSTS FOR QUALITY IMPROVEMENT

The problems described above have exposed several impediments to the reliable delivery of high-quality care, including the lack of information regarding provider or institutional performance, the weakness of incentives for QI, the difficulty for practicing physicians to stay abreast of evidence-based medicine, and the absence of system support (such as information technology) for quality. Each will need to be addressed in order to make substantial gains in the quality of care.

The first step in QI begins with *quality measurement.* Fifteen years ago, there were only a handful of generally accepted quality measures, such as whether patients with acute myocardial infarction received aspirin or beta-blockers. More recently, scores of such measures have been promulgated by a variety of organizations, including payers (such as the Centers for Medicare & Medicaid Services [CMS]), accreditors and regulators (such as the Joint Commission), and medical societies (Table 3-3). (In the United States, an organization called the National Quality Forum exists largely to review proposed measures and endorse those that meet prespecified validity criteria.[20]) These measures have identified many opportunities for improvement among individual physicians, practices, and hospitals.

Given the enormous amount of new literature published each year, no individual physician can possibly remain abreast of all the evidence-based advances in a given field. *Practice guidelines,* such as those for the care of community-acquired pneumonia or for deep venous thrombosis prophylaxis, aim to synthesize evidence-based best practices into sets of summary recommendations. Although some providers deride guidelines as "cookbook medicine," there is increasing agreement that standardizing best practices is ethically and clinically appropriate; in fact, so-called *High Reliability Organizations* "hard wire" such practices whenever possible (Chapter 15). The major challenges for guideline developers are the need to keep guidelines updated as new knowledge accumulates[21] and the difficulties in developing guidelines that are relevant to the care of patients with multiple, potentially overlapping illnesses.[22] *Clinical pathways* are similar to guidelines, but attempt to articulate a series of steps, usually temporal (on day 1, do the following; on day 2; and so on). They are generally more useful for stereotypical processes such as

Table 3-3   EXAMPLES OF PUBLICLY REPORTED QUALITY MEASURES

Acute myocardial infarction and chest pain measures
  Aspirin at arrival (both inpatient and outpatient measure)
  Aspirin at discharge
  ACE inhibitor or ARB for LVS dysfunction
  Fibrinolytic agent received within 30 min of hospital arrival (both inpatient and outpatient measure)
  Percutaneous coronary intervention (PCI) received within 90 min of hospital arrival
  Smoking cessation advice/counseling
  Median time to fibrinolysis (outpatient measure only)
  Median time to transfer to another facility for acute coronary intervention (outpatient measure only)
  Median time to ECG (outpatient measure only)

Heart failure measures
  Evaluation of LVS function
  ACE inhibitor or ARB for LVS dysfunction
  Discharge instructions
  Smoking cessation advice/counseling

Pneumonia measures
  Initial antibiotic timing
  Pneumococcal vaccination
  Influenza vaccination
  Blood culture performed in the ED prior to initial antibiotic received in hospital
  Appropriate initial antibiotic selection
  Smoking cessation advice/counseling

Surgical care improvement/surgical infection prevention measures
  Prophylactic antibiotic received within 1 h of surgical incision (both inpatient and outpatient measure)
  Prophylactic antibiotics discontinued within 24 hours after surgery end time
  Prophylactic antibiotic selection
  Surgery patients with recommended venous thromboembolism prophylaxis ordered
  Surgery patients who received appropriate venous thromboembolism prophylaxis within 24 hours prior to surgery
    to 24 hours after surgery
  Cardiac surgery patients with controlled 6 AM postoperative blood glucose
  Surgery patients with appropriate hair removal
  Surgery patients on a beta blocker prior to arrival who received a beta-blocker during the perioperative period
  Inpatients whose urinary catheters were removed within 2 days after surgery to reduce the risk of infection

Children's asthma care
  Children receiving reliever medication (like albuterol) while hospitalized for asthma
  Children receiving systemic corticosteroid medication (oral and IV medication that reduces inflammation and
    controls symptoms) while hospitalized for asthma
  Children and their caregivers receiving a home management plan of care document while hospitalized for asthma

ACE, angiotensin-converting enzyme; ARB, angiotensin-receptor blocker; LVS, left ventricular systolic. (Reproduced with permission from the Hospital Quality Alliance and the Centers for Medicare & Medicaid Services (CMS). Available at: http://www.hospitalcompare.hhs.gov/staticpages/for-professionals/poc/Technical-Appendix.aspx#POC3.)

the postoperative management of patients after cardiac bypass surgery or hip replacement.

THE CHANGING QUALITY LANDSCAPE

Although one could argue that professionalism should be sufficient incentive to provide high-quality care, our recent recognition that the unwavering provision of such care depends on a system organized to reliably translate research into practice means that it will take significant investments (i.e., in developing guidelines, physician education, hiring case managers or clinical pharmacists, building information systems, and more) to deliver optimal care. The traditional payment system, which compensates physicians and hospitals equally whether quality is superb or appalling, provides no incentive to make the requisite investments.

This is changing rapidly, with a blizzard of initiatives to support and catalyze QI activities. Virtually all involve several steps: defining reasonable quality measures (evidence-based measures that capture appropriate structures, processes, or outcomes), measuring the performance of providers or systems, and using these results to promote change. Although each of these steps comes with challenges, the final one has probably created the greatest degree of uncertainty and been the subject of the most experimentation.

The first step in the series of activities designed to promote QI involves *selecting appropriate measures.* For local QI activities, it may be fine to use process measures that seem plausibly connected to an outcome of interest, even if the evidence connecting the two is not bulletproof. It is also often appropriate to use measures captured through self-report by the involved providers, even while recognizing the inherent biases in such data. Although we all aspire to perfect measurement, "don't let the perfect be the enemy of the good" is a reasonable rule for many local QI projects.

On the other hand, it makes sense to insist on higher standards for measures that are being used for public reporting or pay-for-performance programs. My colleagues and I have called these high-stake assessments "*Accountability Measures*" and proposed four criteria that they should meet (Table 3-4).[23]

This distinction is of more than academic interest. Jha and colleagues have shown that even if a provider checks a box attesting that he or she provided discharge counseling to patients with heart failure (the process measure), there is no correlation to readmission rates (the outcome), probably because the quality of such counseling varies widely.[24] Moreover, after Medicare instituted a quality measure related to the timing of initial antibiotic administration for patients with pneumonia (the "Four Hour Rule"), subsequent studies demonstrated that many emergency department (ED) patients who were given

Table 3-4	**PROPOSED CRITERIA FOR "ACCOUNTABILITY MEASURES" ADDRESSING PROCESSES OF CARE**

1. There is a strong evidence base showing that the care process leads to improved outcomes.
2. The measure accurately captures whether the evidence-based care process has, in fact, been provided.
3. The measure addresses a process that has few intervening care processes that must occur before the improved outcome is realized.
4. Implementing the measure has little or no chance of inducing unintended adverse consequences.

From Chassin MR, Loeb JM, Schmaltz SP, et al. Accountability measures—using measurement to promote quality improvement. *N Engl J Med* 2010;363:683–688. Reproduced with permission.

antibiotics by rushed physicians later proved not to have pneumonia, or any infection, at all.[25] It is clear that we have much to learn about which measures to target, how to collect the data, and how to promote improvement at a reasonable cost and with a minimum of unanticipated consequences.[26]

Once we settle on appropriate measures, the next steps involve *promoting and supporting improvement* and making it stick. Although one might hope that clear feedback will generate meaningful improvement in a provider's performance, experience has shown that this strategy leads to only modest change. Increasingly, a more aggressive strategy of *transparency* (disseminating the results of quality measures to key stakeholders) is becoming the norm. With simple transparency, the hope is that providers will find the public dissemination of their quality gaps of sufficient concern to motivate improvement. Further, many believe that patients (or their proxies, such as third-party payers) will begin to use such data to make choices about where patients receive care. To date, although there is little evidence that patients are using such data to make purchasing decisions, studies *have* shown impressive improvements in some publicly reported quality measures, supporting the premise that transparency itself may generate change.[23] Berwick, James, and Coye's framework (Figure 3-1) is useful for considering the two interwoven pathways—selection by patients or purchasers, and change undertaken by the provider organization—through which measurement and transparency can stimulate improvement.[27]

The newest strategy to motivate improvement is to tie payments for service to quality performance (*Pay for Performance,* or "P4P").[28] Although P4P is conceptually attractive, it also raises a host of questions: Are quality data accurate? Should payments go to best performers or to those with the great-

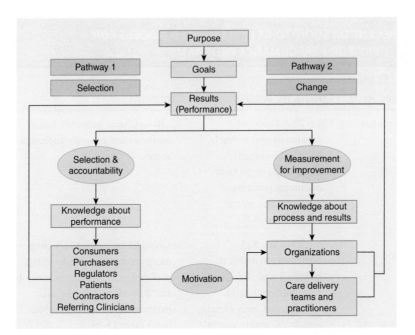

Figure 3-1 ▪ The figure demonstrates the two interwoven pathways (selection and change) by which measurement of performance measures can lead to improvement. (From Committee on Quality of Health Care in America, Institute of Medicine. *Crossing the Quality Chasm: A New Health System for the 21st Century.* Washington, DC: National Academy Press, 2001. Reproduced with permission.)

est improvements? Do existing measures adequately assess quality in patients with complex, multisystem disease? and does P4P erode professionalism or create undue focus on measurable practices and relative inattention to other important processes that are not being compensated?[28,29] At this writing, various flavors of P4P (Table 3-5[11,30–33]) are being implemented, and tested, in a variety of settings. Early evidence from these experiments indicates that P4P may produce only a little more change than that generated by transparency alone (Figure 3-2); the jury is still out on whether this marginal benefit (if it in fact exists) is enough to overcome the concerns cited above.[29,34]

QUALITY IMPROVEMENT STRATEGIES

Whether the motivation is ethics, embarrassment, or economics, the next question is how to actually improve the quality of care. There is no simple answer. In general, most institutions and physicians with success in this area

Table 3-5   **RECENT OR SOON-TO-BE IMPLEMENTED MODELS FOR PAY-FOR-PERFORMANCE PROGRAMS**

Program	Location: Sponsor (Year Introduced)	Criteria for Bonus/Penalty	Comments
Value-based Purchasing[11]	US: CMS (2012)	Up to 2% of hospital reimbursement withheld, and can be earned back, based on mixture of clinical processes/outcomes and patient satisfaction scores	70–30 weighting between clinical measures and patient satisfaction scores
Meaningful Use[30]	US: CMS (2011–12)	Approximately $25 billion in payments to hospitals and physicians for implementing IT systems that meet certain standards; within several years, this will change to reimbursement penalties for those lacking IT	Meaningful use criteria including using computerized order entry, performing drug–drug interaction and drug-allergy checks, and maintaining up-to-date problem lists (Table 13–5)
Readmission Penalties[31]	US: CMS (2012)	Hospitals with excess numbers of readmissions will see their reimbursements cut	Up to 3% of Medicare payments will be withheld for those in highest quartile of readmissions
"No Pay for Errors"[32]	US: CMS and some private payers (2009)	Hospitals that previously received extra payments for certain complicating conditions will no longer receive these payments if these conditions are deemed preventable	Examples of these conditions are certain hospital-associated infections, pressure ulcers, and retained surgical objects. Relatively small amount of money at risk
Primary Care Pay for Performance Program[33]	UK: National Health Service (2004)	GPs received bonuses based on performance on more than 100 ambulatory quality measures	GPs could earn approximately 25% bonus based on performance

CMS, Centers for Medicare & Medicaid Services; GP, general practitioners; IT, information technology; UK, United Kingdom; US, United States.

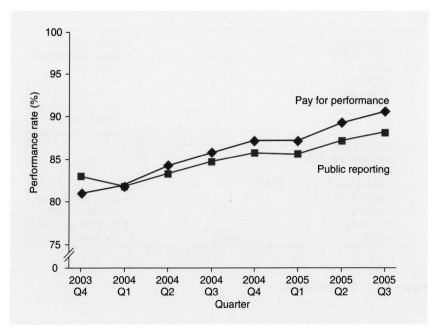

Figure 3-2 ▪ Relative performance in two groups of hospitals that either participated in a pay for performance program (in addition to having their data publicly reported) vs. those hospitals subject to public reporting alone. The rate is the percentage of patients given the specified care on 10 process measures in 3 conditions (acute myocardial infarction, congestive heart failure, and pneumonia). (From Lindenauer PK, Remus D, Roman S, et al. Public reporting and pay for performance in hospital quality improvement. *N Engl J Med* 2007;356:486–496. Reproduced with permission.)

use a variation of the "*Plan-Do-Study-Act*" (PDSA) cycle (Figure 3-3), recognizing that QI activities must be carefully planned and implemented, that their impact needs to be measured, and that the results of these activities need to be fed back into the system in a continuously iterative process of improvement. A number of more complex and sophisticated methods (Lean, Six Sigma, Toyota Production System) have been developed in the business, manufacturing, and engineering worlds, and have been adapted to healthcare, often (but not always) successfully.[35,36] A detailed discussion of these methods is beyond the scope of this book; interested readers are referred to several excellent resources.[37–39]

In addition to the PDSA cycle, several other tactics are useful. For QI practices that require predictable repetition, efforts to "*hard wire*" the practice or use alternative providers who focus on the activity are often beneficial. For example, the strategy most likely to increase the rate of pneumococcal

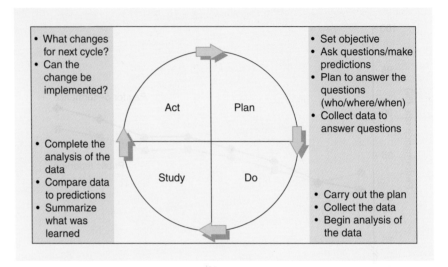

Figure 3-3 ▪ The PDSA cycle.

vaccination of hospitalized patients with pneumonia is to embed it in a standard order set (either paper-based or computerized).[40] Having a nurse remove the patient's shoes before the doctor enters the room can increase rates of diabetic foot examinations in outpatient practice. Empowering critical care nurses or respiratory therapists to follow a weaning protocol safely shortens the time patients with respiratory failure spend on mechanical ventilators.[41]

In some areas, though, QI involves much more complex and interdependent activities. In these circumstances, bringing teams together to examine their practices and participate in a PDSA cycle is the most likely path to success. For example, a group of cardiac surgeons in the northeastern United States participated in a multicenter QI project in which they observed each other's care, agreed on best practices, scrutinized each other's outcomes, and suggested improvement strategies. The result: a 24% reduction in cardiac surgery mortality.[42] This kind of approach is likely to be facilitated by team training and is in keeping with what we have come to understand about improvement in complex adaptive systems of care (Chapters 2 and 15).[43]

COMMONALITIES AND DIFFERENCES BETWEEN QUALITY AND PATIENT SAFETY

Although patient safety is a subset of the larger issue of quality of care, it is important to appreciate the sometimes subtle differences between the two areas, particularly when it comes to measuring performance and changing practices and systems.

Mr. S, a 74-year-old man, is admitted to the hospital with severe sub-sternal chest pain. In the ED, his electrocardiogram (ECG) shows the ST elevation typical of a significant myocardial infarction. In this hospital, ST-elevation myocardial infarctions are managed with emergent balloon angioplasty, and there is strong evidence linking "door-to-balloon times" to ultimate outcome. There is a delay in reaching the cardiologist on call; when he finally arrives an hour later, the cardiac catheterization lab is not prepared for the proce-dure, leading to another delay. The cardiologist, Dr. G, orders a dose of metoprolol, a beta-blocker. Dr. G's handwriting is difficult to read, but the pharmacist is reluctant to page the doctor, who is known for his "difficult personality." So the pharmacist takes his best guess at the prescription and dispenses a dose of metformin, a medicine for diabetes. Ultimately, the mistake is recognized and the correct medi-cine is administered as the patient is being wheeled up for his angio-plasty. The door-to-balloon time is 150 minutes, well above the goal of 90 minutes or less. The patient survives, but is left with a moderate amount of heart damage (ejection fraction 35%, normal 55%–70%) and mildly symptomatic heart failure.

This case illustrates both quality and safety problems. The administration of the wrong medicine (metformin instead of metoprolol) is clearly an error. Future approaches to preventing such errors would likely include computeriza-tion, standardization, and changes in culture to ensure that the pharmacist would promptly call the physician to clarify an ambiguous order. But the prolonged door-to-balloon time also represents a quality problem, a failure in the process of care. There were no overt errors in this process, it just took far longer than it should have because of lack of coordination, planning, and training. The com-bined result of both kinds of problems was a poor outcome.

Differentiating these quality and safety problems is important as we con-sider their causes and how best to prevent them. Let's assume that the patient's insurer was interested in measuring the quality and safety of care in this hospital. It would be relatively easy to implement a transparent, auditable process to docu-ment the door-to-balloon time. Ditto for whether the patient received aspirin, a beta-blocker, or a flu shot at discharge. Turning to outcomes, it would be straight-forward to figure out whether Mr. S and similar patients were alive or dead at the time of discharge (though remember that we'd need some pretty sophisticated case-mix adjustment to be sure that our outcome assessment wasn't unfairly dis-advantaging hospitals or doctors that attract sicker patients). Public reporting of door-to-balloon times, perhaps accompanied by higher reimbursement for better performance (via P4P), would likely spur improved performance.

But how could this insurer learn of Mr. S's medication error? It is dif-ficult to imagine a transparent, auditable and efficient system that does not depend on self reporting by the nurse, pharmacist, or physician to capture the error. Moreover, a strategy of public reporting (or P4P) for medication errors might well leave providers reluctant to report them, causing the system to be unaware that such errors were occurring and ill prepared to generate the shared knowledge—as well as the money and will—to fix them.

The process of fixing both problems (door-to-balloon times and medication errors) might be relatively similar, in that both are likely to require changes in core processes (*all patients with chest pain will receive ECGs within the first 5 minutes of arriving in the ED*; *all prescriptions will include medication name, dose, and indication*), thoughtful implementation of technology (perhaps an automatic ECG reader for the chest pain protocol; CPOE for the medication error), and changes in culture (an unwavering commitment to change by system leaders; simulation training to improve door-to-balloon time performance; teamwork training to improve physician–pharmacist communication and dampen down hierarchies for the medication error).[44]

The bottom line is that patients have a right to expect care that is *both* high quality and safe. The IOM report on medical errors, *To Err is Human,* helped catalyze a national push to improve safety, and has led to important changes in culture, training, regulation, and technology.[45] However, because measuring safety tends to depend largely on providers' self-report (although this may change over time with the computerization of medical records and refinements in measurement strategies such as trigger tools [Chapters 1 and 14]), the twin strategies of transparency and differential payment are more likely to improve quality than safety.[46] Happily, the two endeavors have enough commonalities (the need for improved information systems, standardization, and simplification, use of multidisciplinary teams, and improvement cycles) that QI initiatives will often result in better safety. Other cornerstones of patient safety, such as the creation of a safety culture (Chapter 15), may be largely independent of QI efforts and will require a distinct focus. And all of these quality and safety improvement activities are relevant to the increasingly important work of removing waste and unnecessary cost from our healthcare system.

| VALUE: CONNECTING QUALITY | (AND SAFETY) TO THE COST OF CARE

Outside the world of healthcare, we base most of our purchasing decisions on our perception of *value*: quality divided by cost. Who among us is rich enough to always buy the very best thing, or frugal enough to always buy the least expensive one? Much of the focus of our lives as consumers is spent trying to determine the value of the things we're considering buying—whether it's a car, a house, a café mocha, or a college education—by weighing the measured (or perceived) quality against the cost. As we do this, we ask a simple question: is the item or service worth the price?

Healthcare decisions have traditionally not been made this way (I sometimes refer to this as "healthcare exceptionalism"), partly because of the limited ability of patients (and their doctors, for that matter) to make rational judgments about the quality of a given physician, surgeon, or hospital, and partly because one of the functions of healthcare insurance is to shield us from shouldering the full cost of our purchasing decisions. In other words, when you're buying your Starbucks coffee or an Audi sedan, you're well aware of the price and are in a perfect position to judge whether the quality (and safety, in the case of the car) is worth it. But in healthcare, the service is often "covered" or the patient is responsible for only a portion of the cost.

Much of the decade-long revolution in quality measurement and reporting can be seen as an effort to provide patients (or other interested parties, such as, in the United States, employers or insurers or, in countries with single-payer systems, the government) with the information they need to make rational decisions about healthcare value. This framework becomes even more important as the costs of healthcare continue to rise, crowding out resources for other worthwhile private and public pursuits. Increasingly, efforts to improve quality, safety, and patient satisfaction are not taking place in a cost-agnostic vacuum. Rather, healthcare providers and organizations will be pushed relentlessly to improve both the numerator *and the denominator* of the value equation.[12]

In this environment, we can already see the incentives shifting, from promoting the best care to promoting the best care *at the lowest cost.* Both Medicare's "value-based purchasing" and "no pay for errors" initiatives—in which anything but perfect performance leads to reimbursement cuts rather than additional payments for top performers—may well be early indications of the shape of the "pay-for-performance" initiatives of the future.[11,32]

KEY POINTS

- Safety is usually considered a subset of quality, but it is more difficult to measure, in part because identification of incidents often depends on self-reports by caregivers.
- Quality measurement is best thought of in terms of "Donebedian's Triad": structure, process, or outcomes. Each type of measure has advantages and disadvantages when compared with the others.
- Measures being employed for public reporting and pay for performance ("Accountability Measures") must meet a higher standard than those used for internal QI.

- There is tremendous activity in the healthcare marketplace promoting transparency (i.e., public reporting) and differential payments based on performance ("pay for performance"). The latter efforts are taking on multiple forms, including so-called "value-based purchasing" and "no pay for errors" initiatives.
- Cost pressures in the United States and elsewhere mean that the healthcare system's target will no longer be quality or safety alone, but value— quality (including safety, access, and the patient's experience) divided by cost.

REFERENCES

1. Committee on Quality of Health Care in America, Institute of Medicine. *Crossing the Quality Chasm: A New Health System for the 21st Century.* Washington, DC: National Academy Press; 2001.
2. Donabedian A. The quality of care. How can it be assessed? *JAMA* 1988;260: 1743–1748.
3. Shojania KG, Showstack J, Wachter RM. Assessing hospital quality: a review for clinicians. *Eff Clin Pract* 2001;4:82–90.
4. Kerr EA, Krein SL, Vijan S, et al. Avoiding pitfalls in chronic disease quality measurement: a case for the next generation of technical quality measures. *Am J Manag Care* 2001;7:1033–1043.
5. Echt, D, P Liebson, L Mitchell, et al. Mortality and morbidity in patients receiving encainide, flecainide, or placebo: The Cardiac Arrhythmia Suppression Trial. *N Engl J Med* 1991;324:781–788.
6. Grady D, Herrington D, Bittner V, et al. Cardiovascular disease outcomes during 6.8 years of hormone therapy: Heart and Estrogen/progestin Replacement Study follow-up (HERS II). *JAMA* 1998;280:605–613.
7. The AIM-HIGH Investigators. Niacin in patients with low HDL cholesterol levels receiving intensive statin therapy. *N Engl J Med* 2011;365:2255–2267.
8. Ferris TG, Torchiana DF. Public release of clinical outcomes data—online CABG report cards. *N Engl J Med* 2010;363:1593–1595.
9. Cleary PD, McNeil BJ. Patient satisfaction as an indicator of quality care. *Inquiry* 1988;25:25–36.
10. Weissman JS, Schneider EC, Weingart SN, et al. Comparing patient-reported hospital adverse events with medical record review: do patients know something that hospitals do not? *Ann Intern Med* 2008;149:100–108.
11. Ferman JH. Value-based purchasing program here to stay: payments will be based on performance. *Health Exec* 2011;26:76, 78.
12. Porter ME. What is value in health care? *N Engl J Med* 2010;363:2477–2481.

13. Lilford R, Pronovost P. Using hospital mortality rates to judge hospital performance: a bad idea that just won't go away. *BMJ* 2010;340:955–957.

14. Wennberg JE, Freeman JL, Culp WJ. Are hospital services rationed in New Haven or over-utilised in Boston? *Lancet* 1987;1:1185–1189.

15. Committee on Understanding and Eliminating Racial and Ethnic Disparities in Health Care, 2003, Institute of Medicine. *Unequal Treatment: Confronting Racial and Ethnic Disparities in Health Care.* Washington, DC: National Academy Press; 2003.

16. McGlynn EA, Asch SM, Adams J, et al. The quality of health care delivered to adults in the United States. *N Engl J Med* 2003;348:2635–2645.

17. Higashi T, Shekelle PG, Adams JL, et al. Quality of care is associated with survival in vulnerable older patients. *Ann Intern Med* 2005;143:274–281.

18. Bradley EH, Herrin J, Elbel B, et al. Hospital quality for acute myocardial infarction: correlation among process measures and relationship with short-term mortality. *JAMA* 2006;296:72–78.

19. Fonarow GC, Abraham WT, Albert NM, et al. Association between performance measures and clinical outcomes for patients hospitalized with heart failure. *JAMA* 2007;297:61–70.

20. In conversation with … Janet Corrigan. *AHRQ WebM&M* (serial online), April 2010. Available at: http://webmm.ahrq.gov/perspective.aspx?perspectiveID=85.

21. Lin GA, Redberg RF, Anderson HV, et al. Impact of changes in clinical practice guidelines on assessment of quality of care. *Med Care* 2010;48:733–738.

22. Boyd CM, Darer J, Boult C, et al. Clinical practice guidelines and quality of care for older patients with multiple comorbid diseases: implications for pay for performance. *JAMA* 2005;294:716–724.

23. Chassin MR, Loeb JM, Schmaltz SP, et al. Accountability measures—using measurement to promote quality improvement. *N Engl J Med* 2010;363:683–688.

24. Jha AK, Orave EJ, Epstein AM. Public reporting of discharge planning and rates of readmissions. *N Engl J Med* 2009;361:2637–2645.

25. Wachter RM, Flanders SA, Fee C, et al. Public reporting of antibiotic timing in patients with pneumonia: lessons from a flawed performance measure. *Ann Intern Med* 2008;149:29–32.

26. Wachter RM. Expected and unanticipated consequences of the quality and information technology revolutions. *JAMA* 2006;295:2780–2783.

27. Berwick DM, James B, Coye MJ. Connections between quality measurement and improvement. *Med Care* 2003;41:I-30–I-38.

28. Fisher ES. Paying for performance—risks and recommendations. *N Engl J Med* 2006;355:1845–1847.

29. Epstein A. Pay for performance at the tipping point. *N Engl J Med* 2007;356:515–517.

30. Blumenthal D, Tavenner M. The "Meaningful Use" regulation for electronic health records. *N Engl J Med* 2010;363:501–504.

31. Epstein AM. Revisiting readmissions—changing the incentives for shared accountability. *N Engl J Med* 2009;360:1457–1459.

32. Wachter RM, Foster NE, Dudley RA. Medicare's decision to withhold payment for hospital errors: the devil is in the details. *Jt Comm J Qual Patient Saf* 2008;34:116–123.

33. Campbell SM, Reeves D, Kontopantelis E, et al. Effects of pay for performance on the quality of primary care in England. *N Engl J Med* 2009;361:368–378.

34. Lindenauer PK, Remus D, Roman S, et al. Public reporting and pay for performance in hospital quality improvement. *N Engl J Med* 2007;356:486–496.

35. Pham HH, Ginsburg PB, McKenzie K, et al. Redesigning care delivery in response to a high-performance network: the Virginia Mason Medical Center. *Health Aff (Millwood)* 2007;26:w532–w544.

36. Kelly EW, Kelly JD, Hiestand B, et al. Six Sigma process utilization in reducing door-to-balloon time at a single academic tertiary care center. *Prog Cardiovasc Dis* 2010;53:219–226.

37. Graban M. *Lean Hospitals: Improving Quality, Patient Safety, and Employee Satisfaction.* New York: Productivity Press; 2008.

38. Liker J. *The Toyota Way.* New York: McGraw-Hill; 2003.

39. Butler G, Caldwell C, Poston N. *Lean-Six Sigma for Healthcare, Second Edition: A Senior Leader Guide to Improving Cost and Throughput.* Milwaukee: ASQ Quality Press; 2009.

40. Schedlbauer A, Prasad V, Mulvaney C, et al. What evidence supports the use of computerized alerts and prompts to improve clinicians' prescribing behavior? *J Am Med Inform Assoc* 2009;16:531–538.

41. Marelich GP, Murin S, Battistella F, et al. Protocol weaning of mechanical ventilation in medical and surgical patients by respiratory care practitioners and nurses: effect on weaning time and incidence of ventilator-associated pneumonia. *Chest* 2000;118:459–467.

42. O'Connor GT, Plume SK, Olmstead EM, et al. A regional intervention to improve the hospital mortality associated with coronary artery bypass graft surgery. The Northern New England Cardiovascular Disease Study Group. *JAMA* 1996;275:841–846.

43. Plesk P. Redesigning health care with insights from the science of complex adaptive systems. Appendix B in: Committee on Quality Health Care in America, Institute of Medicine. *Crossing the Quality Chasm: A New Health System for the 21st Century.* National Academy Press; 2001:309–322.

44. Curry LA, Spatz E, Cherlin E, et al. What distinguishes top-performing hospitals in acute myocardial infarction mortality rates? A qualitative study. *Ann Intern Med* 2011;154:384–390.

45. Kohn LT, Corrigan JM, Donaldson MS, eds. *To Err is Human: Building a Safer Health System.* Washington, DC: National Academy Press, 2000.

46. Pronovost PJ, Miller MR, Wachter RM. Tracking progress in patient safety: an elusive target. *JAMA* 2006;296:696–699.

ADDITIONAL READINGS

Brennan TA, Gawande A, Thomas E, et al. Accidental deaths, saved lives, and improved quality. *N Engl J Med* 2005;353:1405–1409.

Christensen CM, Grossman JH, Hwang J. *The Innovator's Prescription: A Disruptive Solution for Health Care.* New York: McGraw-Hill; 2009.

Eddy DM. Clinical decision making: From theory to practice. Connecting value and costs: whom do we ask, and what do we ask them? *JAMA* 1990;264:1737–1739.

Fisher ES, Wennberg DE, Stukel TA, et al. The implications of regional variations in Medicare spending. Part 1: the content, quality, and accessibility of care. *Ann Intern Med* 2003;138:273–287.

Fisher ES, Wennberg DE, Stukel TA, et al. The implications of regional variations in Medicare spending. Part 2: health outcomes and satisfaction with care. *Ann Intern Med* 2003;138:288–298.

Gawande A. Annals of medicine: the bell curve—what happens when patients find out how good their doctors really are. *New Yorker* Dec 6, 2004: Reporting & Essays.

Gawande A. Annals of medicine: the cost conundrum—what a Texas town can teach us about health care. *New Yorker* June 1, 2009: Reporting & Essays.

Greco PJ, Eisenberg JM. Changing physicians' practices. *N Engl J Med* 1993; 329: 1271–1274.

Horn SD. Performance measures and clinical outcomes. *JAMA* 2006;296:2731–2732.

McClellan M, McKethan AN, Lewis JL, et al. A national strategy to put accountable care into practice. *Health Aff (Millwood)* 2010;29:982–990.

Millenson ML. *Demanding Medical Excellence. Doctors and Accountability in the Information Age.* Chicago, IL: University of Chicago Press; 1997.

Ransom ER, Joshi MS, Nash DB, Ransom SB, eds. *The Healthcare Quality Book, Second Edition.* Chicago: Health Administration Press; 2008.

TYPES OF
MEDICAL ERRORS

MEDICATION ERRORS | 4

SOME BASIC CONCEPTS, TERMS, AND EPIDEMIOLOGY

In June 1995, a middle-aged man named Ramon Vasquez went to see his physician in Odessa, Texas, to investigate his chest pain. His physician, suspecting angina, prescribed a medication. The actual prescription is reproduced in Figure 4-1.

Here's a quiz. Do you think the highlighted portion of the prescription is for:

a. Plendil, a calcium channel blocker sometimes used to treat angina?
b. Isordil, a long-acting nitrate also used to treat angina?
c. Zestril, an angiotensin-converting enzyme inhibitor used to treat high blood pressure and heart failure?

So what did you think? I once asked an audience of hospitalists to interpret this prescription. Half said it was Plendil, one-third Isordil, and the rest Zestril.

The physician actually intended to prescribe 120 tablets of Isordil, at its typical dose of 20 mg by mouth (po) every (Q) 6 hours. Ramon Vasquez's pharmacist read the prescription as Plendil, and instructed the patient to take a 20-mg pill every 6 hours. Unfortunately, the usual starting dose of Plendil is 10 mg/day, making this an eightfold overdose. A day later, Mr. Vasquez was critically ill from low blood pressure and heart failure. He died within the week.

The modern pharmaceutical armamentarium represents one of healthcare's great advances. There are now highly effective agents to treat most common maladies: high blood pressure and cholesterol, diabetes, heart disease, cancer, stroke, acquired immunodeficiency syndrome (AIDS), and more. Taken correctly, the benefits of these medications far outweigh their side effects, though the latter remains a concern even when medications are prescribed and taken correctly.

Figure 4-1 ▪ Ramon Vasquez's prescription.

But the growth in medications (there are now more than 10,000 prescription drugs and biologicals—and 300,000 over-the-counter products—available in the United States[1]) has led to a huge increase in the complexity of the medication prescribing and administration process. It has been estimated that at least 5% of hospital patients experience an *adverse drug event* (ADE; harm experienced by a patient as a result of a medication, from either a side effect or the consequence of an error) at some point during hospitalization. Another 5–10% experience a potential ADE, meaning that they nearly took the wrong medicine or the wrong dose but didn't, often thanks to a last minute catch or dumb luck.[2] When patients are on high-risk medications such as warfarin, insulin, and heparin, errors are particularly common: in a national sample of hospitalized Medicare patients, one in seven receiving heparin experienced an ADE.[3] The cost of preventable medication errors in U.S. hospitals has been estimated at $16.4 billion annually.[4]

Things are no safer outside the hospital. Nearly 1 in 20 hospital admissions can be traced to problems with medications, many of them preventable.[5] When a large group of outpatients on a variety of medications was followed for 3 months, about one in four suffered an ADE, many of them serious.[6] The cost of ambulatory preventable medication errors is nearly $5 billion annually,[7] bumping the total cost of medication errors to over $20 billion each year.[4]

Although many discussions about medication errors focus on the famous illegibility of physicians' handwriting, two studies have shown that doctors' handwriting is no worse than that of many other professionals,[7,8] and—notwithstanding the tragic case of Ramon Vasquez—bad handwriting is not a common cause of medication errors. In fact, many steps along the medication prescribing and administration pathway are vulnerable to mistakes. To illustrate these steps, let's follow the life of an inpatient prescription (in a hospital without computerized order entry or bar code medication administration):

- A physician handwrites a prescription in the "Doctors' Orders" section of the chart.
- The clerk removes a carbon copy of the order and faxes it to the pharmacy, while a nurse transcribes the order into the Medication Administration Record (MAR).
- A pharmacist receives the faxed copy, reads it, and retypes the medication, dose, and frequency into the pharmacy's computer system, which generates labels and a bill and helps track inventory.
- The pharmacist manually transfers the medication (if a pill) from a large bottle into "unit doses"—either cups or a shrink-wrapped container. Intravenous medication may require specialized mixing.
- The medication is delivered to the patient's floor; the label includes the name of the medication and the patient's name. The medicine may be delivered on a cart wheeled to the floor, or through a manual transport or pneumatic tube system.
- The nurse goes to the MAR, sees that the patient is due for a medication, searches the medication cart for it, and walks to the patient's room with the medication (along with different medications for her other patients).
- The nurse enters the patient's room, confirms the patient's identity, checks the medication, and administers it.

Believe it or not, I have simplified this process to avoid taking up too much space. Several hospitals have found that there are actually about *50–100 steps* between a doctor's decision to order a medicine and the delivery of the medicine to the patient. The outpatient process is simpler, but only by a bit. There, the doctor usually gives the patient a paper prescription to carry to a pharmacy. Not only can there be errors in the prescription itself (wrong medicine, wrong dose, illegible prescription, failure to consider allergies or drug–drug, drug–disease, or drug–diet interactions), the administration of the medication (generally a mistake in the pharmacy), or a failure to monitor properly (forgetting to check electrolytes and creatinine in a patient started on a diuretic and angiotensin-converting enzyme inhibitor), but also a new source of errors is introduced: patients themselves (e.g., failure to follow instructions properly or storing the medications in incorrect bottles; Chapter 21).[9] With all these steps, a statistical law takes its toll: in a 50-step process in which each step is done correctly 99% of the time, the chance that at least one error will occur is a staggering 39%!

> *Sarah Geller was a 68-year-old woman who had undergone a cardiac bypass operation. After a stormy postoperative course she seemed to be on the road to recovery. However, on the morning of her planned transfer out of the intensive care unit (ICU), she suffered a grand mal seizure. This shocked her caregivers: she had no seizure history and was not on any epileptogenic medications. They drew some blood tests, and emergently wheeled her to the computed tomography (CT) scanner to rule out the possibility of a stroke or intracerebral hemorrhage. While she was in transit, the lab paged the doctors to report that Geller's serum glucose was undetectable. Despite multiple infusions of glucose, she never recovered from her coma. In the subsequent investigation, it was determined that her bedside tray in the ICU contained vials of both heparin (used to "flush" her intravenous lines to keep them open) and insulin. The vials were of similar size and shape (Figure 4-2). The nurse, intending to flush Ms. Geller's line with heparin, had inadvertently administered a fatal dose of insulin.[10]*

As this case demonstrates, solutions to the problem of medication errors will need to tackle both the prescribing and the administration phase[1,2] (Figure 4-3). Many of the solutions will be technological: the role of computerized provider order entry (CPOE), computerized decision support, and bar

Figure 4-2 ▪ Heparin and insulin vials on a bedside tray.

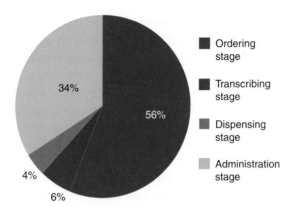

- ■ Ordering stage
- ■ Transcribing stage
- ■ Dispensing stage
- ▨ Administration stage

34%

56%

4%

6%

Figure 4-3 ■ Medication errors, by stage of the medication process. (Reproduced with permission from Bates DW, Cullen DJ, Laird N, et al. Incidence of adverse drug events and potential adverse drug events. Implications for prevention. ADE Prevention Study Group. *JAMA* 1995;274:29–34. Copyright © 1995 American Medical Association. All rights reserved.)

coding and/or radio-frequency identification (RFID) systems will be discussed in Chapter 13. The remainder of this chapter will focus on solutions more specific to the medication prescribing and administration process: standardization, vigilance and the "Five Rights," double checks, preventing interruptions and distractions, unit dosing, removal of risky medications from certain settings, the role of clinical pharmacists, and meeting the challenges of look-alike, sound-alike medications. A final section will review the main strategy to avoid medication errors at the time of transitions: medication reconciliation.

STRATEGIES TO DECREASE MEDICATION ERRORS

Standardization and decreasing ambiguity

> *Betsy Lehman, a popular Boston Globe health columnist, was hospitalized for recurrent breast cancer at Dana-Farber Cancer Institute in 1994. Her experimental protocol called for her to receive an unusually high dose of cyclophosphamide (a chemotherapy agent), followed by a bone marrow transplant. The ordering physicians wrote a prescription: "cyclophosphamide 4 g/sq m over four days," intending that she receive a total of 4 g/m² of body surface area spread out over 4 days. Instead, the nurses administered the total dose (4 g/m²) on each of the 4 days, a fourfold overdose. She died within a month.*

The Lehman case, one of the catalysts for the modern patient safety movement (Table 1-1), can be seen as an argument for computerization and decision support. It would be easy to envision a computer system preprogrammed with the correct dose of chemotherapy that either presented that dose as a default option to the physicians or automatically alarmed when someone prescribed an out-of-range dose.[11] But the case also screams out for standardization: general agreements on inviolable ways of communicating certain orders that would be understandable to everyone.[12] For example, a hospital could mandate that all medications given over multiple days *must* have the daily dose written each day. Or that high-risk medications could only be ordered one day at a time.

One source of ambiguity has been the long-standing use of abbreviations for certain medications. In 2004, the Joint Commission prohibited hospitals from using a group of "*high-risk abbreviations*" (Table 4-1), insisting that the full name of these medications and instructions ("morphine sulfate," not "MS04"; "Insulin 10 Units," not "Insulin 10 U") be spelled out. One of the advantages of CPOE will be to further standardize nomenclature and markedly limit the use of abbreviations. However, as will be further discussed in Chapter 13, CPOE has the capacity to create new classes of medication errors if it is not well designed and implemented.[13,14] For example, unless

Table 4-1	THE JOINT COMMISSION'S "DO NOT USE" LIST	
Do Not Use	**Potential Problem**	**Use Instead**
U (unit)	Mistaken for "0" (zero), the number "4" (four), or "cc"	Write "unit"
IU (International Unit)	Mistaken for IV (intravenous) or the number 10 (ten)	Write "International Unit"
Q.D., QD, q.d., qd (daily)	Mistaken for each other	Write "daily"
Q.O.D., QOD, q.o.d, qod (every other day)	Period after the Q mistaken for "I" and the "O" mistaken for "I"	Write "every other day"
Trailing zero (X.0 mg)	Decimal point is missed	Write X mg
Lack of leading zero (.X mg)		Write 0.X mg
MS	Can mean morphine sulfate or magnesium sulfate	Write "morphine sulfate"
MSO_4 and $MgSO_4$	Confused for one another	Write "magnesium sulfate"

Reproduced with permission from http://www.jointcommission.org/PatientSafety/DoNot UseList/.

Table 4-2 **THE "FIVE RIGHTS" OF MEDICATION ADMINISTRATION***
Right patient
Right route
Right dose
Right time
Right drug

*Some have suggested additions to the original list of "Five Rights," including: right documentation, right action, right form, right response, and the right of a patient to refuse a medication.[16]

sophisticated decision support is built into the system, a provider intending to prescribe "penicillin" can easily select the anti-inflammatory agent "penicillamine" from an alphabetical computerized pick list.[15]

Vigilance and the "Five Rights" of medication administration

While many advances in medication safety have come from system changes such as automation and double checks, individual caregivers are responsible for doing what they can to ensure the safety of their patients. One long-standing nursing principle is known as the *"Five Rights"* (Table 4-2), highlighting the five checks that a nurse is expected to make before administering a medication to a patient. Recently, some have argued for additional checks, including right documentation, right action (i.e., the medication is being given for the correct indication), right form (i.e., oral vs. intravenous, can the pill be safely crushed?), and right response (i.e., the nurse should monitor the patient's response to the medication).[16] Some add still another: the right of a patient to refuse a medication. Although these additional rights have not yet become standard practice, they further illustrate the tremendous challenges of correct medication administration and the limitations of human vigilance as a safety bulwark.

Double checks

Other high-risk industries (nuclear power, aviation, the armed services) have long used double, and even triple, checks to ensure that critical processes are executed correctly. Patient safety, for its part, has come a long way relatively quickly. Until recently, in most hospitals the only process with standardized and inviolable independent double checks was blood administration (in which two nurses confirm ABO blood types prior to a transfusion). Thankfully, most hospitals now have built-in double checks for chemotherapy[12] and other high-risk medications. However, even when double checks are required by policy, it is critical to ensure that they are truly independent. It is very easy (natural, in fact) for the second check to become lackadaisical, in essence a rubber stamp, thereby providing false reassurance rather than truly increased safety.

Preventing interruptions and distractions

Each step in the medication prescribing, preparation, and administrative process is subject to error. While automation is being introduced into every phase, the vast majority of medication deliveries still involve humans in each of those phases. For example, even in a hospital with computerized order entry, the physician still needs to decide on the medication and dosage, a pharmacist needs to take the order and dispense the medication to the floor, and the nurse needs to collect the correct medication from a dispensing machine and deliver it to the patient.

Each of these steps is subject to mistakes, and recent research has quantified the extent to which distractions and interruptions increase the probability of errors (see also Chapter 7).[17] Most of the research has focused on the nursing portion of this chain, although there is little reason to believe that prescribing physicians[18,19] or pharmacists are any less susceptible to the hazards of interruptions and distractions.

One time–motion study of nurses preparing and administering medications found an average of 1.2 interruptions during every medication pass.[20] In a memorable example, it took over 2 hours for a nurse to retrieve one particular medication from a storage device, because the device forced the nurse to close all 25 drawers each time she wanted to retrieve the medication. Even the process of administering high-risk medications, such as chemotherapy, is frequently interrupted.[21] In one study, every time a nurse was interrupted during the preparation and administration process, there was a 12% increase in clinical errors.[22]

Emerging evidence is demonstrating that decreasing or eliminating distractions and interruptions can improve medication safety. In one hospital, nurses were given a protected hour during which they were not to be disturbed by telephone calls or pages. While the study did not isolate this particular intervention from several others, it did find a significant decrease in medication errors.[23] Another hospital created a "No Interruption Zone" (marked off by red tape on the floor) to indicate that a critical care nurse was not to be interrupted. (The principle here is similar to that of the "sterile cockpit"—an aviation standard that prohibits cockpit crews from engaging in anything but mission-critical conversation when the airplane's altitude is below 10,000 ft.[19]) The establishment of the No

Interruption Zone was associated with a reduction in both interruptions and administration errors.[24]

Before we get too excited about such interventions, it's worth heeding the cautionary note of Rivera-Rodriguez and Karsh, who point out that certain interruptions are crucial to the delivery of high quality and safe care.[25] They argue against banning interruptions outright, as interventions need to account for the complexity of healthcare systems. This is an important argument to consider—it's easy to see how certain strategies to eliminate interruptions could lead to unintended consequences and "squeezed balloons."

Obviously, one cure for interruptions and distractions would be to remove humans from the medication prescribing/delivery process. While automation is likely to do that to some degree, people will remain active participants in the medication chain for the foreseeable future. This makes continued attention to, and innovations in, this area essential.

Unit dosing

This refers to the packaging of medications in ready-to-use units that are prepared in the pharmacy and then delivered to the clinical floor. Unit dosing was developed in the 1960s, replacing the old method in which the pharmacy sent large bottles of pills or intravenous medications to a floor, expecting that the nurses would perform the mixing or dispensing. Studies have generally found that unit-dose administration is associated with fewer medication errors, and the practice has now become nearly ubiquitous in American hospitals.[26] Many pharmacy systems now include automatic dispensing machines, which are usually computerized and often linked to centralized inventory control systems.[27,28]

Removal of medications from certain settings

The most widely cited example of this strategy is the removal of concentrated potassium from patient care areas. Because of the dangers of intravenous potassium overdoses (such as stopping the heart, as when potassium is used in capital punishment), such removal seems like a good idea. Rather than having the nurses add potassium to their intravenous solutions on the floor, the new system depends on potassium being added to intravenous bags by pharmacists before the premixed bags are sent to the ward.

This approach is an example of a more general strategy called *forcing functions* (Chapters 2 and 7): technical or physical obstacles designed to decrease the probability of error in error-prone circumstances or environments. Forcing functions are designed to anticipate common human errors and make harm from them impossible by blocking either the error or its consequences. As mentioned in Chapter 2, the most widely cited example of a forcing function was the reengineering of automobile braking systems in the 1980s to make it impossible to shift a car into reverse when the driver's foot was off the brake.

The removal of concentrated potassium from clinical units would seem to be such a forcing function, and thus a logical safety solution. Yet even this seemingly simple strategy was beset by unintended consequences, as many nurses found that it took too long for their intravenous drips to arrive from the pharmacy. Because potassium was still allowed in the ICUs (it often needs to be given emergently there), floor nurses began pilfering potassium from ICU stashes and hoarding it, creating an even more chaotic and potentially unsafe situation.[29] The message behind this experience is not that keeping dangerous medications such as potassium on the floor is a good idea (it probably isn't), but rather that frontline workers often thwart apparently "commonsensical safety fixes" when the fixes get in the way of their perceived ability to do their jobs, a process known as a "*workaround.*"[30,31] Safety planners need to seek out such actual or potential workarounds through focus groups and observations of providers doing their daily work, lest they create an "underground economy" in unsafe practices (Chapter 7).

The use of clinical pharmacists

Of all the strategies employed to try to decrease medication errors, the insertion of clinical pharmacists into the medication prescribing and administration processes is one of the most powerful (of course, this is in addition to having pharmacists read prescriptions and dispense medications, both core functions). For example, in one classic study, clinical pharmacists became part of an ICU team in an academic medical center. They educated the physicians and trainees, rounded with the teams, and intervened when they saw a medication error in the making. The intervention resulted in a nearly threefold decrease in the frequency of ADEs, which led to less patient harm and significant cost savings.[32] More recent studies have found impressive reductions in preventable ADEs and inappropriate medication use when pharmacists rounded with teams on general medical wards and were integrated into emergency departments.[33–35] Unfortunately, in the United States, the high cost and a national shortage of pharmacists has led these strategies to be relatively underemployed.

Meeting the challenge of look-alike, sound-alike medications

Table 4-3 shows a list of common medications that have been the subject of sound-alike, look-alike errors. Although the U.S. Food and Drug

Table 4-3 MEDICATIONS THAT HAVE BEEN THE SUBJECT OF SOUND-ALIKE, LOOK-ALIKE ERRORS	
Generic Drug Names*	**Brand Names**
Acetohexamide/acetazolamide	Adderall/Inderal
Amiodarone/amrinone[†]	Alupent/Atrovent[†]
Bupropion/buspirone	Ambien/Amen
Chlorpromazine/chlorpropamide	Asacol/Os-Cal
Clomiphene/clomipramine	Cardizem/Cardiem
Cyclosporine/cycloserine	Celebrex/Celexa/Cerebyx
Daunorubicin/doxorubicin	Dynacin/DynaCirc
Dimenhydrinate/diphenhydramine	Flomax/Fosamax; Flomax/Volmax
Dobutamine/dopamine[†]	Indinavir/Denavir
Glipizide/glyburide[†]	Lamictal/Lomotil/Lamisil
Hydralazine/hydroxyzine	Lanoxin/Lonox
Methylprednisolone/methyltestosterone	Levbid/Lopid/Lithobid
Nicardipine/nifedipine[†]	Levoxyl/Luvox
Prednisone/prednisolone	Lovenox/Lotronex
Sulfadiazine/sulfisoxazole	Nizoral/Nasarel/Neoral
Tolazamide/tolbutamide	Remeron/Zemuron
Vinblastine/vincristine[†]	Vioxx/Zyvox
	Zyrtec/Zyprexa

*In 2001, the U.S. FDA began requiring the manufacturers of many of these products to use "tall man" lettering (e.g., clomiPHENE and clomiPRAMINE) on their labels. A table that shows these changes can be found in Reference 36.

†Drugs have similar action or indication (e.g., both glipizide and glyburide are oral hypoglycemics prescribed to type 2 diabetics).

Reproduced with permission from Cohen MR. The 2-week itch. *AHRQ WebM&M* (serial online); 2003. Available at: http://webmm.ahrq.gov/case.aspx?caseID=10.

Administration (FDA) now tries, during its drug approval process, to minimize the possibility that a new medication name will be confused with an old one, with 10,000 agents in the pharmacopoeia some problems are inevitable. Among the most confusing examples: the anticonvulsant Cerebyx and the anti-inflammatory Celebrex, the antidepressant Zyprexa and the antihistamine Zyrtec, and the mood stabilizer Lamictal and the antifungal Lamisil.

There are a number of strategies to help minimize the risk of confusion, including the user of "tall man" lettering for the suffixes of drugs that begin with the same prefix, such as "clomiPHENE" and "clomiPRAMINE."[36] But eradicating this problem entirely will require technological help, including bar coding administration systems[37] and computerized order entry with decision support.[38] For example, one can imagine a system that would ask for each medication's indication, and balk if the indication was "seizures" and the chosen medication was Celebrex (instead of Cerebyx) (see Chapter 13).

Medication reconciliation

This chapter has emphasized medication safety when the patient is static: in an ICU bed, on a medical floor, or visiting a doctor in a clinic. But the greatest opportunities for errors in the medication process likely come when patients are transitioning from one setting to another (see also Chapter 8): being admitted to or discharged from the hospital, going from their primary care physician's office to that of a specialist, transferring out of the ICU to the floor, or going from the floor to the operating room. Studies have shown that unintended medication discrepancies occur in about 30% of patients at the time of admission[39] (about 40% of these have moderate or severe potential for harm[40]), a similar percentage when they transfer from one hospital site to another,[41] and in 14% of cases at hospital discharge.[42]

Medication reconciliation is the process of reviewing a patient's complete medication regimen on both ends of a care transition in an effort to avoid unintended inconsistencies.[43] While many physicians have long asked their patients to bring their "old meds" to their clinic appointments (often called a "brown bag review"), medication reconciliation has become formalized relatively recently. The search for optimal methods of performing reconciliation took on some urgency when, in 2004, the Institute for Healthcare Improvement included it among the recommended practices in its 100,000 Lives Campaign (Table 20-2).[44] The following year, the Joint Commission named "med rec" as one of its National Patient Safety

Goals, and in 2006 the organization added it as a requirement for hospital accreditation.

Unfortunately, while medication reconciliation has great face validity, the methods for accomplishing it have varied widely and research on it has produced mixed results. The methods have included having pharmacists perform the entire process, involving patients (particularly ambulatory patients) in their own reconciliation, and embedding the process in electronic systems. One study involving pharmacists demonstrated improved clinical outcomes and reductions in ADEs,[45] and another found that admission medication reconciliation led to a reduction in ADEs caused by incorrect medication changes at the time of admission.[46] The use of an electronic tool to facilitate medication reconciliation led to fewer potential ADEs at the time of hospital discharge.[47] On the other hand, one study conducted in four academic primary care clinics found that half of the medication lists remained incomplete after a medication reconciliation intervention, and most still contained errors.[48]

While research is beginning to illustrate some best practices in medication reconciliation, uncertainty about what really works remains and most successful studies illustrate beneficial effects on potential ADEs rather than true patient harm. Many institutions have seen their med rec initiatives stall because of disagreements on crucial issues, such as whose job it is to perform the reconciliation.[49] In light of this uncertainty, in 2009 the Joint Commission announced that, while it would continue to assess how institutions managed medication risks at the point of care transitions, it would no longer formally score medication reconciliation during its accreditation surveys. The challenges of medication reconciliation vividly illustrate how difficult it is to implement even relatively "simple" fixes in highly complex systems of care (Chapter 2).

Conservative prescribing

It is worth emphasizing one final point before leaving the topic of medication errors. One key to minimizing these errors is to limit the use of medications to when they are truly indicated—the potential benefits exceed the risks. As one example of this principle, elderly hospitalized patients who received medications considered inappropriate (such as prolonged use of proton pump inhibitors, aspirin in patients without a history of cardiovascular disease, or sedatives and opiates in patients with a history of falls) have a nearly twofold increase in their odds of an adverse event during the hospitalization.[50] Schiff et al. have outlined a series of principles for *conservative prescribing* (Table 4-4), and they are well worth following.[51]

Table 4–4 PRINCIPLES OF CONSERVATIVE PRESCRIBING

Think beyond drugs

Seek nondrug alternatives first

Consider potentially treatable underlying causes of problems rather than just treating the symptoms with a drug

Look for opportunities for prevention rather than focusing on treating symptoms or advanced disease

Use the test of time as a diagnostic and therapeutic trial whenever possible

Practice more strategic prescribing

Use only a few drugs and learn to use them well

Avoid frequent switching to new drugs without clear, compelling evidence-based reasons

Be skeptical about individualizing therapy

Whenever possible, start treatment with only one drug at a time

Maintain heightened vigilance regarding adverse effects

Have a high index of suspicion for adverse drug effects

Educate patients about possible adverse effects to ensure that they are recognized as early as possible

Be alert to clues that you may be treating or risking withdrawal symptoms

Approach new drugs and new indications cautiously and skeptically

Learn about new drugs and new indications from trustworthy, unbiased sources

Do not rush to use newly marketed drugs

Be certain that the drug improves actual patient-centered clinical outcomes rather than just treating or masking a
surrogate marker

Be vigilant about indications creep

Do not be seduced by elegant molecular pharmacology or drug physiology

Beware of selective reporting of studies

Work with patients for a more deliberative shared agenda

Do not hastily or uncritically succumb to patient requests for drugs, especially drugs that they have
heard advertised

Avoid mistakenly prescribing additional drugs for refractory problems, failing to appreciate the potential
for patient nonadherence

Avoid repeating prescriptions for drugs that a patient has previously tried unsuccessfully or that caused
an adverse reaction

Discontinue treatment with drugs that are not working or are no longer needed

Work with patients' desires to be conservative with medications

Consider longer-term, broader effects

Think beyond short-term beneficial drug effects to consider longer-term benefits and risks

Look for opportunities to improve prescribing systems, changes that can make prescribing and
medication use safer

KEY POINTS

- With the explosive growth in available medications, ADEs (both side effects and medication errors) are one of the most common threats to patient safety.
- Errors can occur at any point in the medication chain, particularly in the prescribing and administration stages. For medications taken in the ambulatory environment, patient-related errors and inadequate monitoring are also common.
- Information technology is likely to decrease medication errors, including prescribing errors (through CPOE and computerized decision support) and administration errors (through bar coding and other identification techniques). Unintended consequences are common, however, and should be anticipated.
- In addition to these information technology–related solutions, other important medication safety strategies include: standardization, checking the "Five Rights," double checks, preventing unnecessary distractions and interruptions, unit dosing, removal of high-risk medications from certain settings, engaging clinical pharmacists, specific strategies to mitigate the risks of look-alike, sound-alike medications, and performing medication reconciliation at the time of care transitions.
- Another important way to avoid medication errors is to follow principles of conservative prescribing, avoiding the inappropriate use of medications.

| REFERENCES

1. Aspden P, Wolcott J, Bootman JL, et al., eds.; Committee on Identifying and Preventing Medication Errors. *Preventing Medication Errors: Quality Chasm Series.* Institute of Medicine. Washington, DC: The National Academy Press; 2007.
2. Bates DW, Cullen DJ, Laird N, et al. Incidence of adverse drug events and potential adverse drug events. Implications for prevention. ADE Prevention Study Group. *JAMA* 1995;274:29–34.
3. Classen DC, Jaser L, Budnitz DS. Adverse drug events among hospitalized Medicare patients: epidemiology and national estimates from a new approach to surveillance. *Jt Comm J Qual Patient Saf* 2010;36:12–21, AP1–AP9.
4. *Preventing Medication Errors: A $21 Billion Opportunity.* Washington, DC: National Priorities Partnership and National Quality Forum; December 2010. Available at: www.qualityforum.org/NPP/docs/Preventing_Medication_Error_CAB.aspx.
5. Winterstein AG, Sauer BC, Hepler CD, et al. Preventable drug-related hospital admissions. *Ann Pharmacother* 2002;36:1238–1248.

6. Gandhi TK, Weingart SN, Borus J, et al. Adverse drug events in ambulatory care. *N Engl J Med* 2003;348:1556–1564.

7. Berwick DM, Winickoff DE. The truth about doctors' handwriting: a prospective study. *BMJ* 1996;313:1657–1658.

8. Schneider KA, Murray CW, Shadduck RD, et al. Legibility of doctors' handwriting is as good (or bad) as everyone else's. *Qual Saf Health Care* 2006;15:445.

9. Shojania KG. Safe medication prescribing and monitoring in the outpatient setting. *CMAJ* 2006;174:1257–1258.

10. Bates DW. Unexpected hypoglycemia in a critically ill patient. *Ann Intern Med* 2002;137:110–116.

11. Collins CM, Elsaid KA. Using an enhanced oral chemotherapy computerized provider order entry system to reduce prescribing errors and improve safety. *Int J Qual Health Care* 2011;23:36–43.

12. Jacobson JO, Polovich M, McNiff KK, et al.; American Society of Clinical Oncology; Oncology Nursing Society. American Society of Clinical Oncology/Oncology Nursing Society chemotherapy administration safety standards. *Oncol Nurs Forum* 2009;36:651–658.

13. Sittig DF, Singh H. Defining health information technology-related errors: new developments since 'to err is human'. *Arch Intern Med* 2011;171:1281–1284.

14. Koppel R, Metlay JP, Cohen A, et al. Role of computerized physician order entry systems in facilitating medication errors. *JAMA* 2005;293:1197–1203.

15. Flynn EA. A troubling amine. *AHRQ WebM&M* (serial online); 2006. Available at: http://webmm.ahrq.gov/case.aspx?caseID=136.

16. Elliott M, Liu Y. The nine rights of medication administration: an overview. *Br J Nurs* 2010;19:300–305.

17. Biron AD, Loiselle CG, Lavoie-Tremblay M. Work interruptions and their contribution to medication administration errors: an evidence review. *Worldviews Evid Based Nurs* 2009;6:70–86.

18. Magrabi F, Li SY, Day RO, et al. Errors and electronic prescribing: a controlled laboratory study to examine task complexity and interruption effects. *J Am Med Inform Assoc* 2010;17:575–583.

19. Broom MA, Capek AL, Carachi P, et al. Critical phase distractions in anesthesia and the sterile cockpit concept. *Anesthesia* 2011;66:175–179.

20. Elganzouri ES, Standish CA, Androwich I. Medication Administration Time Study (MATS): nursing staff performance of medication administration. *J Nurs Adm* 2009;39:204–210.

21. Trbovich P, Prakash V, Stewart J, et al. Interruptions during the delivery of high-risk medications. *J Nurs Adm* 2010;40:211–218.

22. Westbrook JI, Woods A, Rob MI, et al. Association of interruptions with an increased risk and severity of medication administration errors. *Arch Intern Med* 2010;170:683–690.

23. Kliger J. Giving medication administration the respect it is due. Comment on: "Association of interruptions with an increased risk and severity of medication administration errors." *Arch Intern Med* 2010;170:690–692.

24. Anthony K, Wiencek C, Bauer C, et al. No interruptions please: impact of a no interruption zone on medication safety in intensive care units. *Crit Care Nurse* 2010;30:21–29.

25. Rivera-Rodriguez AJ, Karsh BT. Interruptions and distractions in healthcare: review and reappraisal. *Qual Saf Health Care* 2010;19:304–312.

26. Murray MD, Shojania KG. Unit-dose drug distribution systems. In: Shojania KG, Duncan BW, McDonald KM, et al., eds. *Making Health Care Safer: A Critical Analysis of Patient Safety Practices.* Evidence Report/Technology Assessment No. 43, AHRQ Publication No. 01-E058. Rockville, MD: Agency for Healthcare Research and Quality; 2001.

27. Murray MD. Automated medication dispensing devices. In: Shojania KG, Duncan BW, McDonald KM, et al., eds. *Making Health Care Safer: A Critical Analysis of Patient Safety Practices.* Evidence Report/Technology Assessment No. 43, AHRQ Publication No. 01-E058. Rockville, MD: Agency for Healthcare Research and Quality; 2001.

28. Chapuis C, Roustit M, Bal G, et al. Automated drug dispensing system reduces medication errors in an intensive care setting. *Crit Care Med* 2010;38:2275–2281.

29. Potassium may no longer be stocked on patient care units, but serious threats still exist! *ISMP Medication Safety Alert!* Acute care ed. October 4, 2007;12:1–2.

30. Spear SJ, Schmidhofer M. Ambiguity and workarounds as contributors to medical error. *Ann Intern Med* 2005;142:627–630.

31. Halbesleben JRB, Savage GT, Wakefield DS, et al. Rework and workarounds in nurse medication administration process: implications for work processes and patient safety. *Health Care Manage Rev* 2010;35:124–133.

32. Leape LL, Cullen DJ, Clapp MD, et al. Pharmacist participation on physician rounds and adverse drug events in the intensive care unit. *JAMA* 1999;282:267–270.

33. Kucukarslan SN, Peters M, Mlynarek M, et al. Pharmacists on rounding teams reduce preventable adverse drug events in hospital general medicine units. *Arch Intern Med* 2003;163:2014–2018.

34. Bladh L, Ottosson E, Karlsson J, et al. Effects of a clinical pharmacist service on health-related quality of life and prescribing of drugs: a randomised controlled trial. *BMJ Qual Saf* 2011;20:738–746.

35. Brown JN, Barnes CL, Beasley B, et al. Effect of pharmacists on medication errors in an emergency department. *Am J Health Syst Pharm* 2008;65:330–333.

36. ISMP updates its list of drug name pairs with tall man letters. *ISMP Medication Safety Alert!* Acute care ed. November 18, 2010;15:1–3.

37. Poon EG, Keohane CA, Yoon CS, et al. Effect of bar-code technology on the safety of medication administration. *N Engl J Med* 2010;362:1698–1707.

38. Garg AX, Adhikari NK, McDonald H, et al. Effects of computerized clinical decision support systems on practitioner performance and patient outcomes: a systematic review. *JAMA* 2005;293:1223–1238.

39. Tam VC, Knowles SR, Cornish PL, et al. Frequency, type and clinical importance of medication history errors at admission to hospital: a systematic review. *CMAJ* 2005;173:510–515.

40. Cornish PL, Knowles SR, Marchesano R, et al. Unintended medication discrepancies at the time of hospital admission. *Arch Intern Med* 2005;165:424–429.

41. Bell CM, Rahimi-Darabad P, Orner AI. Discontinuity of chronic medications in patients discharged from the intensive care unit. *J Gen Intern Med* 2006; 21: 937–941.

42. Forster AJ, Murff HJ, Peterson JF, et al. The incidence and severity of adverse events affecting patients after discharge from the hospital. *Ann Intern Med* 2003;138:161–167.

43. Patient safety primers: medication reconciliation. *AHRQ Patient Safety Network.* Available at: http://psnet.ahrq.gov/primer.aspx?primerID=1.

44. Berwick DM, Calkins DR, McCannon CJ, et al. The 100,000 Lives Campaign: setting a goal and a deadline for improving health care quality. *JAMA* 2006;295:324–327.

45. Schnipper JL, Kirwin JL, Cotugno MC, et al. Role of pharmacist counseling in preventing adverse drug events after hospitalization. *Arch Intern Med* 2006;166:565–571.

46. Boockvar KS, Blum S, Kugler A, et al. Effect of admission medication reconciliation on adverse drug events from admission medication changes. *Arch Intern Med* 2011;171:860–861.

47. Schnipper JL, Hamann C, Ndumele CD, et al. Effect of an electronic medication reconciliation application and process redesign on potential adverse drug events: a cluster-randomized trial. *Arch Intern Med* 2009;169:771–780.

48. Nassaralla CL, Naessens JM, Hunt VL, et al. Medication reconciliation in ambulatory care: attempts at improvement. *Qual Saf Health Care* 2009;18:402–407.

49. Poon EG. Medication reconciliation: whose job is it? *AHRQ WebM&M* (serial online), September 2007. Available at: http://webMM.ahrq.gov/case.aspx?caseID=158.

50. Hamilton H, Gallagher P, Ryan C, et al. Potentially inappropriate medications defined by STOPP criteria and the risk of adverse drug events in older hospitalized patients. *Arch Intern Med* 2011;171:1013–1019.

51. Schiff GD, Galanter WL, Duhig J, et al. Principles of conservative prescribing. *Arch Intern Med* 2011;171:1433–1440.

ADDITIONAL READINGS

Bates DW, Spell N, Cullen DJ, et al. The costs of adverse drug events in hospitalized patients. *JAMA* 1997;277:307–311.

Bell CM, Brener SS, Gunraj N, et al. Association of ICU or hospital admission with unintentional discontinuation of medications for chronic diseases. *JAMA* 2011;306:840–847.

Cohen MR, ed. *Medication Errors.* 2nd ed. Washington, DC: American Pharmaceutical Association; 2006.

Coleman EA, Smith JD, Raha D, et al. Posthospital medication discrepancies: prevalence and contributing factors. *Arch Intern Med* 2005;165:1842–1847.

Kaboli PJ, Hoth AB, McClimon BJ, et al. Clinical pharmacists and inpatient medical care: a systematic review. *Arch Intern Med* 2006;166:955–964.

Leape LL, Kabcenell A, Gandhi TK, et al. Reducing adverse drug events: lessons from a breakthrough series collaborative. *Jt Comm J Qual Improv* 2000;26:321–331.

McDowell SE, Mt-Isa S, Ashby D, et al. Where errors occur in the preparation and administration of intravenous medicines: a systematic review and Bayesian analysis. *Qual Saf Health Care* 2010;19:341–345.

Weingart SN, Wilson RM, Gibberd RW, et al. Epidemiology of medical error. *BMJ* 2000;320:774–777.

SURGICAL ERRORS | 5

▌SOME BASIC CONCEPTS AND TERMS

More than 20 million people undergo surgery every year in the United States alone. In the past, surgery could be extremely dangerous, in part because of the risks of the surgery itself (bleeding, infection), and in part because of the high risks of anesthesia. Because of major safety improvements in both of these areas, surgeries today are extremely safe, and anesthesia-related deaths are rare.[1] Advances in surgery, anesthesia, and postoperative care have led to major declines in mortality in disorders generally treated by surgery, such as diseases of the gallbladder and appendix.[2]

Nevertheless, a number of troubling surgical safety issues persist. This chapter will deal with some of the more problematic issues directly related to surgery: anesthesia-related safety complications, wrong-site and wrong-patient surgery, retained foreign bodies, and surgical fires. I will end the chapter with a brief discussion of nonsurgical procedural safety.

Of course, surgery is not immune to medication errors (Chapter 4), diagnostic errors (Chapter 6), teamwork and communication errors (Chapter 9), and nosocomial infections, including surgical site infections (Chapter 10). These issues will be covered in their respective chapters, although some elements that are more specific to surgery—such as the use of the surgical checklist—will be touched on here. Early enthusiasm for the use of perioperative beta-blockers has waned after several studies in the past decade found surprisingly high rates of harm.[3,4] Interested readers are referred to the latest American College of Cardiology/American Heart Association guidelines.[5] For our purposes, suffice it to say that the general principles surrounding treating targeted patients with proper medications are likely to comport with similar discussions elsewhere in the book (e.g., venous thromboembolism prophylaxis, Chapter 11).

As with medication errors, in which problems from the intervention are grouped under a broad term ("adverse drug events") that includes both errors and side effects (Chapter 4), some surgical complications occur despite impeccable care, while others are caused by errors. Surgeries account for a relatively high percentage of both adverse events and preventable adverse events. For example, one of the major chart review studies of adverse events (the

Utah–Colorado study) found that 45% of all adverse events were in surgical patients; of these, 17% resulted from negligence and 17% led to permanent disability. Looked at another way, 3% of patients who underwent an operation suffered an adverse event, and half of these were preventable.[6]

The field of surgery has always taken safety extremely seriously. The first efforts to measure complications of care and approach them scientifically were developed by Boston surgeon Ernest Codman in the early twentieth century. Codman's "End-Result Hospital"—following every patient for evidence of errors in treatment and disseminating the results of this inquiry—was both revolutionary and highly controversial[7–9] (Appendix III). Nevertheless, the American College of Surgeons soon began inspecting hospitals (in 1918), an effort that served as the forerunner of the Joint Commission (Chapter 20). More recently, the person arguably most responsible for putting safety on the radar screen of modern medicine was another surgeon, Dr. Lucian Leape.[10,11] And the field of surgery has pioneered the use of comparative data (most prominently in the form of the National Surgical Quality Improvement Program[12]) and regional collaboratives (such as in the Northern New England Cardiovascular Disease Study Group[13]) to promote performance improvement.

Despite these remarkable contributions, surgery, like the rest of medicine, has traditionally approached safety as a matter of individual excellence: a complication was deemed to represent a failing by the surgeon. Our new focus on systems improvement is allowing surgery to make major advances in safety.

VOLUME–OUTCOME RELATIONSHIPS

Beginning with a 1979 study by Luft et al. that demonstrated a relationship between higher volumes and better outcomes for certain surgeries, a substantial literature has generally supported the commonsensical notion that "practice makes perfect" when it comes to procedures.[14] The precise mechanism of this relationship has not been elucidated, but it seems to hold for both the volume of individual operators (e.g., the surgeon, the interventional cardiologist) and the institution (e.g., the hospital or surgicenter).[15]

Although much of the volume–outcome relationship probably owes to the fact that well-functioning teams take time to gel—learning to anticipate each others' reactions and preferences—there also seems to be a learning curve for procedural competence. One of the best-studied examples is that of laparoscopic cholecystectomy, a technique that essentially replaced the more dangerous and costly open cholecystectomy in the early 1990s. As "lap choley" emerged as the preferred procedure for gallbladder removal, tens of thousands of practicing surgeons needed to learn the procedure well after the completion of their formal training, providing an organic test of the volume–outcome curve.

The findings were sobering. One early study of lap choleys showed that injuries to the common bile duct dropped almost 20-fold once surgeons had at least a dozen cases under their belts.[16] After that, the learning curve flattened, but not by much: the rate of common bile duct injury on the 30th case was still 10 times higher than the rate after 50 cases.

One can assume that most graduates of today's surgical residencies are well trained in the techniques of laparoscopic surgery. But in the early days of a new procedure, patients have no such reassurance. A 1991 survey found that only 45% of 165 practicing surgeons who had participated in a 2-day practical course on laparoscopic cholecystectomy felt the workshop had left them adequately prepared to start performing the procedure. Yet three-quarters of these surgeons reported that they implemented the new procedure immediately after returning to their practices.[17]

Obviously, part of the solution to the volume–outcome and learning curve conundrums will lie in new training models, including the use of realistic simulation (Chapter 17). In fact, one study found that surgical residents who underwent simulation training until they reached a predefined level of proficiency were three times less likely to commit technical errors during laparoscopic cholecystectomy than those who received traditional training.[18] In addition, some surgical and procedural specialties are now requiring minimum volumes for privileging and board certification, and a major coalition of payers (the Leapfrog Group) promotes high-volume centers as one of its safety standards under the banner of "evidence-based hospital referral" (Table 5-1). Certain states or insurers are insisting on minimum volumes or channeling patients to higher volume providers; institutions that achieve good outcomes and have high volumes are sometimes dubbed "Centers of Excellence."

Although such policies appear attractive at first, they are not without their own risks. First, patients may not be anxious to travel long distances to receive care from high-volume providers or institutions. Second, volumes that are *too* high may actually compromise quality by overtaxing institutions or physicians. Finally, many of the procedures being discussed, such as cardiac or transplant surgery, are relatively lucrative. Losing them could threaten the economic viability of low-volume institutions, which often cross-subsidize nonprofitable services (care of the uninsured, trauma care) with profits from the well-reimbursed surgeries.

This is not to say that channeling patients to high-volume (or better yet, demonstrably safer or higher quality[19]) doctors and practices is a mistake, but rather that it is a complex maneuver that requires thoughtful consideration of both expected and unforeseen consequences.

PATIENT SAFETY IN ANESTHESIA

Although it is often stated that the modern patient safety movement began in late 1999 with the publication of *To Err is Human*,[20] the field of anesthesia is a noteworthy exception. Anesthesia began focusing on safety a generation earlier, and its success story holds lessons for the rest of the patient safety field.

Table 5-1 THE LEAPFROG GROUP'S VOLUME STANDARDS*	
Treatment or Procedure	Recommended Annual Volumes: Hospitals/Surgeons
Coronary artery bypass graft	≥450/100
Percutaneous coronary intervention	≥400/75
Aortic valve replacement	≥120/22
Bariatric surgery	≥125/20
Abdominal aortic aneurysm repair	≥50/8
Esophagectomy	≥13/2
Pancreatic resection	≥11/2
High-risk delivery (expected birth weight <1500 g, gestational age <32 weeks, or prenatal diagnosis of major congenital anomaly)	Neonatal ICU with annual count of very low-birth-weight babies ≥50

*In 2003, the Leapfrog Group added selected process and outcome measures to the minimum volume requirements cited above.

Reproduced with permission from http://www.leapfroggroup.org/media/file/Leapfrog-Evidence-Based_Hospital_Referral_Fact_Sheet.pdf and http://www.leapfroggroup.org/media/file/Leapfrog-Surgeon_Volume_Fact_Sheet.pdf.

In 1972, a young engineer named Jeff Cooper began work at the Anesthesia Bioengineering Unit at Massachusetts General Hospital (MGH). Like Codman 60 years earlier, what he saw at MGH bothered him: mistakes were common, cover-ups were the norm, and systems to prevent errors were glaringly absent. Even worse, many procedures and environments appeared to be all but designed to promote errors. For example, he noticed that turning the dial clockwise increased the dose of anesthetic in some anesthesia machines, and decreased it in others. After delivering a lecture entitled "The Anesthesia Machine: An Accident Waiting to Happen," Cooper and his colleagues began looking at procedures and equipment through a human factors lens (Chapter 7), using the technique of "critical incident analysis" to explore all causative factors for mistakes.[21–23]

Around the same time, anesthesiology was in the midst of a malpractice crisis characterized by terrific acrimony and skyrocketing premiums. Other researchers, recognizing the possibility that there might be error patterns, began a careful review of settled malpractice cases for themes and lessons ("*closed-case analysis*").[24] And they found such patterns, in the form of poor machine design, lack of standardization, lax policies and procedures, poor education, and more.

The research and insights from Cooper's work and the closed-case analyses were important, but they needed to be brought into the mainstream, particularly among physicians. Luckily, as so often happens, the right person emerged at the right time. Ellison "Jeep" Pierce assumed the presidency of the American Society of Anesthesiologists in 1983. Energized by the experience of a friend's daughter who died under anesthesia during a routine dental procedure, Pierce conceived of a foundation to help support work to make care safer—in fact, he probably coined the term "patient safety" in founding the Anesthesia Patient Safety Foundation (APSF).[25] APSF, working closely with other professional, healthcare, and industry groups, helped push the field forward, beginning by convincing caregivers that there was a real problem and that it was soluble with the right approach.[26,27]

What lessons from anesthesia are relevant to our broader efforts to improve overall patient safety?[1,28,29] First, safety requires strong leadership, with a commitment to openness and a willingness to embrace change. Second, learning from past mistakes is an essential part of patient safety. In the case of anesthesia, the closed-case reviews led to key insights. Third, although technology is not the complete answer to safety, it must be a part of the answer. In anesthesia, the thoughtful application of oximetry, capnography, and automated blood pressure monitoring has been vital. Fourth, where applicable, the use of human factors engineering and forcing functions can markedly enhance safety (Chapter 7). For example, changing the anesthesia tubing so that the incorrect gasses could not be hooked up was crucial; this was a far more effective maneuver than trying to educate or remind anesthesiologists about the possibility of mix-ups. Finally, anesthesia was in the throes of a malpractice crisis and had a number of highly visible errors reported in the media. Sparks like these are often necessary to disrupt the inertia and denial that can undermine so many safety efforts. In the 1980s, anesthesiologists paid exorbitant rates for malpractice insurance—among the highest in the medical profession. Now that errors causing patient harm are so unusual, today's rates fall in the midrange of all specialties, a good example of the "business case for safety."

WRONG-SITE/WRONG-PATIENT SURGERY

In 1995, Willie King, a 51-year-old diabetic man with severe peripheral vascular disease, checked into a hospital in Tampa, Florida, for amputation of a gangrenous right leg. The admitting clerk mistakenly entered into the computer system that Mr. King was there for a left *below-the-knee amputation. An alert floor nurse caught the error after seeing a printout of the day's operating room (OR) schedule; she called the OR to correct the mistake. A scrub nurse made a handwritten correction to the printed schedule, but the computer's schedule was not changed. Since this computer schedule was the source of subsequent printed copies, copies of the incorrect schedule were distributed around the OR and hospital. King's surgeon entered the OR, read the wrong procedure off one of the printed schedules, prepped the wrong leg, and then began to amputate it. The error was discovered partway through the surgery, too late to save the left leg. Of course, the gangrenous right leg still needed to be removed, and a few weeks later it was, leaving King a double amputee.*

Events like these are so egregious that they have been dubbed "Never Events"—meaning that they should never occur under any circumstances (Appendix VI). And who could possibly disagree? While one major study estimated the incidence of wrong-site or wrong-patient surgery to be approximately 1 in every 100,000 operations,[30] other studies—particularly those that also considered outpatient surgery and nonsurgical procedures—have given higher estimates.[31,32] And in one survey of approximately 1000 hand surgeons, 20% admitted to having operated on the wrong site at least once in their career, and an additional 16% had prepared to operate on the wrong site but caught themselves just in time.[33]

When one hears of wrong-site or wrong-patient procedures, it is difficult to resist the instinct to assign blame, usually to the operating surgeon. Yet we know there must be something more at play than simply a careless surgeon or nurse. The answer, as usual, is Swiss cheese (Chapter 2) and bad systems. Appreciating this makes clear the need for a multidimensional approach aimed at preventing the inevitable human slips from causing terrible harm.

The Joint Commission has promoted the use of the *Universal Protocol* to prevent wrong-site and wrong-patient surgery and procedures (Table 5-2). In essence, the Protocol acknowledges that single solutions to this problem are destined to fail, and that robust fixes depend on multiple overlapping layers of protection. Several elements of the Universal Protocol merit further comment.

At first glance, *sign-your-site*—the surgeon marks the surgical site in indelible ink after verifying the correct site—would appear to be a particularly strong solution. But the early history of sign-your-site demonstrates that even reasonable safety solutions are destined to fail without strong standard policies and enforcement protocols. In the mid-1990s, before the Joint Commission or surgical professional societies entered the fray, a number of well-meaning orthopedic surgeons began to use markings to help ensure that they operated on the correct surgical site. Unfortunately, without a standardized approach, the result would

Table 5-2   THE JOINT COMMISSION'S "UNIVERSAL PROTOCOL FOR PREVENTING WRONG-SITE, WRONG-PROCEDURE, AND WRONG-PERSON SURGERY"

Conduct a preprocedure verification process

1. Implement a preprocedure process to verify the correct procedure, for the correct patient, at the correct site. *Note*: The patient is involved in the verification process when possible

2. Identify the items that must be available for the procedure and use a standardized list to verify their availability. At a minimum, these items include the following:

   - Relevant documentation (e.g., history and physical, signed procedure consent form, nursing assessment, and preanesthesia assessment)
   - Labeled diagnostic and radiology test results (e.g., radiology images and scans, or pathology and biopsy reports) that are properly displayed
   - Any required blood products, implants, devices, and/or special equipment for the procedure
     Note: The expectation of this element of performance is that the standardized list is available and is used consistently during the preprocedure verification. It is not necessary to document that the standardized list was used for each patient

3. Match the items that are to be available in the procedure area to the patient

Mark the procedure site

1. Identify those procedures that require marking of the incision or insertion site. At a minimum, sites are marked when there is more than one possible location for the procedure and when performing the procedure in a different location would negatively affect quality or safety
   Note: For spinal procedures, in addition to preoperative skin marking of the general spinal region, special intraoperative imaging techniques may be used for locating and marking the exact vertebral level

2. Mark the procedure site before the procedure is performed and, if possible, with the patient involved

3. The procedure site is marked by a licensed independent practitioner who is ultimately accountable for the procedure and will be present when the procedure is performed. In limited circumstances, the licensed independent practitioner may delegate site marking to an individual who is permitted by the organization to participate in the procedure and has the following qualifications:

   - An individual in a medical postgraduate education program who is being supervised by the licensed independent practitioner performing the procedure, who is familiar with the patient, and who will be present when the procedure is performed
   - A licensed individual who performs duties requiring a collaborative agreement or supervisory agreement with the licensed independent practitioner performing the procedure (i.e., an advanced practice registered nurse [APRN] or physician assistant [PA]), who is familiar with the patient, and who will be present when the procedure is performed
     Note: The hospital's leaders define the limited circumstances (if any) in which site marking may be delegated to an individual meeting these qualifications

4. The method of marking the site and the type of mark is unambiguous and is used consistently throughout the hospital
   Note: The mark is made at or near the procedure site and is sufficiently permanent to be visible after skin preparation and draping. Adhesive markers are not the sole means of marking the site

5. A written, alternative process is in place for patients who refuse site marking or when it is technically or anatomically impossible or impractical to mark the site (e.g., mucosal surfaces or perineum)

(continued)

Table 5-2   THE JOINT COMMISSION'S "UNIVERSAL PROTOCOL FOR PREVENTING WRONG-SITE, WRONG-PROCEDURE, AND WRONG-PERSON SURGERY" (*continued*)

Mark the procedure site

Note: Examples of other situations that involve alternative processes include:

- Minimal access procedures treating a lateralized internal organ, whether percutaneous or through a natural orifice
- Teeth
- Premature infants, for whom the mark may cause a permanent tattoo

A time out is performed before the procedure

1. Conduct a time out immediately before starting the invasive procedure or making the incision
2. The time out has the following characteristics:
   - It is standardized, as defined by the hospital
   - It is initiated by a designated member of the team
   - It involves the immediate members of the procedure team, including the individual performing the procedure, the anesthesia providers, the circulating nurse, the operating room technician, and other active participants who will be participating in the procedure from the beginning
3. When two or more procedures are being performed on the same patient, and the person performing the procedure changes, perform a time out before each procedure is initiated
4. During the time out, the team members agree, at a minimum, on the following:
   - Correct patient identity
   - The correct site
   - The procedure to be done
5. Document the completion of the time out

   Note: The hospital determines the amount and type of documentation.

have been nearly comical if it wasn't so scary: some surgeons placed an "X" on the surgical site (as in "X marks the spot"), while others placed an "X" on the *opposite* limb (as in "don't cut here"). Although there were no documented cases of wrong-site surgery resulting from this anarchy, the implementation of standard rules was crucial (under the Universal Protocol, the surgical site is the only one to be marked). Even today, the effectiveness of site marking depends on its correct implementation (Figure 5-1).[34] We have also learned that the same strategies that help prevent laterality errors (right vs. left arm) may not work for other types of wrong-site surgery, such as incorrect spinal level errors.[35]

    Another key element in the Universal Protocol is the *time out*, during which the entire surgical team is supposed to huddle and briefly discuss and agree upon the patient's name and intended procedure. This too seems like a robust safety solution, a fail-safe step sure to catch any errors that eluded prior protections. Yet we have come to recognize how dependent this step is on having a culture of safety (Chapters 9 and 15), one in which people low in the hierarchy are

Figure 5-1 ■ Clinical example of correct versus incorrect modalities of surgical site marking. **(A)** This patient was scheduled for a surgical procedure on his right forearm. The intern marked and initialed the site on the dressing, which came off prior to surgery (1). The resident corrected the mistake by marking the surgical site on skin, using a regular pen (2). Neither the marking nor the initials are legible (2). Finally, the site was again marked and initialed by the attending surgeon with a permanent marker (3). **(B)** During the surgical preparation, the site marking with the regular pen was washed off immediately (2), whereas the permanent marker remained visible throughout the surgical preparation (3). This example emphasizes the crucial importance of using a permanent marker and large and legible letters, and signing the marking with the surgeon's initials. "YES" is the designated, standardized identifier for the correct surgical site at Denver Health Medical Center. (Reproduced with permission from Stahel PF, Mehler PS, Clarke TJ, et al. The 5th anniversary of the "Universal Protocol": pitfalls and pearls revisited. *Patient Saf Surg* 2009;3:14. [Original figure available from PubMed Central at: http://www.ncbi.nlm.nih.gov/pmc/articles/PMC2712460/figure/F1/.])

comfortable raising their concerns "up the authority gradient." Without a safe culture and good communication, interventions such as time outs can be robotic and perfunctory, providing the illusion, rather than the reality, of safety.[31]

While the components of the Universal Protocol made sense and likely led to some improvements in surgical safety, this is yet another example (like medication reconciliation, discussed in Chapter 4) in which a more holistic approach, one that respected the challenges of achieving meaningful changes within complex adaptive systems (Chapter 2), was needed.[34] The past several years have seen a number of successful experiments that embedded the core processes (such as sign-your-site and preoperative time outs and briefings[36]) within a broader set of activities designed to create a culture of safety, encourage communication, increase situational awareness, and focus all of the members of the surgical team on the task at hand.[37,38]

The first such effort was an eight-hospital international study that combined the use of the World Health Organization's Surgical Safety Checklist (Figure 5-2) with a variety of other activities designed to improve teamwork

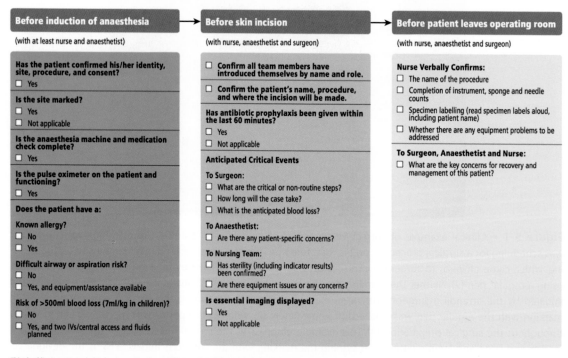

Before induction of anaesthesia

(with at least nurse and anaesthetist)

Has the patient confirmed his/her identity, site, procedure, and consent?
☐ Yes

Is the site marked?
☐ Yes
☐ Not applicable

Is the anaesthesia machine and medication check complete?
☐ Yes

Is the pulse oximeter on the patient and functioning?
☐ Yes

Does the patient have a:

Known allergy?
☐ No
☐ Yes

Difficult airway or aspiration risk?
☐ No
☐ Yes, and equipment/assistance available

Risk of >500ml blood loss (7ml/kg in children)?
☐ No
☐ Yes, and two IVs/central access and fluids planned

Before skin incision

(with nurse, anaesthetist and surgeon)

☐ **Confirm all team members have introduced themselves by name and role.**

☐ **Confirm the patient's name, procedure, and where the incision will be made.**

Has antibiotic prophylaxis been given within the last 60 minutes?
☐ Yes
☐ Not applicable

Anticipated Critical Events

To Surgeon:
☐ What are the critical or non-routine steps?
☐ How long will the case take?
☐ What is the anticipated blood loss?

To Anaesthetist:
☐ Are there any patient-specific concerns?

To Nursing Team:
☐ Has sterility (including indicator results) been confirmed?
☐ Are there equipment issues or any concerns?

Is essential imaging displayed?
☐ Yes
☐ Not applicable

Before patient leaves operating room

(with nurse, anaesthetist and surgeon)

Nurse Verbally Confirms:
☐ The name of the procedure
☐ Completion of instrument, sponge and needle counts
☐ Specimen labelling (read specimen labels aloud, including patient name)
☐ Whether there are any equipment problems to be addressed

To Surgeon, Anaesthetist and Nurse:
☐ What are the key concerns for recovery and management of this patient?

This checklist is not intended to be comprehensive. Additions and modifications to fit local practice are encouraged.   Revised 1 / 2009   © WHO, 2009

Figure 5-2 ■ The World Health Organization's Surgical Safety Checklist. (Available at: http://whqlibdoc.who.int/publications/2009/9789241598590_eng_Checklist.pdf. Reproduced by permission.)

and communication.[39] While its results—a nearly 50% decrease in deaths and complications, at both rich and poor hospitals—were impressive, the findings have been questioned in light of the study's before-and-after design, the absence of controls for confounding variables, and the fact that the outcomes did not correlate with the degree of compliance with the intervention.[40]

Reassuringly, an even more comprehensive surgical safety intervention (this one involved 11 distinct checklists applied by caregivers along the surgical continuum) was implemented at six teaching hospitals in the Netherlands.[41] Patients at participating hospitals had 30% fewer complications and a nearly 50% lower mortality rate than those at control institutions. As in the seminal study in Michigan ICUs (Chapter 10)—in which a checklist-based intervention resulted in major decreases in central line–associated bloodstream infections, leading many people to focus on the checklist as a magic bullet[42,43]—both the WHO and Netherlands study authors emphasized the importance of culture change and teamwork as key success factors.[39,41] In fact, the WHO investigators subsequently demonstrated that improvements in safety culture correlated with the improved surgical outcomes.[44] Moreover, a study of the implementation of teamwork training (along with checklists) in 74 Veterans Affairs hospitals found a striking improvement in surgical mortality, along with evidence of a dose–response curve.[45]

It is clear that checklists are part of the answer, but only part. Because issues related to checklists, teamwork, and culture have become so central to the entire field of patient safety, I will discuss them more fully in Chapter 15.

RETAINED SPONGES AND INSTRUMENTS

In October 2002, a Canadian woman repeatedly tripped the alarm on a metal detector as she attempted to board a flight in Regina, Saskatchewan. On a closer search, the detector wand continued to bleep as it was passed over her abdomen. Since security personnel were unable to identify anything metallic on her person, they let her board her flight to Calgary. The woman wondered whether the episode was related to the recurrent stomach pain she'd been experiencing since her abdominal surgery four months earlier. After her trip, she saw her doctor, who ordered an abdominal x-ray. Shockingly, it showed the outline of a metal retractor, a tool used by the surgical team months earlier. The surgeons had inadvertently left the object behind when they closed up, which was no small feat—the retractor was a foot long and 2 inches wide, practically the size of a crowbar.

The term "retained sponge" (also called "gossypibomas," from the Latin "gossypium" [cotton] and "boma" [place of concealment][46]) is often used as a catchall phrase for all manner of surgical paraphernalia left behind after surgery. A review by Gawande et al. of 54 patients with retained foreign bodies over a 16-year period found that roughly two-thirds were actual sponges—square or rectangular bits of absorbent gauze designed to soak up blood in the operative field—while the remaining one-third were surgical instruments.[47] This frequency corresponds to an overall "retained sponge" rate of about 1 per 10,000 surgeries, which works out to at least one case each year for a typical large hospital in the United States. Because the study drew its sample from malpractice cases, the problem is undoubtedly more common than this published estimate. In fact, a more recent study found a retained foreign object rate of 1 per 5500 operations.[48] Determining actual incidence figures is made more challenging by the fact that the average retained surgical sponge is discovered seven years after the surgery.[49]

Unlike many other safety problems, the retained sponge/instrument problem would seem to be preventable by the thoughtful implementation of systematic, mechanical solutions. In the 1940s, manufacturers produced sponges with loops that were attached to a 2-in metal ring. The ring then hung outside the operative field while the sponges were placed inside the field. When the operation was over, the nurse simply harvested the sponges by gathering the rings—the way a trail of fishing hooks is pulled out of the water by reeling in the line. Clever as this sounds, surgeons found the ring system unwieldy, and many simply cut the rings off: a classic example of a *routine rule violation* (Chapter 15).[50] By the 1960s, manufacturers tried another approach, producing surgical sponges with an embedded radiopaque thread (Figure 5-3A) meant to show up on x-rays (Figure 5-3B). But obtaining a postoperative x-ray on every patient is impractical, so the x-ray solution usually comes into play many months later, when a patient has persistent postoperative pain and the doctors are trying to figure out why.

To laypeople, leaving a sponge or tool behind may seem like a particularly boneheaded error—until you remember that complex or emergency surgeries often require dozens, even hundreds, of sponges (along with scores of other instruments and needles), often placed under considerable time pressure. This is one reason surgical teams have long used *"sponge, sharp, and instrument counts."* The standard protocol requires four separate counts: when the instruments are set up and the sponges are unpacked, when the surgery begins and the items are called for and used, at the time of closure, and during external suturing. Unfortunately, the chaotic and pressured circumstances in most busy ORs and the frequent changes in personnel,[51] coupled with the reluctance of the nurses to admit (consciously or not) to the fallacy of an earlier count, create situations in which the counts fail. In the most startling finding of Gawande et al., while one-third of the retained sponge cases had not been subject to a documented count, two-thirds of the cases were.[47] And in about half the cases, there were actually *multiple*

Figure 5-3 ▪ Surgical sponge **(A)** with an embedded radiopaque thread, shown on x-ray **(B)**.

counts documented to be in agreement. This means that every sponge and instrument was accounted for, despite the fact that one would turn up later—rather inconveniently—in a patient's abdomen.

The real lesson from all of this is that what appears to be a perfectly logical safety practice often turns out to be highly imperfect. Because sponge counts of any kind are inherently unreliable, some experts have recommended taking an x-ray of every surgical site before the field is sutured. Even if x-rays were free and patients and staff were willing to put up with the procedure, keeping anesthetized surgical patients on the table any longer than strictly necessary creates its own problems. Partly for this reason, Gawande and his colleagues recommend x-rays only in high-risk cases: those involving emergency surgery, prolonged surgery, surgery that required a real-time change in clinical strategy, and surgery on obese patients. Even this plan has gaps, because radiopaque markers are subtle and can be overlooked on x-rays.[48]

Ultimately, the best solution to the retained sponge problem probably lies in new technology. Some companies have developed bar-coded sponges to aid in the counting process,[51] while others have embedded their sponges with radio-frequency ID tags that cause a detector wand to *beep* when the surgeon waves it over the field before closure.[52] Still others have built automatic "sponge counters," resembling tollbooth coin machines, which can be loaded up and checked after every surgery. Although the experience with these technologies is still limited, institutions utilizing them have reported positive results. In a decision-analytic model, both the bar-coded sponge and radio-frequency-tagged sponge systems appear to be more cost-effective than either sponge counting or programs of universal or selective postprocedure radiographs (bar coding is less expensive than radio-frequency tagging, but probably takes more nursing time to use).[53] It seems likely that one or several of these technological solutions will be ready for widespread implementation soon, hopefully rendering gossypibomas a historical curiosity.

SURGICAL FIRES

Surgical fires are unusual but frightening and potentially deadly. It has been estimated that there are between 50 and 200 such fires annually in the United States, leading to morbidity in 20% of cases (often severe, including tracheal or pulmonary burns) and one or two deaths.[46,54]

The genesis of surgical fires, one-third of which involve the airways, is the confluence of what has been called the *fire safety triangle*: an ignition source (such as electrocautery and lasers), a fuel source (e.g., gauze, drapes, even endotracheal tubes [Figure 5-4]), and oxidizers (usually oxygen but sometimes

Figure 5-4 ■ Demonstration of rocket-like flames shooting from an endotracheal tube caused by laser ignition of the tube with 100% oxygen flowing. (Courtesy of ECRI Institute; reproduced with permission. Original figure available at: http://www.patientsafetyauthority.org/ADVISORIES/AdvisoryLibrary/2007/mar4(1)/Publishing Images/4_fig2.JPG. Copyright 2011 ECRI Institute. www.ecri.org. 5200 Butler Pike, Plymouth Meeting, PA 19462. 610–825–6000.)

nitrous oxide). Concerns about OR fires were very high in the distant past, but interest (and risk) waned with the ending of the era of flammable anesthetics about 25 years ago. The recent uptick in concern likely relates to the more frequent use of cautery and lasers in the OR, and more aggressive use of oxygen in anesthetized patients.[55]

A series of prevention maneuvers has been recommended, addressing all three elements of the triangle.[54] They include: ignition sources should be stored away from the patients and their tips should be visualized while hot, time should be allowed for alcohol-based prep solutions to dry prior to draping patients, oxygen concentrations should be kept to the lowest safe amount, and cautery around the airway should be used sparingly and only after the anesthesiologist is warned so that he or she can turn down the oxygen.

In case of a fire in the OR or procedural suite, all personnel should be immediately notified. For fires involving the airway, the flow of gas should be turned off and the airway cooled with normal saline. For fires in other locations, smothering with water, saline, or by physical means is advised; use of a carbon dioxide fire extinguisher should be reserved for persistent flames.

SAFETY IN NONSURGICAL BEDSIDE PROCEDURES

While most of the attention regarding procedural safety has focused on surgical operations, there is growing recognition that nonsurgical procedures carry risks as well. As we turn our attention to bedside procedures, it is worth appreciating some differences between the two domains. One big one: the OR is (on a good day) an organized system of care, where policies and procedures can be enacted and measured, and individual participants can be given responsibility for compliance (i.e., "The circulating nurse will not allow the procedure to begin until the time out has been completed"). On the other hand, some procedures (such as thoracentesis and central line placement) may involve only a single physician and his or her patient, offering fewer opportunities for independent double checks.

Complication rates for certain bedside procedures are surprisingly high. For example, 6% of thoracenteses result in a pneumothorax, one-third of which require chest tube placement.[56] Central venous catheter placement can be very risky, with complication rates (arterial laceration, pneumothorax, thrombosis, and infection) exceeding 15%.[57] Paracentesis, lumbar puncture, and arthrocentesis are somewhat safer, but all have significant risks.[58,59]

Strategies to decrease the risks of procedures fall into several categories: education and skill building, policies and practices to decrease overall process risks such as wrong-patient and wrong-site procedures, adjunctive technologies, and organizational changes.

There is abundant evidence that our traditional academic strategy of "see one, do one, teach one" is both ineffective and unethical (Chapter 17). As one window into this, studies have shown that many residents remain uncomfortable with certain procedures even after being charged with supervising them for their junior colleagues.[60] Most of the advances in the area of *education and skill building* have come through the development of formal curricula and competency-based assessment strategies—including forbidding learners from performing procedures independently until they have been deemed competent.[61,62] (The use of simulation to enhance both teaching and assessment of procedures is further discussed in Chapter 17.) There are now a number of Web-based aids (the videos produced by the *New England Journal of Medicine* are the best I've seen[63]) that demonstrate correct technique and pitfalls far better than a static textbook chapter or monograph ever could.

Bedside procedures are at risk for the same kinds of *wrong-site and wrong-patient errors* that I discussed earlier. In fact, a study of 132 self-reported wrong-site or wrong-patient events found that similar numbers came from nonoperative procedures as formal surgeries.[64] The Joint Commission requires the bedside proceduralist to perform the same Universal Protocol for bedside procedures as is required for major surgical operations.[65,66] While it is permissible for an individual proceduralist to go through the Protocol alone, bringing another person in the room for an independent check is a sound practice. Barsuk et al. reengineered the procedure process—including adding requirements for procedural kits (which included relevant checklists) to be signed out by nurses from locked storage cabinets (a forcing function, Chapter 7) and that nurses be present at all procedures—and found that compliance with the Universal Protocol skyrocketed, from 16% to 94%.[67]

Adjunctive technologies can be quite helpful. The most important is *bedside ultrasound*, whose use drastically lowers the rates of pneumothorax after thoracentesis and both pneumothorax and subsequent infection (the latter improvement likely owing to fewer sticks) after central line placement.[56,57] Learning to use bedside ultrasound correctly is not trivial, and teaching this skill should be integrated into the educational program described above.[61,62] Of course, other technologies may more directly improve the safety of certain procedures. For example, the availability of peripherally inserted central catheters (*PICC lines*) has obviated the need for subclavian or jugular puncture in some patients who require access to the central circulation.

Finally, some hospitals have developed dedicated *procedure services* to improve the safety of procedures. These services are staffed by a limited number of physicians (frequently hospitalists) who receive additional training in the relevant procedures and commit to spending significant time on the service. Early data support the premise that such services enhance safety and patient satisfaction,[68–70] probably via several mechanisms: narrowing the number of providers and thereby ensuring that those performing procedures are skilled and have high volumes, allowing for implementation of standard policies and protocols, and freeing clinicians from other distractions while performing procedures. In teaching hospitals, the procedure service not only ensures the safety of individual procedures but also takes on responsibility for educating trainees, in matters ranging from the angle of insertion of the needle to correct hygiene practices, and from the proper use of ultrasound to when a procedure is *not* indicated or too risky and needs to be referred to a more specialized provider (i.e., interventional radiologist). In my judgment, these services represent a major advance in patient safety and should be implemented widely.

KEY POINTS

- Patient safety issues in surgery include those common to other fields (e.g., medication errors, healthcare-associated infections, readmissions, communication mishaps), and also several specific to surgery (e.g., wrong-site surgery, retained sponges, OR fires).

- Evidence for a volume–outcome relationship in many surgical areas argues for new types of simulator training.
- Anesthesia embraced the importance of many patient safety principles (systems thinking, human factors engineering, learning from mistakes, standardization) earlier than any other field in medicine, and has amassed the most impressive safety record.
- A comprehensive application of the "Universal Protocol" (including "sign-your-site" and the preprocedural "time out"), coupled with teamwork training and the use of checklists, is currently the best strategy to prevent wrong-site and wrong-patient errors and has been demonstrated to improve surgical outcomes.
- Retained sponges and other surgical instruments is an uncommon safety hazard. Sponge counts and x-rays have traditionally been the main preventive strategies, but prevention will ultimately depend on more robust detection technologies.
- Surgical fires result from the interaction of the three elements of the fire safety triangle (ignition source, fuel source, and oxidizers). They can be prevented with adherence to a series of safety maneuvers addressing each element of the triangle.
- Nonsurgical procedures, such as thoracentesis and central line placement, carry significant risks. Robust competency-based training, proper adjunctive use of bedside ultrasound, implementing checklists and time outs, and a dedicated procedure service can decrease these risks significantly.

REFERENCES

1. Gaba DM. Anaesthesiology as a model for patient safety in health care. *BMJ* 2000; 320:785–788.
2. Milamed DR, Hedley-Whyte J. Contributions of the surgical sciences to a reduction of the mortality rate in the United States for the period 1968 to 1988. *Ann Surg* 1994;219:94–102.
3. Lindenauer PK, Pekow P, Wang K, et al. Perioperative beta-blocker therapy and mortality after major noncardiac surgery. *N Engl J Med* 2005;353:349–361.
4. POISE Study Group, Devereaux PJ, Yang H, et al. Effects of extended-release metoprolol succinate in patients undergoing non-cardiac surgery (POISE trial): a randomised controlled trial. *Lancet* 2008;371:1839–1847.
5. American College of Cardiology Foundation/American Heart Association Task Force on Practice Guidelines. 2009 ACCF/AHA focused update on perioperative beta blockade incorporated into the ACC/AHA 2007 guidelines on perioperative cardiovascular evaluation and care for noncardiac surgery. *J Am Coll Cardiol* 2009;54:e13–e118.

6. Thomas EJ, Studdert DM, Burstin HR, et al. Incidence and types of adverse events and negligent care in Utah and Colorado. *Med Care* 2000;38:261–271.

7. Sharpe VA, Faden AI. *Medical Harm: Historical, Conceptual and Ethical Dimensions of Iatrogenic Illness.* Cambridge, England: Cambridge University Press; 1998.

8. Neuhauser D. John Williamson and the terrifying results of the medical practice information demonstration project. *Qual Saf Health Care* 2002;11:387–389.

9. Vincent C. *Patient Safety.* 2nd ed. London: Elsevier; 2010.

10. Leape LL. Error in medicine. *JAMA* 1994;272:1851–1857.

11. Leape LL. An interview with Lucian Leape. *Jt Comm J Qual Saf* 2004;30:653–658.

12. Rowell KS, Turrentine FE, Hutter MM, et al. Use of national surgical quality improvement program data as a catalyst for quality improvement. *J Am Coll Surg* 2007;204:1293–1300.

13. O'Connor GT, Plume SK, Olmstead EM, et al. A regional intervention to improve the hospital mortality associated with coronary artery bypass graft surgery. The Northern New England Cardiovascular Disease Study Group. *JAMA* 1996;275:841–846.

14. Luft HS, Bunker JP, Enthoven AC. Should operations be regionalized? The empirical relation between surgical volume and mortality. *N Engl J Med* 1979;301:1364–1369.

15. Eggli Y, Halfon P, Meylan D, et al. Surgical safety and hospital volume across a wide range of interventions. *Med Care* 2010;48:962–971.

16. Moore MJ, Bennett CL. The learning curve for laparoscopic cholecystectomy. The Southern Surgeons Club. *Am J Surg* 1995;170:55–59.

17. Morino M, Festa V, Garrone C. Survey on Torino courses. The impact of a two-day practical course on apprenticeship and diffusion of laparoscopic cholecystectomy in Italy. *Surg Endosc* 1995;9:46–48.

18. Ahlberg G, Enochsson L, Gallagher AG, et al. Proficiency-based virtual reality training significantly reduces the error rate for residents during their first 10 laparoscopic cholecystectomies. *Am J Surg* 2007;193:797–804.

19. Shahian DM. Improving cardiac surgery quality—volume, outcome, process? *JAMA* 2004;291:246–248.

20. Kohn L, Corrigan J, Donaldson M, eds. *To Err is Human: Building a Safer Health System.* Committee on Quality of Health Care in America, Institute of Medicine. Washington, DC: National Academy Press; 2000.

21. Cooper JB, Newbower RS, Long CD, et al. Preventable anesthesia mishaps: a study of human factors. *Anesthesiology* 1978;49:399–406.

22. Cooper JB, Long CD, Newbower RS, et al. Critical incidents associated with intraoperative exchanges of anesthesia personnel. *Anesthesiology* 1982;56:456–461.

23. Cooper JB, Newbower RS, Kitz RJ. An analysis of major errors and equipment failures in anesthesia management: considerations for prevention and detection. *Anesthesiology* 1984;60:34–42.

24. Caplan RA, Posner KL, Ward RJ, et al. Adverse respiratory events in anesthesia: a closed claims analysis. *Anesthesiology* 1990;72:828–833.

25. Pierce EC. 40 years behind the mask: safety revisited. *Anesthesiology* 1996;29:965–975.

26. Gawande A. *Complications: A Surgeon's Notes on an Imperfect Science.* New York, NY: Metropolitan Books; 2002.

27. Cooper JB. The APSF: 20-year anniversary of the first patient safety organization—past, present & future. *APSF Newsletter.* Spring 2007;22:1, 3.

28. Lagasse RS. Anesthesia safety: model or myth? A review of the published literature and analysis of current original data. *Anesthesiology* 2002;97:1609–1617.

29. Cooper JB. Getting into patient safety: a personal story. *AHRQ WebM&M* (serial online); August 2006. Available at: http://webmm.ahrq.gov/perspective.aspx?perspectiveID=29.

30. Kwaan MR, Studdert DM, Zinner MJ, et al. Incidence, patterns, and prevention of wrong-site surgery. *Arch Surg* 2006;141:353–358.

31. Seiden SC, Barach P. Wrong-side/wrong-site, wrong-procedure, and wrong-patient adverse events: are they preventable? *Arch Surg* 2006;141:931–939.

32. Neily J, Mills PD, Eldridge N, et al. Incorrect surgical procedures within and outside of the operating room. *Arch Surg* 2009;144:1028–1034.

33. Meinberg EG, Stern PJ. Incidence of wrong-site surgery among hand surgeons. *J Bone Joint Surg Am* 2003;85-A(2):193–197.

34. Stahel PF, Mehler PS, Clarke TJ, et al. The 5th anniversary of the "Universal Protocol": pitfalls and pearls revisited. *Patient Saf Surg* 2009;3:14.

35. Mody MG, Nourbakhsh A, Stahl DL, et al. The prevalence of wrong level surgery among spine surgeons. *Spine* 2008;33:194–198.

36. Allard J, Bleakley A, Hobbs A, et al. Pre-surgery briefings and safety climate in the operating theater. *BMJ Qual Saf* 2011;20:711–717.

37. Weick KE. The collapse of sensemaking in organizations: the Mann Gulch disaster. *Adm Sci Q* 1993;38:628–652.

38. Healey AN, Nagpal K, Moorthy K, et al. Engineering the system of communication for safer surgery. *Cogn Tech Work* 2011;13:1–10.

39. Haynes AB, Weiser TG, Berry WR, et al.; for the Safe Surgery Saves Lives Study Group. A surgical safety checklist to reduce morbidity and mortality in a global population. *N Engl J Med* 2009;360:491–499.

40. Birkmeyer JD. Strategies for improving surgical quality—checklists and beyond. *N Engl J Med* 2010;363:1963–1965.

41. de Vries EN, Prins HA, Crolla RM, et al.; SURPASS Collaborative Group. Effect of a comprehensive surgical safety system on patient outcomes. *N Engl J Med* 2010;363:1928–1937.

42. Pronovost P, Needham D, Berenholtz S, et al. An intervention to decrease catheter-related bloodstream infections in the ICU. *N Engl J Med* 2006;355:2725–2732.

43. Bosk CL, Dixon-Woods M, Goeschel CA, et al. Reality check for checklists. *Lancet* 2009;374:444–445.

44. Haynes AB, Weiser TG, Berry WR, et al.; Safe Surgery Saves Lives Study Group. Changes in safety attitude and relationship to decreased postoperative morbidity and mortality following implementation of a checklist-based surgical safety intervention. *BMJ Qual Saf* 2011;20:102–107.

45. Neily J, Mills PD, Young-Xu Y, et al. Association between implementation of a medical team training program and surgical mortality. *JAMA* 2010;304:1693–1700.

46. Zahiri HR, Stromberg J, Skupsky H, et al. Prevention of 3 "never events" in the operating room: fires, gossypiboma, and wrong-site surgery. *Surg Innov* 2011;18:55–60.

47. Gawande AA, Studdert DM, Oray EJ, et al. Risk factors for retained instruments and sponges after surgery. *N Engl J Med* 2003;348:229–235.

48. Cima RR, Kollengode A, Garnatz J, et al. Incidence and characteristics of potential and actual retained foreign object events in surgical patients. *J Am Coll Surg* 2008; 207:80–87.

49. Wan W, Le T, Riskin L, et al. Improving safety in the operating room: a systematic literature review of retained surgical sponges. *Curr Opin Anaesthesiol* 2009;22:207–214.

50. de Saint Maurice G, Auroy Y, Vincent C, et al. The natural lifespan of a safety policy: violations and system migration in anaesthesia. *Qual Saf Health Care* 2010;19: 327–331.

51. Greenberg CC, Diaz-Flores R, Lipsitz SR, et al. Bar-coding surgical sponges to improve safety: a randomized controlled trial. *Ann Surg* 2008;247:612–616.

52. Cima RR, Kollengode A, Clark J, et al. Using a data-matrix–coded sponge counting system across a surgical practice: impact after 18 months. *Jt Comm J Qual Patient Saf* 2011;37:51–58.

53. Regenbogen SE, Greenberg CC, Resch SC, et al. Prevention of retained surgical sponges: a decision-analytic model predicting relative cost-effectiveness. *Surgery* 2009; 145:527–535.

54. Caplan RA, Barker SJ, Connis RT, et al.; for American Society of Anesthesiologists Task Force on Operating Room Fires. Practice advisory for the prevention and management of operating room fires. *Anesthesiology* 2008;108:786–801.

55. Landro L. In just a flash, simple surgery can turn deadly. *Wall Street Journal.* February 18, 2009:D1.

56. Gordon CE, Feller-Kopman D, Balk EM, et al. Pneumothorax following thoracentesis: a systematic review and meta-analysis. *Arch Intern Med* 2010;170:332–339.

57. McGee DC, Gould MK. Preventing complications of central venous catheterization. *N Engl J Med* 2003;348:1123–1133.

58. De Gottardi A, Thevenot T, Spahr L, et al. Risk of complications after abdominal paracentesis in cirrhotic patients: a prospective study. *Clin Gastroenterol Hepatol* 2009;7:906–909.

59. Sempere AP, Berenguer-Ruiz L, Lezcano-Rodas M, et al. Lumbar puncture: its indications, contraindications, complications and technique. *Rev Neurol* 2007;45:433–436.

60. Mourad M, Kohlwes J, Maselli J; MERN Group, Auerbach AD. Supervising the supervisors—procedural training and supervision in internal medicine residency. *J Gen Intern Med* 2010;25:351–356.

61. Dong Y, Suri HS, Cook DA, et al. Simulation-based objective assessment discerns clinical proficiency in central line placement: a construct validation. *Chest* 2010;137: 1050–1056.

62. Barsuk JH, McGaghie WC, Cohen ER, et al. Use of simulation-based mastery learning to improve the quality of central venous catheter placement in a medical intensive care unit. *J Hosp Med* 2009;4:397–403.

63. Available at: http://www.nejm.org/multimedia/medical-videos.

64. Stahel PF, Sabel AL, Victoroff MS, et al. Wrong-site and wrong-patient procedures in the universal protocol era: analysis of a prospective database of physician self-reported occurrences. *Arch Surg* 2010;145:978–984.

65. The Joint Commission. *Universal Protocol*; 2010. Available at: http://jointcommission.org/assets/1/18/UP_Poster.pdf.

66. Norton E. Implementing the universal protocol hospital-wide. *AORN J* 2007;85: 1187–1197.

67. Barsuk JH, Brake H, Caprio T, et al. Process changes to increase compliance with the Universal Protocol for bedside procedures. *Arch Intern Med* 2011;171:947–949.

68. Mourad M, Auerbach AD, Maselli J, et al. Patient satisfaction with a hospitalist procedure service: is bedside procedure teaching reassuring to patients? *J Hosp Med* 2011;6:219–224.

69. Smith CC, Gordon CE, Feller-Kopman D, et al. Creation of an innovative inpatient medical procedure service and a method to evaluate house staff competency. *J Gen Intern Med* 2004;19:510–513.

70. Lucas BP, Asbury JK, Wang Y, et al. Impact of a bedside procedure service on general medicine inpatients: a firm-based trial. *J Hosp Med* 2007;2:143–149.

ADDITIONAL READINGS

Ali M, Osborne A, Bethune R, et al. Preoperative surgical briefings do not delay operating room start times and are popular with surgical team members. *J Patient Saf* 2011;7:138–142.

Birkmeyer NJ, Dimick JB, Share D, et al. Hospital complication rates with bariatric surgery in Michigan. *JAMA* 2010;304:435–442.

Bosk CL. *Forgive and Remember: Managing Medical Failure.* 2nd ed. Chicago, IL: University of Chicago Press; 2003.

Encinosa WE, Hellinger FJ. The impact of medical errors on ninety-day costs and outcomes: an examination of surgical patients. *Health Serv Res* 2008;43:2067–2085.

Gawande A. *Better: A Surgeon's Notes on Performance.* New York, NY: Metropolitan Books; 2007.

Gawande A. *The Checklist Manifesto: How to Get Things Right.* New York: Metropolitan Books; 2009.

Leonardi MJ, McGory ML, Ko CY. Publicly available hospital comparison web sites: determination of useful, valid, and appropriate information for comparing surgical quality. *Arch Surg* 2007;142:863–869.

Makary MA, Sexton JB, Freischlag JA, et al. Patient safety in surgery. *Ann Surg* 2006;243:628–635.

Neily J, Mills PD, Eldridge N, et al. Incorrect surgical procedures within and outside of the operating room: a follow-up report. *Arch Surg* July 18, 2011 [Epub ahead of print].

PA-PSRS Patient Saf Advis. Beyond the count: preventing the retention of foreign objects. *PA-PSRS Patient Saf Advis* June 2009;6:39–45.

Ring DC, Herndon JH, Meyer GS. Case 34-2010: a 65-year-old woman with an incorrect operation on the left hand. *N Engl J Med* 2010;363:1950–1957.

Sexton JB, Makary MA, Tersigni AR, et al. Teamwork in the operating room: frontline perspectives among hospitals and operating room personnel. *Anesthesiology* 2006; 105:877–884.

DIAGNOSTIC ERRORS | 6

SOME BASIC CONCEPTS AND TERMS

The modern patient safety movement has emphasized medication errors, handoff errors, infections, and surgical errors; all of these areas are amenable to technological (e.g., computerized order entry), procedural (e.g., double checks), and policy (e.g., "sign-your-site") solutions. Diagnostic errors have been less well emphasized, in part because they are more difficult to measure and to fix.

Interestingly, this relative inattention to diagnostic errors began from the very start of the patient safety movement.[1] In the landmark Institute of Medicine report *To Err is Human*,[2] the term "medication errors" is mentioned 70 times, while "diagnostic errors" comes up only twice. This is ironic, since diagnostic errors accounted for 17% of preventable errors in the Harvard Medical Practice Study,[3] the source of the IOM estimate of 44,000 to 98,000 yearly deaths from medical mistakes (the "jumbo jet a day" figure that helped launch the safety movement; Chapter 1). A systematic review of autopsy studies conducted over four decades found that nearly 1 in 10 patients suffered a major antemortem diagnostic error, a figure that has fallen only slightly (the best recent estimate is about 5%) despite all of today's advanced imaging and laboratory techniques.[4] Diagnostic error remains the most common reason for a paid malpractice claim in ambulatory patients.[5]

At first glance, diagnostic errors would seem to represent human failings—pure failures of cognition. And it is true that, perhaps more than any other area in patient safety, the training and skills of the diagnostician remain of paramount importance. However, in keeping with our modern understanding of patient safety, there *are* system fixes that can decrease the frequency and consequences of diagnostic mistakes. In this chapter, I will discuss the cognitive as well as the process failures (such as failure to transfer the results of a crucial laboratory or radiologic study to the correct provider in a timely way) that give rise to diagnostic errors.

MISSED MYOCARDIAL INFARCTION: A CLASSIC DIAGNOSTIC ERROR

Annie Jackson, a 68-year-old African-American woman with mild diabetes, high blood pressure, and elevated cholesterol, presented to the emergency department after 30 minutes of squeezing chest discomfort. An ECG was quickly obtained. The ER physician, Dr. Zoe Bennett, studied the tracing and saw some nonspecific changes in the ST and T segments—not entirely normal but not the ST-segment elevations that are classic for acute myocardial infarction (MI). On exam, she found mild tachycardia, clear lungs, and mild tenderness over the lower part of the patient's sternum. She considered the latter discovery quite reassuring (after all, such tenderness would be more characteristic of a musculoskeletal process than a heart attack), but also ordered a troponin (a biomarker released by damaged heart cells). It came back mildly elevated, again not in the range specific for MI but not normal either. Nevertheless, she made a diagnosis of costochondritis (inflammation of the sternum–rib joint), prescribed an anti-inflammatory agent and bed rest, and released Ms. Jackson from the emergency department. She died later that night, a victim of an untreated MI.

We can only guess which cognitive error caused Dr. Bennett to release Annie Jackson from the ER.[6] Perhaps because Ms. Jackson was a woman, she underestimated her chance of having a heart attack. She almost certainly relied too heavily on chest wall tenderness for her diagnosis—it is unusual, but not unheard of, in MI patients. She also overemphasized the lack of clear evidence on the ECG and troponin tests. Although they were "nonspecific," both were clearly abnormal and thus justified admission. Maybe she was just exhausted after a long day at work.[7]

We do know, however, that this particular error—sending patients home with heart attacks—is distressingly common and frequently lethal. Nearly 1 in 25 patients with MIs are mistakenly sent home, and these patients have a much higher death rate than MI victims who are correctly diagnosed and hospitalized.[8] Because missed MI is the best-studied diagnostic error, I will use it to make several broader points about these errors.

In the 1970s, researchers began studying the problem of missed MIs and quickly concluded that many errors were related to patient characteristics. Physicians were more likely to send patients home despite worrisome histories or abnormal data when the patients were in groups traditionally believed to be at lower risk for MI, such as younger patients (under age 55) and women. Nonwhites were also mistakenly sent home more often, raising the question of racial bias, conscious or unconscious, among caregivers.[8] In one particularly sobering study, 720 physicians were shown videotapes of actors playing patients with chest pain that could have been heart related.[9] Four actors, each speaking precisely the same script, appeared on the videos: a white man, a white woman, a black man, and a black woman. Regardless of their own race and ethnicity, the physicians were far more likely to recommend cardiac catheterization for the white male than for the black female. Similar variations in diagnostic and therapeutic practices have been seen elsewhere in medicine, catalyzing vigorous efforts to address these *"healthcare disparities."*[10]

Researchers found that physician-specific differences were also at play. For example, one study showed that senior physicians were significantly more likely than their younger colleagues to correctly hospitalize chest pain patients (those with real MIs).[11] Were the older physicians better diagnosticians? Perhaps not—the older physicians were also more likely to hospitalize patients *without* heart attacks. In other words, with experience came risk aversion. Another study showed that risk aversion was not simply a function of age. One hundred and nineteen physicians completed a questionnaire assessing their attitudes toward risk. Doctors who appeared to be risk seekers (e.g., those who like fast cars and sky diving) were four times more likely to send the same chest pain patient home than the risk avoiders.[12]

One could easily look at cases like Annie Jackson's and see careless doctoring, a blown diagnosis, and a fatal mistake. But by now, hopefully, you're approaching this case with a more systems-focused mindset, thinking: How can we improve our ability to diagnose patients who come to the ER with a constellation of symptoms, findings, and risk factors that may yield ambiguous results but can be life-threatening? Too often, without a systematic approach, the clinical decision—to admit or discharge the patient—is based on the physician's faulty reasoning, which in turn may be traced to poor training, inadequate experience, personal and professional bias, fuzzy thinking brought on by overwork and fatigue, or even the physician's own tolerance for risk.

COGNITIVE ERRORS: ITERATIVE HYPOTHESIS TESTING, BAYESIAN REASONING, AND HEURISTICS

As cognitive psychologists began to study how physicians think, they found that even well-trained doctors can engage in faulty thinking because they take cognitive shortcuts, reinforced by a professional culture that rewards the appearance of certainty.[13,14] This means that preventing diagnostic errors is likely to depend on understanding how physicians approach diagnostic decisions, and providing them with tools (either cognitive or adjunctive, such as information technology) to help them make correct decisions more often.

Beginning in the 1970s, several researchers began to try to understand how great diagnosticians think. Led by Dr. Jerome Kassirer (later the editor of the *New England Journal of Medicine*), they observed the diagnostic reasoning of dozens of clinicians, and found that the good ones naturally engaged in a process called *iterative hypothesis testing*.[15] This means that, after hearing the initial portion of a case, they immediately began thinking about possible scenarios to explain the facts, modifying their opinions as more information became available. For example, a skilled physician presented with the case of a 57-year-old man with 3 days of chest pain, shortness of breath, and light-headedness responds by thinking, "The worst thing this could be is a heart attack or blood clot to the lungs. I need to ask a few more questions to see if the chest pain bores through to the back, which would make me worry about an aortic dissection. I'll also ask about typical cardiac symptoms, such as sweating and nausea, and see if the pain is squeezing or radiates to the left arm or jaw. But even if it doesn't, I'll certainly get an ECG to be sure no cardiac event has occurred. If he also reports a fever or cough, I might begin to suspect pneumonia or pleurisy. The chest x-ray should help sort that out."

Every answer the patient gives and each positive or negative finding on the physical examination (*yes, there is a fever*; *no, the spleen is not enlarged*) triggers an automatic, almost intuitive recalibration of the probability of the various alternatives. The skilled diagnostician does this so effortlessly that novices often struggle as they try to understand the science that underlies the expert's decision to embrace certain facts (the clear lung fields in the patient with dyspnea markedly elevate the probability of pulmonary embolism since this would be highly unusual in severe heart failure) while discarding others (the lack of an S_3 gallop—a subtle and often absent finding—does little to dissuade the expert from the possibility of heart failure).

We now recognize that much of this art consists of applying an unconscious, intuitive version of *Bayes' theorem*, developed by the eighteenth-century British theologian-turned-mathematician Thomas Bayes.[16] In essence, Bayes' theorem says that any medical test must be interpreted from two perspectives. The first is: How accurate is the test? That is, how often does it give right or wrong answers? The second is: How likely is it that this patient has the disease the test is looking for? Bayesian reasoning is why it is foolish to screen apparently healthy 35-year-old executives with a cardiac treadmill test (or, for that matter, a "heart scan"), because positive results will mostly be false positives. Conversely, a 65-year-old smoker with high cholesterol who develops squeezing chest pain when shoveling snow has about a 95% chance of having significant coronary artery disease. In this case, a negative treadmill test lowers this probability to only about 80%, so the clinician who reassures the patient that the normal treadmill means his heart is fine is making a terrible, and potentially fatal, mistake.

In addition to misapplications of iterative hypothesis testing and failure to appreciate the implications of Bayesian reasoning, we now understand that many diagnostic errors are caused by cognitive shortcuts ("*heuristics*") that clinicians take, often in the name of efficiency.[17] For example, many errors occur when clinicians are too quick to pronounce judgment, and then defend that turf too vigorously despite the emergence of contradictory evidence.[13,14] This is human nature, of course; we tend to see what we expect to see rather than than what's actually in front of our eyes. By the way, did you notice the word "than" used twice in a row in the previous sentence? Even when we don't intend to do it, our brains can take cognitive shortcuts to get us to our goal—whether it's finishing a sentence or discharging a patient from the ER.

This particular cognitive bias, known as "anchoring" (or "premature closure"), is only one of the many pitfalls that underlie many diagnostic errors. Other common biases include the availability heuristic, framing effects, and blind obedience (Table 6-1).[22] Practicing physicians were first introduced to these concepts in the past decade, although the concepts have long been

Table 6-1 **SELECTED COGNITIVE BIASES LEADING TO MISSED DIAGNOSES, AND CORRECTIVE STRATEGIES**			
Circumstance and Pitfall	**Classic Definition**	**Corrective Strategies**	**Example**
Availability heuristic	Judging by ease of recalling past cases	Verify with legitimate statistics ("If you hear hoof beats, think about horses, not zebras")	A patient with crushing chest pain was incorrectly treated for myocardial infarction, despite indications that an aortic dissection was present[18]
Anchoring heuristic (premature closure)	Relying on initial impressions	Reconsider in light of new data or second opinion, consider extremes ("If the patient dies unexpectedly, what would it be from?")	Repeated positive blood cultures with *Corynebacterium* were dismissed as contaminants; the patient was eventually diagnosed with *Corynebacterium* endocarditis[19]
Framing effects	Being swayed by subtle wording	Examine case from alternative perspectives ("Let's play devil's advocate ...")	A heroin-addicted patient with abdominal pain was treated for opiate withdrawal, but proved to have bowel perforation[20]
Blind obedience	Showing undue deference to authority or technology	Reconsider when authority is more remote (in case of human authority); assess test accuracy (in case of technology)	A false-negative rapid test for *Streptococcus* pharyngitis resulted in a delay in diagnosis[21]

Adapted and reproduced with permission from Redelmeier DA. Improving patient care. The cognitive psychology of missed diagnoses. *Ann Intern Med* 2005;142:115–120; *Patient Safety Primer: Diagnostic Errors*. AHRQ Patient Safety Network. Available at: http://psnet.ahrq.gov/primer.aspx?primerID=12.

applied to other domains in which decisions need to be made under conditions of uncertainty, ranging from battlefields to Wall Street.

Over the past decade, researchers began to study these biases in health-care. In one interesting study, internal medicine residents were presented with a series of cases in which the diagnosis was known.[23] The researchers then presented additional cases with similar symptoms but different correct diagnoses. The residents were more likely to offer (mistaken) diagnoses drawn from the first cases in the subsequent cases, clear evidence of availability bias. The researchers repeated the exercise after asking residents to engage in *reflective practice*, a process that lies at the core of a skill known as *metacognition* (thinking about one's own thinking).[24] The impact of availability bias was lessened considerably, offering hope that some errors related to faulty application of heuristics can be prevented.

There is also some evidence that experienced clinicians are more likely to remain flexible and avoid premature closure than inexperienced ones,[25] which gives hope that this competency can be inculcated (although it seems unlikely that classroom training will ever match the impact of receiving feedback about a missed diagnosis in a real patient).[22] There is also emerging evidence that a clinician's emotional state can influence the risk of committing diagnostic errors.[7] While few of us are able to change our emotional state at will, sensitizing clinicians to this relationship (*I realize that I'm angry. I'd better slow down and rethink this or ask a colleague for help*) may help prevent some errors.

IMPROVING DIAGNOSTIC REASONING

In Chapter 13, we will explore the role of computerized decision support and more general use of information technology in helping physicians to be smarter diagnosticians. At this juncture, suffice it to say that such computerized adjuncts are likely to help clinicians make better, more evidence-based decisions, but will not for the foreseeable future replace the clinician's mind as the main diagnostic workhorse.

Can our cognitive biases be overcome? Perhaps more than any area in clinical medicine, when diagnosing patients we need to learn from our mistakes and to deepen our understanding of clinical reasoning. As with most errors, the answer will come through systems thinking, but here this means better systems for training physicians to avoid common diagnostic speed bumps (Table 6-1). As Canadian safety expert and emergency medicine physician Pat Croskerry puts it:

One uniquely distinguishing characteristic of those who make high-quality decisions is that they can largely free themselves from the common pitfalls to which novices are vulnerable. A rite of passage in all disciplines of medicine is learning about clinical pitfalls that have been identified by the discipline's experts. This [says] in effect, "Here is a typical error that will be made, and here is how to avoid it."[17]

Interestingly, in the case of the chest pain triage decision (a decision that early researchers hoped to perfect through a combination of electronic decision support and a better appreciation of diagnostic pitfalls), most experts have concluded that the quest for diagnostic certainty is futile. In a number of research studies, even the best algorithms could not reliably identify patients whose actual risk of MI was so low that it was safe to send them home—especially when the penalty for even occasional failure can be a tragic death and a multimillion-dollar lawsuit. So the real progress in chest pain triage has come not from honing our diagnostic abilities, but rather from developing new ways (usually involving repeated cardiac biomarker tests and a predischarge treadmill test) to "rule out MI" inexpensively over a reasonably short (6–12 hours) observational period.[26] In essence, we have abandoned our quest for diagnostic perfection and accepted instead the more mundane task of managing our uncertainty safely by resolving it quickly and inexpensively.

Yet the studies cited earlier offer some hope that clinicians' cognitive abilities can be improved—by teaching trainees about heuristics and providing opportunities for reflective practice, giving physicians feedback about diagnoses they got right and wrong, and encouraging participation in M&M and similar conferences in which diagnostic errors are dissected and reviewed. Trowbridge's 12 tips for teaching avoidance of diagnostic errors (Table 6-2) seem like a useful starting point for these educational efforts.[27]

In light of the emerging popularity of checklists in other parts of the safety field (Chapters 5 and 15), some authorities have even advocated the use of diagnostic checklists—both general checklists that prompt clinicians to collect complete data and engage in metacognition (Table 6-3) and specific ones that force consideration of "do not miss" diagnoses when faced with certain symptoms or signs such as chest pain or tachycardia.[28] The theory behind diagnostic checklists emerges out of cognitive psychology's "dual-process" model of thinking and reasoning (Figure 6-1), which states that clinicians engage in both Type 1 (fast, reflexive, intuitive, and largely subconscious) and Type 2 (analytic, slow, deliberate, and requiring focused attention) thinking.[29] Checklists might help prevent Type 1 errors by forcing physicians to slow down and overcome their innate diagnostic overconfidence.[13,14] While this is an elegant model and an appealing idea, the effectiveness of this approach and its acceptability to clinicians has not yet been tested.[30]

Table 6-2 TWELVE TIPS FOR TEACHING AVOIDANCE OF DIAGNOSTIC ERRORS

1. Explicitly describe heuristics and how they affect clinical reasoning
2. Promote the use of "diagnostic time outs"
3. Promote the practice of "worst-case scenario medicine"
4. Promote the use of a systematic approach to common problems
5. Ask why
6. Teach and emphasize the value of the clinical exam
7. Teach Bayesian theory as a way to direct the clinical evaluation and avoid premature closure
8. Acknowledge how the patient makes the clinician feel
9. Encourage learners to find clinical data that don't fit with a provisional diagnosis; ask "What can't we explain?"
10. Embrace zebras
11. Encourage learners to slow down
12. Admit one's own mistakes

Reproduced with permission from Trowbridge RL. Twelve tips for teaching avoidance of diagnostic errors. *Med Teach* 2008;30:496–500.

Table 6-3 PROPOSED GENERAL DIAGNOSTIC CHECKLIST

❑ Obtain your own complete medical history
❑ Perform a focused and purposeful physical exam
❑ Generate initial hypotheses and differentiate these with additional history, physical exam, and diagnostic tests
❑ Pause to reflect—take a diagnostic "time out"
  ○ Was I comprehensive?
  ○ Did I consider the inherent flaws of heuristic thinking?
  ○ Was my judgment affected by any other bias?
  ○ Do I need to make the diagnosis now, or can I wait?
  ○ What is the worst-case scenario?
❑ Embark on a plan, but acknowledge uncertainty and ensure a pathway for follow-up

Reproduced with permission from Ely JW, Graber ML, Croskerry P. Checklists to reduce diagnostic error. *Acad Med* 2011;86:307–313. © 2011 Association of American Medical Colleges. Published by Lippincott Williams & Wilkins, Inc.

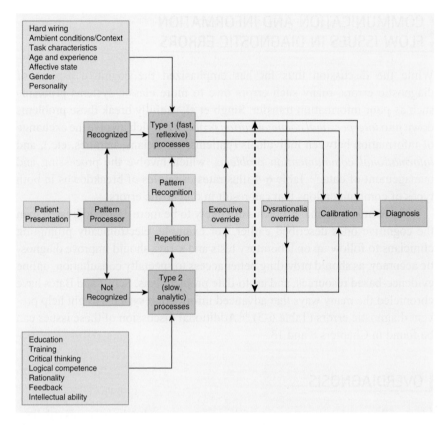

Figure 6-1 ■ A model for diagnostic reasoning based on dual-process theory. Type 1 thinking can be influenced by multiple factors, many of them subconscious (specific biases, emotional reaction toward or previous experiences with the patient or any of the diagnoses being considered), and is therefore represented as multiple channeled. On the other hand, Type 2 processes are single channeled and linear. Type 2 override of Type 1 ("executive override") occurs when physicians take a time out to reflect on their thinking, possibly with the help of checklists. In contrast, Type 1 thinking may irrationally override Type 2 ("dysrationalia override") when physicians insist on going their own way, such as when they ignore evidence-based clinical decision rules that can usually outperform them. "Calibration" represents the degree to which the perceived and actual diagnostic accuracy correspond. (Adapted with permission from Croskerry P. A universal model for diagnostic reasoning. *Acad Med* 2009;84:1022–1028. © 2011 Association of American Medical Colleges. Published by Lippincott Williams & Wilkins, Inc.)

COMMUNICATION AND INFORMATION FLOW ISSUES IN DIAGNOSTIC ERRORS

While the discussion thus far has emphasized the cognitive aspects of diagnostic errors, many such errors owe to more classic systems problems such as poor information transfer. Singh et al. usefully break these problems down into *interpersonal communication problems*, which involve the exchange of information between individuals (patients, physicians, families, etc.), and *informational communication problems*, which involve the processing and management of data.[31] Table 6-4 illustrates examples of breakdowns in both types of communications that can result in diagnostic errors.

These informational problems are likely to be more easily addressed than the cognitive ones described earlier. For example, electronically prompting clinicians to follow up on laboratory tests and x-rays should improve diagnostic accuracy, as should providing better access to specialty consultation, online evidence-based resources, and up-to-date problem lists. Schiff and Bates have chronicled the many ways that advanced information systems might help prevent diagnostic errors (Table 6-5).[32] Additional discussion of these issues can be found in Chapters 8 and 13.

OVERDIAGNOSIS

Most of the emphasis in the area of diagnostic errors has been in missed diagnoses or wrong diagnoses, but there is a problem with overdiagnosis as well—the detection of abnormalities that will never cause symptoms or death during a patient's lifetime if left alone. This problem may be accelerating because of the growing availability of highly sensitive diagnostic tests to identify small lesions (tumors mostly, but also partial vascular blockages, blood clots, and other lesions) whose clinical importance is unknown. "Because doctors don't know which patients are overdiagnosed," writes Gilbert Welch of Dartmouth, whose work has helped put this issue on the patient safety map, "we tend to treat them all."[33]

For example, we are diagnosing many more cases of prostate and breast cancer than in the past, due to the widespread use of highly sensitive PSA screening and mammography. While it is not certain that aggressive treatment of these early cancers is leading to improved overall outcomes, it is undoubtedly leading to some cases of harm.[34] Similarly, the incidence of pulmonary embolism is rising, probably due to the remarkable ability of computer tomographic pulmonary angiography to find small, and potentially clinically unimportant, emboli.[35]

Table 6-4	**TYPES AND EXAMPLES OF COMMUNICATION BREAKDOWNS THAT CAN LEAD TO DIAGNOSTIC ERRORS**

Examples of communication breakdowns that may result in data gathering–related errors

1. Interpersonal transmission errors: A patient does not inform her physician about a new growth in her breast
2. Interpersonal reception errors: The patient informs his or her physician about a change in his or her mole, but the physician gets distracted by an interruption and fails to perform a complete history and exam
3. Interpersonal acknowledgment errors: The physician informs the patient to return to the clinic after an urgent x-ray, but does not verify that the patient understood. Patient gets lost to follow-up leading to delayed diagnosis
4. Informational transmission errors: A patient calls the nurse two days after a physician visit with continued symptoms of fever and chills; information is recorded appropriately but is lost before it reaches the physician
5. Informational reception errors: Information about a patient's continued symptoms is placed in the physician's message inbox but not dated; physician misunderstands and believes that the note was from two days ago
6. Informational acknowledgment errors: A physician reads an e-mail from a nurse about a recent change in a patient's mole, but does not inform the nurse what to do next. The patient believes that the physician is not too concerned and does not seek care

Examples of communication breakdowns that may result in diagnosis verification–related diagnostic errors

7. Interpersonal transmission errors: A radiologist fails to inform the referring physician about free air noted on a patient's abdominal x-ray
8. Interpersonal reception errors: The laboratory calls the on-call physician on a weekend to inform him or her about the abnormal test results, but the covering physician informs the wrong primary physician. The patient's physician never receives the abnormal test result
9. Interpersonal acknowledgment errors: The laboratory calls the on-call physician at night about a critical test result, but the physician is only partially awake; no action is taken
10. Informational transmission errors: An abnormal radiology report of a potential malignancy is not sent to the primary care physician
11. Informational reception errors: An electronic notification of the abnormal radiology report is sent to the physician via the electronic medical record, but the physician either does not read the alert transmitting the test result or fails to take action on it
12. Informational acknowledgment errors: Physician does not electronically acknowledge the receipt of transmitted abnormal test results. No further action is taken and the results are lost to follow-up

Reproduced with permission from Singh H, Naik AD, Rao R, et al. Reducing diagnostic errors through effective communication: harnessing the power of information technology. *J Gen Intern Med* 2008;23:489–494.

There is another issue at play as well. Diagnoses that previously were largely unknown—restless leg syndrome, fibromyalgia, and low testosterone, for example—became commonplace after pharmaceutical companies with potentially effective treatments began to beseech patients to "ask your doctor" about them. Woloshin and Schwartz call this "disease mongering" and it is likely that it adds to the toll of overdiagnosis and overtreatment.[36]

Table 6-5	LEVERAGING ELECTRONIC CLINICAL DOCUMENTATION TECHNOLOGY TO DECREASE DIAGNOSTIC ERROR RATES
Role for Electronic Documentation	**Goals and Features of Redesigned Systems**
Providing access to information	Ensure ease, speed, and selectivity of information searches; aid cognition through aggregation, trending, contextual relevance, and minimizing of superfluous data
Recording and sharing assessments	Provide a space for recording thoughtful, succinct assessments, differential diagnoses, contingencies, and unanswered questions; facilitate sharing and review of assessments by both patient and other clinicians
Maintaining dynamic patient history	Carry forward information for recall, avoiding repetitive patient querying and recording while minimizing copying and pasting
Maintaining problem lists	Ensure that problem lists are integrated into workflow to allow for continuous updating
Tracking medications	Record medications patient is actually taking, patient responses to medications, and adverse effects to avert misdiagnoses and ensure timely recognition of medication problems
Tracking tests	Integrate management of diagnostic test results into note workflow to facilitate review, assessment, and responsive action as well as documentation of these steps
Ensuring coordination and continuity	Aggregate and integrate data from all care episodes and fragmented encounters to permit thoughtful synthesis
Enabling follow-up	Facilitate patient education about potential red flag symptoms; track follow-up
Providing feedback	Automatically provide feedback to clinicians upstream, facilitating learning from outcomes of diagnostic decisions
Providing prompts	Provide checklists to minimize reliance on memory and directed questioning to aid in diagnostic thoroughness and problem solving
Providing placeholder for resumption of work	Delineate clearly in the record where clinician should resume work after interruption, preventing lapses in data collection and thought process
Calculating Bayesian probabilities	Embed calculator into notes to reduce errors and minimize biases in subjective estimation of diagnostic probabilities
Providing access to information sources	Provide instant access to knowledge resources through context-specific "infobuttons" triggered by keywords in notes that link user to relevant textbooks and guidelines
Offering second opinion or consultation	Integrate immediate online or telephone access to consultants to answer questions related to referral triage, testing strategies, or definitive diagnostic assessments
Increasing efficiency	More thoughtful design, workflow integration, and distribution of documentation burden could speed up charting, freeing time for communication and cognition

Reproduced with permission from Schiff GD, Bates DW. Can electronic clinical documentation help prevent diagnostic errors? *N Engl J Med* 2010;362:1066–1069.

THE POLICY CONTEXT FOR DIAGNOSTIC ERRORS

Since diagnostic reasoning is so central to many physicians' own notion of professionalism, there is a lot of activity (keeping up with the literature, attending courses, tracking down follow-up on patients) that is, at its core, focused on improving diagnostic effectiveness. The fact that these activities are often undertaken voluntarily (although they are sometimes promoted by board certification[37] or continuing education requirements) is impressive.

But the kinds of pressures for quality and safety that are now marbled through the rest of the healthcare system (Chapter 3)—accreditation standards, public reporting, and pay for performance—largely bypass the issue of diagnostic errors. For example, none of the Agency for Healthcare Research and Quality's 25 Patient Safety Indicators (Appendix V), nor the 34 Safe Practices recommended by the National Quality Forum (Appendix VII), assess diagnostic accuracy.[38] Of course, this is linked to the reasons that diagnostic errors received so little attention in the first decade of the safety movement: these errors are difficult to measure and fix.[1]

The risk is that these pressures will cause healthcare delivery organizations, training programs, and caregivers themselves to de-emphasize diagnostic accuracy and the systems that can support it while prioritizing other, potentially less important, aspects of safety, quality, and value. In a policy environment in which hospitals, clinics, and physicians are compensated or lauded for giving the "right treatment" without regard to diagnostic accuracy, organizations and providers may do quite well by giving the "correct treatments" for the wrong diagnoses.

KEY POINTS

- Despite advances in laboratory testing, clinical imaging, and information technology, diagnostic errors remain commonplace. Nevertheless, because they are more difficult to measure and fix than other adverse events, they have been relatively neglected in the patient safety movement.
- Clinicians' diagnostic and therapeutic actions are influenced by both patient-related (e.g., age, gender, race) and clinician-related (e.g., fatigue, past experience, risk tolerance) factors.
- Good diagnosticians correctly apply iterative hypothesis testing and Bayesian reasoning, and avoid cognitive pitfalls and biases, such as anchoring (getting stuck on initial impressions) and the availability heuristic (being unduly influenced by prior cases).

- Improving diagnostic reasoning will involve both computerized decision support and training clinicians to be more effective diagnostic thinkers. Electronic tools that allow for accurate, timely flow of key information will also help.
- Although not traditionally emphasized in the patient safety field, overdiagnosis—prompted by both increasingly sensitive screening tests and corporate marketing—is an important safety problem as well.

REFERENCES

1. Wachter RM. Why diagnostic errors don't get any respect—and what can be done about them. *Health Aff (Millwood)* 2010;29:1605–1610.
2. Kohn L, Corrigan J, Donaldson M, eds. *To Err is Human: Building a Safer Health System*. Committee on Quality of Health Care in America, Institute of Medicine. Washington, DC: National Academy Press; 2000.
3. Leape LL, Brennan TA, Laird N, et al. The nature of adverse events in hospitalized patients. Results of the Harvard Medical Practice Study II. *N Engl J Med* 1991;324: 377–384.
4. Shojania KG. Changes in rates of autopsy-detected diagnostic errors over time: a systematic review. *JAMA* 2003;289:2849–2856.
5. Bishop TF, Ryan AK, Casalino LP. Paid malpractice claims for adverse events in inpatient and outpatient settings. *JAMA* 2011;305:2427–2431.
6. Croskerry P. The importance of cognitive errors in diagnosis and strategies to minimize them. *Acad Med* 2003;78:775–780.
7. Croskerry P, Abbass A, Wu AW. Emotional influences in patient safety. *J Patient Saf* 2010;6:199–205.
8. Lee TH, Rouan GW, Weisberg MC, et al. Clinical characteristics and natural history of patients with acute myocardial infarction sent home from the emergency room. *Am J Cardiol* 1987;60:219–224.
9. Schulman KA, Berlin JA, Harless W, et al. The effect of race and sex on physicians' recommendations for cardiac catheterization. *N Engl J Med* 1999;340:618–626.
10. Agency for Healthcare Research and Quality. *National Healthcare Disparities Report: Summary*. Rockville, MD: Agency for Healthcare Research and Quality; 2010. Available at: http://www.ahrq.gov/qual/nhdr10/nhdr10core.pdf.
11. Ting HH, Lee TH, Soukup JR, et al. Impact of physician experience on triage of emergency room patients with acute chest pain at three teaching hospitals. *Am J Med* 1991;91:401–408.
12. Pearson SD, Goldman L, Orav EJ, et al. Triage decisions for emergency department patients with chest pain: do physicians' risk attitudes make the difference? *J Gen Intern Med* 1995;10:557–564.

13. Friedman CP, Gatti GG, Franz TM, et al. Do physicians know when their diagnoses are correct? Implications for decision support and error reduction. *J Gen Intern Med* 2005;20:334–339.

14. Berner ES, Graber ML. Overconfidence as a cause of diagnostic error in medicine. *Am J Med* 2008;121(suppl 1):S2–S23.

15. Kassirer JP. Teaching clinical medicine by iterative hypothesis testing—let's preach what we practice. *N Engl J Med* 1983;309:921–923.

16. Wachter RM, Shojania KG. Diagnostic errors. In: *Internal Bleeding: The Truth behind America's Terrifying Epidemic of Medical Mistakes.* New York, NY: Rugged Land; 2004.

17. Croskerry P. Achieving quality in clinical decision making: cognitive strategies and detection of bias. *Acad Emerg Med* 2002;9:1184–1204.

18. Graber M. Crushing chest pain: a missed opportunity. *AHRQ WebM&M* (serial online); January 2004. Available at: http://webmm.ahrq.gov/case.aspx?caseID=45.

19. Weinstein MP. Contaminated or not? Guidelines for interpretation of positive blood cultures. *AHRQ WebM&M* (serial online); January 2008. Available at: http://webmm.ahrq.gov/case.aspx?caseID=168.

20. Gordon AJ. Dependence vs. pain. *AHRQ WebM&M* (serial online); July 2008. Available at: http://webmm.ahrq.gov/case.aspx?caseID=179.

21. Kaplan EL. Rapid mis-st(r)ep. *AHRQ WebM&M* (serial online); February 2007. Available at: http://webmm.ahrq.gov/case.aspx?caseID=145.

22. Redelmeier DA. Improving patient care. The cognitive psychology of missed diagnoses. *Ann Intern Med* 2005;142:115–120.

23. Mamede S, van Gog T, van den Berge K, et al. Effect of availability bias and reflective reasoning on diagnostic accuracy among internal medicine residents. *JAMA* 2010;304:1198–1203.

24. Mamede S, Schmidt HG, Rikers R. Diagnostic errors and reflective practice in medicine. *J Eval Clin Pract* 2007;13:138–145.

25. Eva KW, Link CL, Lutfey KE, et al. Swapping horses midstream: factors related to physicians' changing their minds about a diagnosis. *Acad Med* 2010;85: 1112–1117.

26. Goldman L, Kirtane AJ. Triage of patients with acute chest pain and possible cardiac ischemia: the elusive search for diagnostic perfection. *Ann Intern Med* 2003;139: 987–995.

27. Trowbridge RL. Twelve tips for teaching avoidance of diagnostic errors. *Med Teach* 2008;30:496–500.

28. Ely JW, Graber ML, Croskerry P. Checklists to reduce diagnostic error. *Acad Med* 2011;86:307–313.

29. Croskerry P. A universal model for diagnostic reasoning. *Acad Med* 2009;84: 1022–1028.

30. Winters BD, Aswani MS, Pronovost PJ. Commentary: reducing diagnostic errors: another role for checklists? *Acad Med* 2011;86:279–281.

31. Singh H, Naik AD, Rao R, et al. Reducing diagnostic errors through effective communication: harnessing the power of information technology. *J Gen Intern Med* 2008;23:489–494.

32. Schiff GD, Bates DW. Can electronic clinical documentation help prevent diagnostic errors? *N Engl J Med* 2010;362:1066–1069.

33. Welch HG. Overdiagnosis and mammography screening. *BMJ* 2009;339:b1425.

34. Welch HG, Schwartz LM, Woloshin S. *Overdiagnosed. Making People Sick in the Pursuit of Health*. Boston, MA: Beacon Press; 2011.

35. Wiener RS, Schwartz LM, Woloshin S. Time trends in pulmonary embolism in the United States: evidence of overdiagnosis. *Arch Intern Med* 2011;171:831–837.

36. Woloshin S, Schwartz LM. Giving legs to restless legs: a case study of how the media helps make people sick. *PLoS Med* 2006;3:e170.

37. Brennan TA, Horwitz RI, Duffy FD, et al. The role of physician specialty board certification status in the quality movement. *JAMA* 2004;292:1038–1043.

38. Newman-Toker DE, Pronovost PJ. Diagnostic errors—the next frontier for patient safety. *JAMA* 2009;301:1060–1062.

ADDITIONAL READINGS

Gandhi TK, Lee TH. Patient safety beyond the hospital. *N Engl J Med* 2010;363:1001–1003.

Gladwell M. *Blink: The Power of Thinking without Thinking*. New York, NY: Little, Brown and Company; 2005.

Graber M. Diagnostic errors in medicine: a case of neglect. *Jt Comm J Qual Saf* 2005;31:106–113.

Groopman J. *How Doctors Think*. Boston, MA: Houghton Mifflin; 2007.

Kahneman D. *Thinking Fast and Slow*. New York, NY: Farrar, Straus and Giroux; 2011.

Kahneman D, Lovallo D, Sibony O. Before you make that big decision.... *Harv Bus Rev* June 2011;89:50–60, 137.

Kahneman D, Slovic P, Tversky A. *Judgment under Uncertainty: Heuristics and Biases*. Cambridge, England: Cambridge University Press; 1987.

Kassirer JP, Kopelman RI. Cognitive errors in diagnosis: instantiation, classification, and consequences. *Am J Med* 1989;86:433–441.

Klein G. *Sources of Power: How People make Decisions*. Cambridge, MA: Massachusetts Institute of Technology; 1999.

Pauker SG, Wong JB. How (should) physicians think? A journey from behavioral economics to the bedside. *JAMA* 2010;304:1233–1235.

Weingart SN, Saadeh MG, Simchowitz B, et al. Process of care failures in breast cancer diagnosis. *J Gen Intern Med* 2009;24:702–709.

HUMAN FACTORS AND ERRORS AT THE PERSON– MACHINE INTERFACE

7

INTRODUCTION

Until now, we have discussed several paradigm shifts required to improve patient safety. The dominant one, of course, is replacing an environment based on "blame and shame" with one in which safety is viewed as a top priority and systems thinking is employed effectively. Second is an awareness of the impact of culture and relationships on communication and the exchange of information. This chapter will introduce another lens through which to view safety problems: how human factors engineering (HFE) can improve the safety of person–machine interactions and the environment in which healthcare providers work.

To prime ourselves for a discussion of HFE, let us consider the following scenarios:

- An obstetric nurse inadvertently connects an opiate pain medication intended for an epidural catheter into a mother's intravenous line, leading to the patient's death.[1] A subsequent review demonstrated that the bags and lines used for epidural and intravenous infusions were similar in size and shape, leaving nothing other than human vigilance to prevent a bag intended for epidural use from connecting to an IV catheter or hub.
- A hospitalized elderly man dies after a heart attack suffered while in a monitored bed in one of America's top hospitals. A later investigation reveals that the main crisis monitor had been turned off, and multiple lower level alarms—including ones that showed that the patient's heart rate was slowing dangerously for nearly half an hour before his heart stopped—weren't noticed by the busy nursing staff, who had become so inured to frequent false alarms that they suffered from "alarm fatigue."[2]

This chapter was coauthored by Bryan Haughom, MD.

- Modern multichannel infusion pumps are routinely used in the ICU to administer multiple medications and fluids through a single central line (Figure 7-1). This often results in a confusing tangle of tubes that cannot be easily differentiated. No surprise, then, that a busy ICU nurse might adjust the dose of the wrong medication.
- Medications are often stored in vials in doses that are highly concentrated. This means that they frequently need to be carefully diluted before being administered. For example, a vial of phenylephrine contains 10 mg/mL, while the usual IV dose administered to patients is 0.1 mg—one-hundredth of the dose in the vial! Inadvertent administration of full strength phenylephrine can cause a stroke.

Figure 7-1 ■ A modern sea of intravenous drips and lines. Is it any wonder that there are sometimes errors when incorrect medications or rates are administered to a desperately ill patient? (Courtesy of Michael Gropper, MD, PhD, with permission.)

■ An elderly patient dies when a Code Blue team—responding to the call for help after a cardiac arrest—is unable to connect the defibrillator pads to the defibrillator.[3] A subsequent analysis showed that over the years the hospital had accumulated more than a dozen defibrillator models on its floors, so providers were often unfamiliar with the models at hand and incompatibilities were common.[4]

In each of these examples, significant hazards resulted from people interacting with products, tools, procedures, and processes in the clinical environment. One could argue that these errors could have been prevented by more careful clinicians or more robust training. However, as we have already learned, to minimize the chances that fallible humans (in other words, all of us) will cause patient harm, it is critical to apply systems thinking. In the case of person–machine interfaces, this systems focus leads us to consider issues around device design, the environment, and the care processes that accompany device use. The field of HFE provides the tools to accomplish this.

HUMAN FACTORS ENGINEERING

Human factors engineering is an applied science of systems design that is concerned with the interplay between humans, machines, and their work environments.[5,6] Its goal is to assure that devices, systems, and working environments are designed to minimize the likelihood of error and optimize safety. As one of its central tenets, the field recognizes that humans are fallible and that they often overestimate their abilities and underestimate their limitations. Human factors engineers strive to understand the strengths and weaknesses of our physical and mental abilities and use that information to design safer devices, systems, and environments.

HFE is a hybrid field, mixing various engineering disciplines, design, and cognitive psychology. Its techniques have long been used in the highly complex and risky fields of aviation, electrical power generation, and petroleum refining, but its role in patient safety has only recently been appreciated.[7–9] In applying HFE to healthcare, there has been a particular emphasis on the design and use of devices such as intravenous pumps, catheters, computer software and hardware, and the like.

Many medical devices have poorly designed user interfaces that are confusing and clumsy to use.[10,11] According to the U.S. Food and Drug Administration (FDA), approximately half of all medical device recalls between 1985 and 1989 stemmed from poor design. FDA officials, along with other human factors experts, now recognize the importance of integrating human factors principles into the design of medical equipment.[11–13]

In Chapter 2, I introduced the concept of *forcing functions*, design features that prevent the user from taking an action without deliberately considering information relevant to that action. The classic example of a forcing function was the redesign of automobiles that prevented cars from being placed in reverse if the driver's foot was off the brake. In healthcare, forcing functions have been created to make it impossible to connect the wrong gas canisters to an anesthetized patient or prevent patients from overdosing themselves while receiving patient-controlled analgesia (PCA). Although forcing functions are the most straightforward application of HFE, it is important to appreciate other healthcare applications, ranging from improving device design to aiding in device procurement decisions to evaluating processes within the care environment.

For example, many hospitals are now approaching the challenge of increasing the frequency with which providers clean their hands partly as a human factors problem (Chapter 10).[14,15] While these institutions continue to work on education and observation, they also ensure that cleaning gel dispensers are easy to use and strategically located throughout the hospital wards. In fact, a whole field of patient safety–centered hospital and clinic design has emerged, and some buildings have been constructed using human factors principles.[16,17]

Despite these early success stories, HFE remains conspicuously underused as a patient safety tool, for reasons ranging from the lack of well-defined avenues to report and correct design or process flaws within hospitals to the natural tendency of highly trained caregivers to feel that they can outsmart or work around problems.[9] With the dramatic growth in the volume and complexity of man–machine clinical interactions, the probability that human workers will make mistakes has escalated, as has the importance of considering HFE approaches.

USABILITY TESTING AND HEURISTIC ANALYSIS

One of the key tools in HFE is *usability testing*, in which experts observe frontline workers engaging in their task under realistic conditions—either actual patient care or simulated environments that closely replicate reality. Users are observed, videotaped, and asked to "talk through" their thought processes, explaining their actions as well as their difficulties with a given application or device. Engineers then analyze the data in order to fine-tune their design for the users, the chosen tasks, and the work environment.[18]

Software engineers and design firms now see usability testing as an indispensable part of their work, preferring to make modifications at the design stage instead of waiting until errors have become apparent through real-world use. Similarly, many equipment manufacturers and a growing number of healthcare organizations now employ individuals with human factors expertise to advise them on equipment purchasing decisions, modify existing equipment to prevent errors, or identify error-prone equipment and environmental situations.[8,10,11] These trained individuals instinctively approach errors with a human factors mindset, asking questions about usability and possible human factors solutions before considering fixes involving retraining and incentives, interventions that may seem easier than device or environmental redesign but are generally far less effective.

Usability testing can be a complex process, requiring not only human factors experts but also extensive investigatory time and cooperation from users. A less resource-intensive alternative is known as *heuristic analysis*.[11] The term heuristics was first mentioned in Chapter 6 in reference to the cognitive shortcuts that clinicians often take during diagnostic reasoning, shortcuts that can lead to errors. In the context of HFE, though, heuristics have a different connotation: "rules of thumb" or governing principles for device or system design. In heuristic evaluations, the usability of a particular system or device is assessed by applying established design fundamentals such as visibility of system status, user control and freedom, consistency and standards, flexibility, and efficiency of use (Table 7-1).[18,19]

During a heuristic evaluation, experts navigate the user interface searching for usability issues. In essence, analysts try to put themselves in the shoes of the end user, looking for error-prone functions or designs that might ultimately compromise safety. The information gleaned from these analyses becomes feedback to the design teams, who iteratively update and refine the design of prototypes. The ultimate shortcoming of heuristics, however, is that they are only as good as the analyst performing the evaluation. Without putting end users in real-time situations and observing their work, it is difficult to fully unearth problematic design issues. Nevertheless, heuristic evaluations can provide valuable information to a design team, or even to a hospital looking to review devices or systems they already own or are looking to purchase.[8,11]

Inability to truly stand in for the novice is only one problem that designers and engineers have in anticipating all the safety hazards of complex systems. In my interview with him, Donald Norman, the author of the best-selling book, *The Design of Everyday Things*,[20] reflected on another real-world human factors issue:

[As an engineer], you focus too much, and don't appreciate that all the individual elements of your work, when combined together,

Table 7-1 **EXAMPLES OF HEURISTIC PRINCIPLES**	
Visibility of system status	Users should be aware of system status System should provide appropriate feedback as well as appropriate instructions to complete a task
User control and freedom	Users should feel "in control" of a system System should provide clear exits at every step of a task, supply undo as well as redo functions, and avoid irreversible actions
Match between system and world	Language utilized by the system should be that of the end user System should fit within the mental model of the end user
Consistency and standards	User interface and system functions should be consistent
Recognition rather than recall	Users' memory load should be minimized Systems should take advantage of user's inherent tendency to process information in "chunks" as opposed to by rote memory
Flexibility and efficiency of use	Interfaces should be designed to accommodate customizability
Error recovery and prevention	Systems should be designed to prevent errors before they occur If errors do occur, users should be able to recover from them via reversible actions The system should also provide clear steps detailing how to recover
Help and documentation	Help and documentation should be available to users The language used should be appropriate for the end user, avoid jargon

Reproduced with permission from Ginsburg G. Human factors engineering: a tool for medical device evaluation in hospital procurement decision-making. *J Biomed Inform* 2005;38:213–219; Zhang J, Johnson TR, Patel VL, et al. Using usability heuristics to evaluate patient safety of medical devices. *J Biomed Inform* 2003;36:23–30; Kushniruk AW, Patel VL. Cognitive and usability engineering methods for the evaluation of clinical information systems. *J Biomed Inform* 2004;37:56–76.

create a system—one that might be far more error-prone than you would have predicted from each of the individual components. For example, the anesthesiologist may review beforehand what is going to be needed. And so he or she picks up the different pieces of equipment that measure the different things, like the effects of the drugs on the patient. Each instrument actually may be designed quite well, and it may even have been rigorously tested. But each instrument works differently. Perhaps each has an alarm that goes off when something's wrong. Sounds good so far. But when you put it together as a system it's a disaster. Each alarm has a different setting, and the appropriate response to one may be incredibly dangerous for another. When things really go wrong, all the alarms are beeping and the resulting cacophony of sounds means nobody can get any work done. Instead of tending to the patient, you're spending all of your time turning off the alarms. So part of the problem is not seeing it as a system, that things have to work in context. And that these items actually should be talking to each other so that they can help the anesthesiologist prioritize the alarms.[21]

The difficulty of anticipating all these interactions and dependencies is yet another powerful argument for usability testing, not only of individual devices but also of multiple devices as they interact in actual systems.

In addition to their use in the design and purchase of medical devices such as ventilators, programmable IV pumps, defibrillators, and anesthesia equipment, human factors principles should also be utilized in the design and implementation of advanced information technology systems (Chapter 13). With the increasing computerization of healthcare, this interface—between HFE and information technology—is becoming ever more critical, and the growing list of unintended consequences of information technology systems is partly an indictment of our lack of focus on this area.[22,23]

The consequences go well beyond inefficiency and workarounds. One prominent pediatric teaching hospital reported an increase in mortality rates after a commercial computerized provider order entry (CPOE) system went live.[24] Although the findings are controversial and a subsequent study at another hospital (using the same CPOE system) found improved mortality,[25] the authors' description of the problems is a useful cautionary note regarding the hazards of poor design and implementation. For example, they observed:

Before CPOE implementation, physicians and nurses converged at the patient's bedside to stabilize the patient. After CPOE implementation, while one physician continued to direct medical management, a second physician was often needed solely to enter orders into the computer during the first 15 minutes to one hour if a patient arrived in extremis. Downstream from order entry, bedside nurses were no longer allowed to grab critical medications from a satellite medication dispenser located in the ICU because as part of CPOE implementation, all medications, including vasoactive agents and antibiotics, became centrally located within the pharmacy department. The priority to fill a medication order was assigned by the pharmacy department's algorithm. Furthermore, because pharmacy could not process medication orders until they had been activated, ICU nurses also spent significant amounts of time at a separate computer terminal and away from the bedside. When the pharmacist accessed the CPOE system to process an order, the physician and the nurse were "locked out," further delaying additional order entry.[24]

Human factors techniques can also be used to increase the safety of a working environment, such as by standardizing devices within a hospital to make training easier and increase reliability, carefully designing equipment and processes in a pharmacy to ensure that pharmacists always dispense the right drug in the correct dose, and optimizing a clinical work environment by providing adequate lighting, eliminating distractions (including excess noise), and ensuring that care providers receive adequate rest.

APPLYING HUMAN FACTORS ENGINEERING PRINCIPLES

In the end, usability testing and heuristic analysis can be used together or separately to design safe, effective, and intuitive devices for use in complex clinical care situations. Let's now return to the clinical scenarios outlined at the beginning of the chapter. How could HFE principles be applied to prevent these unsafe conditions? Here are some approaches human factors engineers might consider for each scenario:

- To prevent an epidural–intravenous mix-up, a forcing function could ensure that medications intended for epidural use are physically incapable of connecting to intravenous hubs.[26,27] An effective bar-coding system is another obvious solution. (Tragically—and ironically—the hospital where this error occurred *had* a bar-coding system, but its usability and reliability problems were well known and the nurses had learned to use workarounds, particularly in urgent situations.[1,28])
- Alarm fatigue can be mitigated by careful selection of equipment and by implementing policies and procedures developed after consultation with nurses and other caregivers and detailed observations of workflow.[2,29]
- By employing standardized color coding and other techniques, nurses using multichannel infusion pumps can more easily differentiate IV lines.[30]
- Pharmacies can be equipped with high-reliability robotic systems that produce bar-coded unit-dose medications that can be double checked using bar-coding devices at the bedside before they are administered to the patient. Multidose vials are inherently risky and should be avoided where possible.[31]
- The hospital where this error occurred standardized its defibrillators (buying more simple, "goof-proof" ones) and increased the frequency of testing.[3,4,32]

A dramatic case study in the application of HFE to another patient safety problem, adapted from the book *Set Phasers on Stun*,[33] is described in Box 7-1.

HM was a 4-year-old girl with a complex history, including birth defects and cardiac problems. She was no stranger to the hospital, to the telemetry unit, or to its nurses. Nurse K carefully attended to her fragile patient, ensuring that each of the six ECG leads were properly placed on HM's small body. As soon as they were all in place, Nurse K gently folded the bed sheet over HM's frail torso, and tucked her into bed. After properly connecting the ECG leads to the patient, the final step was to plug them into the heart monitor, which would allow the nurses to observe HM's heart rhythm at the nursing station down the hall.

After Nurse K lifted the guardrail on the side of the bed, she grabbed the ECG cord and scanned the head of the bed for the connection to the monitor. As was typical in this unit, there were several machines at the bedside—in this case, including an ECG machine and an IV infusion pump. The cord connected to the ECG leads in her hand had a characteristic six-pin connector at the end. It was designed such that it would fit perfectly with its counterpart. She grabbed the cord that was dangling down next to the heart monitor, lined up the two ends and pushed them together. It didn't even cross her mind that the cord she had just connected could potentially be from something other than the ECG machine. After all, she was a seasoned nurse who handled these machines every day, and they all seemed to have different connecting pins.

Unbeknownst to her she had connected the ECG leads to the IV infusion pump. The cord from the infusion pump matched the size and shape of the six-pin ECG cord reasonably well. The similarity might not have been so dangerous had the infusion pump not been a battery powered portable model. Nurse K had no way to know she had been holding a live electrical wire, with the full electrical current of the IV pump. Connecting the cords delivered a direct shock to the little girl's chest, from which she could not be revived.

Though it may be easy simply to claim that Nurse K should have paid closer attention to the situation, it would be an incomplete analysis. Even if she had been paying attention, would she have avoided this fateful error? We may never know. However, looking at this case through a human factors lens reveals a number of potential pitfalls to which Nurse K fell victim. The most glaring is the similarity between the ECG and IV pump cord. Despite the fact that they weren't perfect matches, they matched closely enough that one

(continued)

> **Box 7-1   A CASE STUDY OF A FATAL ERROR THAT MIGHT HAVE BEEN PREVENTED BY AN HFE APPROACH** (*continued*)
>
> could connect the two. The most powerful HFE solution might be designing the two connections to have unique colors or shapes—the ECG cord round and the IV pump cord square, for example. Perhaps the device industry might be willing to subscribe to a set of standards such that all ECG cords have the same color and shape (ditto for pump cords). Another solution might be to have a warning label on the infusion pump's cord, alerting that it can deliver a direct and potentially fatal current.
>
> Even beyond the design of the devices, what other problems may have led to this child's death? Could the conditions of the room—the setup, the lighting, the ambient noise, or the nurse's workload—have played a role in the outcome? Maybe Nurse K wasn't used to seeing these particular device models in the same room. Maybe the demands of her job and the busy environment of a hospital floor were taking their toll. We'll never know for sure. But it is certain that the thoughtful application of HFE principles to this situation would have made it a safer environment.
>
> ---
>
> Reproduced with permission from Casey S. *Set Phasers on Stun: And Other True Tales of Design, Technology, and Human Error*. 2nd ed. Santa Barbara, CA: Aegean Publishing; 1998.

KEY POINTS

- HFE is the applied science of systems design. It is concerned with the interplay of humans, machines, and their work environments.
- Thoughtful application of HFE principles can help prevent errors at the person–machine interface.
- Usability testing and heuristic analysis aim to identify error-prone devices or systems before they lead to harm.
- The initial focus of HFE in healthcare was on the design of medical devices. Today it is broader, with efforts to try to create safe environments of care (i.e., designing hospital rooms around safety principles) and to decrease errors associated with poorly designed clinical information systems.

REFERENCES

1. Smetzer J, Baker C, Byrne FD, et al. Shaping systems for better behavioral choices: lessons learned from a fatal medication error. *Jt Comm J Qual Patient Saf* 2010;36: 152–163, 1AP–2AP.

2. Kowalczyk L. Patient alarms often unheard, unheeded. *Boston Globe*. February 13–14, 2011. Available at: http://articles.boston.com/2011-02-13/news/29347393_1_alarms-monitors-nurses.

3. Abella BS, Edelson DP. Resuscitation errors: a shocking problem. *AHRQ WebM&M* (serial online); July/August 2007. Available at: http://www.webmm.ahrq.gov/case.aspx?caseID=155.

4. Fairbanks RJ, Caplan SH, Bishop PA, et al. Usability study of two common defibrillators reveals hazards. *Ann Emerg Med* 2007;50:424–432.

5. Weinger MB, Pantiskas C, Wiklund M, et al. Incorporating human factors into the design of medical devices. *JAMA* 1998;280:1484.

6. Schneider PJ. Applying human factors in improving medication-use safety. *Am J Health Syst Pharm* 2002;59:1115–1119.

7. Kohn LT, Corrigan JM, Donaldson MD. *To Err is Human—Building a Safer Health System*. Washington, DC: National Academy Press; 1999.

8. Ginsburg G. Human factors engineering: a tool for medical device evaluation in hospital procurement decision-making. *J Biomed Inform* 2005;38:213–219.

9. Wears RL, Perry SJ. Human factors and ergonomics in the emergency department. *Ann Emerg Med* 2002;40:206–212.

10. Lin L, Isla R, Doniz K, et al. Applying human factors to the design of medical equipment: patient-controlled analgesia. *J Clin Monitor Comput* 1998;14:253–263.

11. Zhang J, Johnson TR, Patel VL, et al. Using usability heuristics to evaluate patient safety of medical devices. *J Biomed Inform* 2003;36:23–30.

12. Food and Drug Administration. *Human Factors*. Available at: http://www.fda.gov/MedicalDevices/DeviceRegulationandGuidance/HumanFactors/default.htm.

13. Sawyer D, Aziz KJ, Backinger CL, et al. *Do it by Design: An Introduction to Human Factors in Medical Devices*. Washington, DC: US Department of Health and Human Services, Public Health Service, Food and Drug Administration, Center for Devices and Radiological Health; 1996.

14. Gawande A. *Better: A Surgeon's Notes on Performance*. New York, NY: Metropolitan Books; 2007.

15. Sax H, Allegranzi B, Uçkay I, et al. 'My five moments for hand hygiene': a user-centred design approach to understand, train, monitor and report hand hygiene. *J Hosp Infect* 2007;67:9–21.

16. Facilities Guidelines Institute, AIA Academy of Architecture for Health. *2006 Guidelines for Design and Construction of Health Care Facilities*. Washington, DC: The American Institute of Architects; 2006.

17. Birnbach DJ, Nevo I, Scheinman SR, et al. Patient safety begins with proper planning: a quantitative method to improve hospital design. *Qual Saf Health Care* 2010;19:462–465.

18. Kushniruk AW, Patel VL. Cognitive and usability engineering methods for the evaluation of clinical information systems. *J Biomed Inform* 2004;37:56–76.

19. Nielsen J. *Usability Engineering*. New York, NY: Academic Press; 1993.

20. Norman DA. *The Design of Everyday Things*. New York, NY: Basic Books; 2002.

21. Norman DA. In conversation with… Donald A. Norman. *AHRQ WebM&M* (serial online); November 2006. Available at: http://webmm.ahrq.gov/perspective.aspx?perspectiveID=33.

22. Ash JS, Sittig DF, Dykstra R, Campbell E, Guappone K. The unintended consequences of computerized provider order entry: findings from a mixed methods exploration. *Int J Med Inform* 2009;78(suppl 1):S69–S76.

23. Sittig DF, Singh H. Defining health information technology–related errors: new developments since 'to err is human'. *Arch Intern Med* 2011;171:1281–1284.

24. Han YY, Carcillo JA, Venkataraman ST, et al. Unexpected increased mortality after implementation of a commercially sold computerized physician order entry system. *Pediatrics* 2005;116:1506–1512.

25. Longhurst CA, Parast L, Sandborg CI, et al. Decrease in hospital-wide mortality rate after implementation of a commercially sold computerized physician order entry system. *Pediatrics* 2010;126:14–21.

26. Epidural-IV route mix-ups: reducing the risk of deadly errors. *ISMP Medication Safety Alert!* Acute care ed. July 3, 2008;13:1–3.

27. Simmons D, Symes L, Guenter P, Graves K. Tubing misconnections: normalization of deviance. *Nutr Clin Pract* 2011;26:286–293.

28. Koppel R, Wetterneck T, Telles JL, Karsh BT. Workarounds to barcode medication administration systems: their occurrences, causes, and threats to patient safety. *J Am Med Inform Assoc* 2008;15:408–423.

29. Gee T, Moorman BA. Reducing alarm hazards: selection and implementation of alarm notification systems. *Patient Saf Qual Healthc* March/April 2011;8:14–17.

30. Porat N, Bitan Y, Shefi D, et al. Use of colour-coded labels for intravenous high-risk medications and lines to improve patient safety. *Qual Saf Health Care* 2009;18:505–509.

31. Vanderveen T. Vial mistakes involving heparin. *AHRQ WebM&M* (serial online); May 2009. Available at: http://webmm.ahrq.gov/case.aspx?caseid=201.

32. Karsh BT, Scanlon M. When is a defibrillator not a defibrillator? When it's like a clock radio… The challenge of usability and patient safety in the real world. *Ann Emerg Med* 2007;50:433–435.

33. Casey SM. *Set Phasers on Stun: And Other True Tales of Design, Technology, and Human Error*. Santa Barbara, CA: Aegean Publishing Company; 1998.

ADDITIONAL READINGS

Cooper JB, Newbower RS, Long CD, et al. Preventable anesthesia mishaps: a study of human factors. *Anesthesiology* 1978;49:399–406.

France DJ, Throop P, Walczyk B, et al. Does patient-centered design guarantee patient safety? Using human factors engineering to find a balance between provider and patient needs. *J Patient Saf* 2005;1:145–153.

Gosbee J. Human factors engineering and patient safety. *Qual Saf Health Care* 2002;11:352–354.

Gosbee J. Human factors engineering can teach you how to be *surprised* again. *AHRQ WebM&M* (serial online); November 2006. Available at: http://webmm.ahrq.gov/perspective.aspx?perspectiveID=32.

Maughan BC, Lei L, Cydulka RK. ED handoffs: observed practices and communication errors. *Am J Emerg Med* 2011;29:502–511.

Spath PL, ed. *Error Reduction in Health Care: A Systems Approach to Improving Patient Safety*. 2nd ed. San Francisco, CA: Jossey-Bass; 2011.

Spear SJ, Schmidhofer M. Ambiguity and workarounds as contributors to medical error. *Ann Intern Med* 2005;142:627–630.

Tenner E. *Why Things Bite Back: Technology and the Revenge of Unintended Consequences*. New York, NY: A.A. Knopf; 1996.

Tonks A. Safer by design. *BMJ* 2008;336:186–188.

TRANSITION AND HANDOFF ERRORS | 8

An 83-year-old man with a history of chronic obstructive pulmonary disease (COPD), gastroesophageal reflux disease, and paroxysmal atrial fibrillation with sick sinus syndrome was admitted to the cardiology service of a teaching hospital for initiation of an antiarrhythmic medication and placement of a permanent pacemaker.

The patient underwent pacemaker placement via the left subclavian vein at 2:30 PM. A routine postoperative single-view radiograph was taken and showed no pneumothorax. The patient was sent to the recovery unit for overnight monitoring. At 5:00 PM, the patient stated he was short of breath and requested his COPD inhaler. He also complained of new left-sided back pain. The nurse found that his oxygenation had dropped from 95% to 88%. Supplemental oxygen was started and the nurse asked the covering physician to see the patient. The patient was on the nurse practitioner (NP)-run non-house staff service; however, the on-call intern provides coverage for patients after the NPs leave for the day.

The intern, who had never met the patient before, examined him and found him already feeling better and with improved oxygenation after receiving the supplemental oxygen. The nurse suggested a stat x-ray be done in light of the recent surgery. The intern concurred and the portable x-ray was completed within 30 minutes. About an hour later, the nurse wondered about the x-ray and asked the covering intern if he had seen it. The intern stated that he was signing out the x-ray to the night float resident, who was coming on duty at 8:00 PM.

Meanwhile, the patient continued to feel well except for mild back pain. The nurse gave him analgesics and continued to monitor his heart rate and respirations. At 10:00 PM, the nurse still hadn't heard anything about the x-ray, so she called the night float resident. The night float had been busy with an emergency but promised to look at the x-ray and advise the nurse if there was any problem. Finally at midnight, the evening nurse signed out to the night shift nurse, mentioning the patient's symptoms and noting that the night float intern had not called with any bad news.

The next morning, the radiologist read the x-ray performed at 6:00 PM and notified the NP that it showed a large left pneumothorax. A chest tube was placed at 2:30 PM, nearly a full day after the x-ray was performed. Luckily, the patient suffered no long-lasting harm from the delay.[1]

SOME BASIC CONCEPTS AND TERMS

In a perfect world, patients would stay in one place and be cared for by a single set of doctors and nurses. But, come to think of it, who would want such a world? Patients get sick, and then get better. Doctors and nurses work shifts, and then go home. Residents graduate from their programs and enter practice. So handoffs—the process of transferring primary authority and responsibility for clinical care from one departing caregiver to another incoming one[2]—and transitions are facts of medical life.

As we all learned when we played the game of "telephone" as kids, every handoff and transition comes with the potential for a "voltage drop" in information. (It also carries the possibility that a new set of eyes or circumstances will lead to a clinical benefit, but our purpose here is not to explore that optimistic scenario.) In fact, handoff and transitional errors are among the most common and consequential errors in healthcare. Despite this, these mistakes received little attention until recently, in part because, by their very nature, they tend to fall between the cracks of professional silos. As we have come to recognize the frequency and impact of handoff and transition errors, we are beginning to learn how to mitigate the harm that often accompanies them.

Healthcare is chock-full of two kinds of transitions and handoffs.[3] The first are *patient related*, as a patient moves from place to place within the healthcare system, either within the same building or from one location to another (Table 8-1). The second are *provider related*, which occur even when patients are stationary (Table 8-2).

Table 8-1   **EXAMPLES OF PATIENT-RELATED TRANSITIONS**
▪ Patient referred from primary care provider to subspecialty consultant
▪ Patient leaves the emergency department to go to the ICU
▪ Patient leaves the ICU to obtain a computed tomography (CT) scan
▪ Patient leaves the hospital to go to a skilled nursing facility

Table 8-2	EXAMPLES OF PROVIDER-RELATED TRANSITIONS (WHEN PATIENT IS STATIONARY)

- Daytime resident signs out to night float resident
- Oncologist's partner covers over a weekend
- Night shift nurse leaves; morning nurse takes over
- Recovery room nurse goes on break

Both kinds of handoffs are fraught with hazards. For example, one study found that 12% of patients experienced preventable adverse events after hospital discharge, most commonly medication errors (Chapter 4).[4] Part of the problem is that nearly half of all discharged patients have test results that are pending at discharge, and many of them (more than half in one study) fall through the cracks.[5] In another study, researchers found that being covered, principally at night, by a different physician was a far better predictor of hospital complications and errors than was the severity of the patient's illness.[6] The same researchers devised a standardized computerized sign-out form and the error rate fell by a factor of 3.[7]

Even if we grant that some transitions are necessary, one might reasonably ask whether healthcare needs to have quite so many of them. The answer is probably yes. Research has demonstrated that patients do worse when nurses work shifts longer than 12 hours, and that intensive care unit (ICU) residents make fewer errors when they work shifts averaging 16 hours instead of the traditional 30–36 hours (Chapter 16).[8,9] Unfortunately, in a 24/7 hospital, implementing these shift limits automatically generates handoffs (Figure 8-1), such as many of the ones in this case (Figure 8-2). Other handoffs emerge when patients receive appropriately specialized care.

Although some might wistfully long for the day when the family doctor saw the patient in the office, the emergency room, the hospital, and the

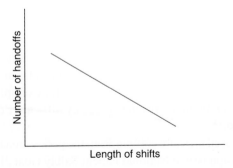

Figure 8-1 ■ The trade-off between shift length and handoffs.

Figure 8-2 ▪ Handoffs in the case that begins this chapter. (Reproduced with permission from Vidyarthi AR. Triple handoff. *AHRQ WebM&M* (serial online); September 2006. Available at: http://www.webmm.ahrq.gov/case.aspx?caseID=134.)

operating and delivery room, most patients now prefer the additional expertise, training, and availability of specialists in sites of care (i.e., emergency department, ICU, and, increasingly, the hospital[10]), procedures (delivering a baby), or diseases (heart attack or stroke). As these specialists become involved in a patient's care, they create transitions and the need for accurate information transfer. So too does a patient's clinical need to escalate the level of care (such as transitioning from hospital floor to step-down unit) or the economic realities that often drive de-escalation (hospital to skilled nursing facility).

The presence of all these handoffs and transitions makes it critical to consider how information is passed between providers and places. Catalyzed in part by the mandated reduction in resident work hours in the United States that began in 2003 (Chapter 16), there has been far more attention paid to handoffs in recent years. In my own hospital, for example, the number of handoffs by internal medicine residents rose by 40% after duty-hours limits were implemented.[11]

There is increased pressure coming from the policy arena as well. In 2006, the Joint Commission issued National Patient Safety Goal 2E (Appendix IV), which required healthcare organizations to "implement a standardized approach to handoff communications including an opportunity to ask and respond to questions." Spurred on by studies demonstrating staggeringly high 30-day readmission rates in Medicare patients (20% overall, nearly 30% in patients with heart failure),[12] in 2012 Medicare began penalizing hospitals with high readmission rates.[13] All of this attention has catalyzed research on handoffs and transitions, giving us a deeper understanding of best practices, which have both structural and interpersonal components.

This chapter will provide a general overview of best practices for person-to-person handoffs and patient transitions, and then focus on one particularly risky transition: hospital discharge. Additional information about handoffs and transitions can be found in the discussion of medication reconciliation (Chapter 4), information technology tools (Chapter 13), and resident duty hours (Chapter 16).

BEST PRACTICES FOR PERSON-TO-PERSON HANDOFFS

Like many other areas of patient safety, the search for best practices in handoffs has led us to examine how other industries and organizations move information around. This search has revealed several elements of effective handoffs: an information system, a predictable and standardized structure, and robust interpersonal communication. In one particularly memorable example, physicians at London's Great Ormond Street Children's Hospital studied Formula 1 motor racing, particularly the pit-stop crews (who switch out a car's tires, gas up the car, clean the vents, and send the car screeching back onto the track—all in seven seconds), for lessons in how to do effective handoffs.[14] The differences in the approaches of the pit-stop crews and the surgical teams were striking. Inspired, Great Ormond hired a human factors expert (Chapter 7) and reengineered the way its teams performed their postoperative handoffs (Table 8-3). The new model resulted in a significant decrease in handoff errors.[15,16]

The Joint Commission's expectations, expressed in its 2006 National Patient Safety Goal, include interactive communications, up-to-date and accurate information, limited interruptions, a process for verification, and an opportunity to review any relevant historical data. Vidyarthi and colleagues developed the mnemonic "ANTICipate" to help structure written sign-outs (Table 8-4). For example, in the case that began the chapter, listing "Tasks" in the form of "if, then" statements might have decreased the ambiguity. The written sign-out might have included: "Check the chest x-ray taken at 6 PM. If clear, call the nurse. If it shows a pneumothorax, call thoracic surgery for possible chest tube." Contingency plans could have taken the form of: "if the patient is short of breath, try an albuterol inhaler (history of COPD), but also consider pneumothorax (patient had recent line placement)."[1]

Safety Theme	Practice	Establishment of Handover Protocol
	Table 8-3 **LESSONS LEARNED FROM FORMULA 1 MOTOR RACING AND AVIATION INDUSTRIES FOR IMPROVING PATIENT HANDOVER FROM SURGERY TO INTENSIVE CARE**	
Leadership	**Formula 1**: the "lollipop" man coordinates the pit stop. **Aviation**: the captain has command and responsibility	**Old**: unclear who was in charge. **New**: anesthetist given overall responsibility for coordinating team, transferred to the intensivist at the end of the handover
Task sequence	**Formula 1 and aviation**: there is a clear rhythm and order to events	**Old**: inconsistent and nonsequential. **New**: three phases defined: (1) equipment and technology handover; (2) information handover; (3) discussion and plan
Task allocation	**Formula 1**: each team member has only one to two clearly defined tasks. **Aviation**: explicit acknowledged allocation of tasks for emergencies	**Old**: informal and erratic. **New**: people allocated tasks: ventilation—anesthetist; monitoring—operating room assistant; drains—nurses. The anesthetist identified and handed information over to the key receiving people
Predicting and planning	**Formula 1**: failure modes and effects analysis (FMEA) used to break down pit stops into individual tasks and risks. **Aviation**: pilots are trained to anticipate the expected, and to plan contingencies	**Old**: risks identified informally and often not acted upon. **New**: a modified FMEA was conducted and senior representatives commented on highest areas of risk. Safety checks were introduced, and the need for a ventilation transfer sheet was identified
Discipline and composure	**Formula 1**: very little verbal communication during a pit stop. **Aviation**: explicit communication strategies used to ensure a calm and organized atmosphere	**Old**: ad hoc and unstructured, with several simultaneous discussions in different areas of the ICU and theaters. **New**: communication limited to the essential during equipment handover. During information handover, the anesthetist and then the surgeon speak alone and uninterrupted, followed by discussion and agreement of the recovery plan
Checklists	**Formula 1 and aviation**: a well-established culture of using checklists	**Old**: none. **New**: a checklist was defined and used as the admission note by the receiving team
Involvement	**Aviation**: crew members of all levels are encouraged and trained to speak up	**Old**: communications primarily within levels (e.g., consultant to consultant or junior to junior). **New**: all team members and grades encouraged to speak up. Built into discussions in phase 3

(continued)

Table 8-3	LESSONS LEARNED FROM FORMULA 1 MOTOR RACING AND AVIATION INDUSTRIES FOR IMPROVING PATIENT HANDOVER FROM SURGERY TO INTENSIVE CARE (continued)	
Safety Theme	**Practice**	**Establishment of Handover Protocol**
Briefing	**Formula 1 and aviation**: well-established cultures of briefing even on race day, and before every flight	**Old and new** (process already in place): planning begins in a regular multidisciplinary meeting, reconfirmed the week before surgery, with further problems highlighted on the day
Situation awareness	**Formula 1**: the "lollipop man" has overall situation awareness at pit stops. **Aviation**: pilots are trained for situation awareness. In difficult circumstances the senior pilot manages the wider aspects of the flight while the other pilot controls the aircraft	**Old**: not previously identified as being important. **New**: the consultant anesthetist and intensivist have responsibility for situation awareness at handover, and regularly stand back to make safety checks
Training	**Formula 1**: a fanatical approach to training and repetition of the pit stop. **Aviation**: training and assessment are regularly conducted in high-fidelity simulators	**Old**: no training existed. **New**: a high turnover of staff requires an alternative approach. The protocol could be learned in 30 minutes. Formal training introduced; laminated training sheets detailing the process are provided at each bedside
Review meetings	**Formula 1**: regular team meetings to review events. **Aviation**: crew are encouraged to debrief after every flight	**Old and new** (already in place): a weekly well-attended clinical governance meeting, where problems/solutions openly discussed

Adapted with permission from Catchpole KR, de Leval MR, McEwan A, et al. Patient handover from surgery to intensive care: using Formula 1 pit-stop and aviation models to improve safety and quality. *Paediatr Anaesth* 2007;17:470–478.

While written sign-outs can take a variety of forms, there is an increasing recognition of the advantages of *computerized sign-out systems* over traditional index cards. At the University of California, San Francisco (UCSF) Medical Center, we developed a computerized sign-out module ("Synopsis"), which resides within the electronic medical record (Figure 8-3). The template standardizes the content of the sign-out and allows multiple providers to see the same data. It also imports certain information from the remainder of the electronic medical record (including administrative information, vital signs, laboratory studies, medication lists, and resuscitation ["code"] status), while allowing for free-text data entry. As one might expect, systems like this

Table 8-4	THE MNEMONIC "ANTICIPATE," HIGHLIGHTING THE ELEMENTS OF A SAFE AND EFFECTIVE HANDOFF
Administrative	Accurate information, such as name and location
New information	A clinical update, including brief history and diagnosis, updated medication and problem list, current baseline status, and recent procedures and significant events
Tasks	The "to do" list, best expressed in "if/then" statements
Illness	The primary provider's assessment of the patient's severity of illness
Contingency plans	Statements that assist in cross-coverage, including things that have and have not worked in the past

Reproduced with permission from Vidyarthi AR. Triple handoff. *AHRQ WebM&M* (serial online); September 2006. Available at: http://www.webmm.ahrq.gov/case.aspx?caseID=134.

Figure 8-3 ■ "Synopsis"—the UCSF Medical Center handoff module embedded in an electronic medical record. (Reproduced with permission.)

improve the quality of sign-outs and decrease the risk of communication-related errors.[7,17,18]

Computers are an essential part of the answer, but only part. Even in healthcare systems that enjoy advanced computerized records, person-to-person communication remains both necessary and potentially error prone (one study of internal medicine residents' sign-outs found omissions and mischaracterizations in nearly one in four information transfers[19]). In civil and military aviation, fields that, like healthcare, depend on the accurate transmittal of information, the so-called *phonetic alphabet* is often used during voice communications. In this system, a standardized word substitutes for a single letter (such as *Alpha* for "A," *Bravo* for "B," *Charlie* for "C," and so on), which permits one person to clarify a bit of information, such as the spelling of a name, without wasting time thinking of words that might have a common reference. Using this same system in a hospital, "Oscar Romeo" for operating room (OR) would never be confused with "Echo Romeo" for ER.

Read backs are also commonly used in aviation and other industries to prevent improperly received messages. For example, a pilot receiving flight plan clearance over the radio from Air Traffic Control always reads it back. In healthcare, we have long used read-back procedures to verify the identity of blood transfusion recipients, but, remarkably, no tradition of read backs for other transfers of risky information existed until the process was mandated by the Joint Commission in 2004 (Appendix IV). It is one measure of our inattention to patient safety that until very recently a physician would have been far more likely to hear the words, "Let me read your order back to you," when calling her local Chinese takeout restaurant than when she called the nurses' station of virtually any American hospital.[20] In one study of 822 telephone calls for critical laboratory test results, read backs caught 29 errors (3.5%), some of them quite serious.[21]

The bottom line is that having a standardized process for provider-to-provider sign-out is essential.[22,23] Sign-outs should take place in a standard place and at a standard time, and the incoming and outgoing personnel must overlap to the degree needed to transmit the relevant information. Ensuring that sign-outs occur in a quiet room, free of distractions, is critical, as is ensuring that both parties have access to the hospital's information system during the process.[24] (On the UCSF medical service, we insist that shift change handoffs occur face-to-face, while end of rotation handoffs, such as when one hospitalist is signing out to another after a 1- to 2-week stint, may take place by telephone, with both parties simultaneously reviewing the electronic health record, sometimes via remote access.)

Beyond these "must do's," there are many variation on the theme. Some units have instituted a *morning briefing* to support reliable communication at shift change.[25] In the ICU, the use of a daily *goal card*—a simple device to ensure that physicians, nurses, and patients focused on the same limited set of goals—led to improved communication and shorter ICU lengths of stay.[26] A dry erase *whiteboard* in patients' rooms can promote communication and teamwork among all of the involved providers.[27] While all of these interventions seem intuitively sensible and relatively straightforward to implement, by now it will not surprise you to learn that they are actually complex changes that should be viewed through a human factors lens (Chapter 7) to be sure they meet their purpose and don't create unintended consequences.[15]

SITE-TO-SITE HANDOFFS: THE ROLE OF THE SYSTEM

Joe Benjamin, a 43-year-old mechanic, came to his local ER with chest pain, and was admitted to the hospital to "rule out MI." Benjamin's ER physician ordered a chest radiograph in addition to the cardiac enzymes and serial electrocardiograms. Since nobody expected Benjamin's x-ray to show anything exciting, and since there was no checklist or protocol to remind anyone to check it, it was forgotten as soon as it was taken. Twelve hours later, after all of the heart attack tests proved negative, Benjamin was discharged. The discharging hospitalist, unaware of the chest x-ray, didn't think to check its results. Meanwhile, the radiologist had reviewed the x-ray and noticed a small lung nodule. He filled out a report for the hospital chart, and sent a version of it to the primary care physician's office, where it was lost.

Two years later, Joe Benjamin developed a chronic cough and a repeat chest x-ray revealed an obvious lung nodule. The radiologist's report read, "The nodule is markedly enlarged compared to the one seen on the x-ray of October 18, 1999." That was the first Benjamin's primary physician had heard of the prior x-ray, and it was too late. Eighteen months later, Joe Benjamin was dead of lung cancer.[20]

In its 2001 report, *Crossing the Quality Chasm: A New Health System for the 21st Century*, the Institute of Medicine compared the U.S. healthcare delivery system to a railroad whose tracks change gauge every few miles:

Health care is composed of a large set of interacting systems—paramedic, emergency, ambulatory, inpatient, and home health care; testing and imaging laboratories; pharmacies; and so forth—that are connected in loosely coupled but intricate networks of individuals, teams, procedures, regulations, communications, equipment, and devices. These systems function within such diverse and diffuse

Table 8-5 A PATIENT/FAMILY DISCHARGE CHECKLIST

You are about to be discharged from the hospital. Please be sure you and/or your family members know the answer to these questions BEFORE you leave:

Do you understand why you were hospitalized, what your diagnosis is, and what treatments you received?

Are there any test results you are still waiting for? Who should you contact for those results?

Has a provider reviewed your medications with you? Do you know which of your home medications to continue, what the current doses are, and which you should stop taking?

Where and when are your follow-up appointments?

What are the warning signs of relapse or medication side effects you should look for?

Who should you contact if you are having difficulties?

Does your primary care physician know you were here and that you are leaving?

Reproduced with permission from Forster A. Discharge fumbles. *AHRQ WebM&M* (serial online); December 2004. Available at: http://webmm.ahrq.gov/case.aspx?caseID=84.

management, accountability, and information structures that the over-all term health system is today a misnomer.[28]

One potential failure point in all of these interlocking systems is the piece of paper, the basic unit of medical record keeping for centuries. Moving paper across healthcare transitions is inherently risky, as it can easily get lost. More-over, several people, separated by place and function, often need to see patient data simultaneously, and each may create new data and observations that must be added to the record. Paper is clearly not the ideal medium for this.

Many of the handoff techniques discussed earlier can help here as well—including the use of read backs, standard communication proto-cols, and checklists (such as for hospital discharge) for patients/families (Table 8-5) and providers (Table 8-6). But part of the problem relates to the absence of integration in most of American medicine. Take, for example, hospital discharge—an inherently risky transition. In the United States, the hospital discharging the patient and the physician receiving the patient are usually not part of the same organization (in most cases, the physician is an independent or small group practitioner). Therefore, the physician's office information system, even if it is computerized, will rarely communi-cate effectively with the hospital's system, and vice versa. This is a formula for a voltage drop at a most critical time.

Integrated systems of care—in which the same organization owns or runs the doctor's office, the nursing home, and the hospital—have great advantages in this regard. Patients who leave a U.S. Veterans Affairs (VA) hospital for a

Table 8-7	KEY ISSUES IDENTIFIED BY A SYSTEMATIC REVIEW ON INTRAHOSPITAL TRANSFERS, ALONG WITH RECOMMENDED IMPROVEMENT STRATEGIES	
Setting	**Key Themes and Challenges**	**Improvement Strategies**
Transportation of critically ill patients	Failure to communicate arrival time and resources required results in delayed or inadequate care	Formalize pretransport coordination process
Discharge of patients from critical care to specialty ward	Ward nurses may lack expertise or confidence in handling critical care patients from the ICU	Introduce an ICU liaison nurse role to facilitate transfer, providing both coordination and clinical support
	Time constraints impede handoff communication during the discharge planning process	Formalize handoff to allow for uninterrupted time to conduct handoff
	Pretransfer communication is critical to ensure resource availability at the receiving ward	Early discharge planning
Transfer of surgical patients	Handoffs are informal and unstructured, leading to inadequate information transfer	Standardize handoff content and structure
	Surgical handoff is particularly poor	Involve all members of multidisciplinary team in handoff
	Work pattern at recovery room is unpredictable; thus, timing of handoff is variable, and handoff takes place amidst other activities	Formalize handoff to allow for uninterrupted time to conduct handoff
Transfers from ED	Content omission was common, in particular communication of the most recent set of vital signs	Standardize handoff content and structure
	Differing approaches to patient care between emergency department (ED) physicians and inpatient teams result in incomplete handoff and interprofessional misunderstandings	Align physicians' view for referrals handoff communication across medical specialties through education and hospital-wide guidelines
	High workload, time constraint, and overcrowding at ED impede handoff communication	Increase staffing level
	Difficulty in assessing information and communicating with providers across units on different shifts	Implement centralized information repository to ease access to patient information

Reproduced with permission from Ong MS, Coiera E. A systematic review of failures in handoff communication during intrahospital transfers. *Jt Comm J Qual Patient Saf* 2011;37:274–284.

One particularly risky transition occurs when a patient leaves his or her hospital floor for an x-ray or other test. Unlike the patient transferring to the ICU, where there is an established nursing intake protocol and the patient has been identified as high risk, many of these intrahospital transports are done haphazardly, with an abrupt decrease in the capabilities of the monitoring personnel and equipment and ambiguity regarding what actions to take in the event of deterioration.[36] One hospital uses a "Ticket to Ride" system, where the ticket—which includes patient identification, stability, and risk information—serves as the communication form between sending and receiving personnel. The transport personnel are responsible for ensuring the nurse completes the ticket, which stays with the patient until return to the home unit. Analysis of over 12,000 transports demonstrated improved transport documentation, higher patient satisfaction with transport, and fewer adverse events.[37] A well-designed checklist would probably serve the same function.

While the risks of intrahospital transfers are obvious, it is also worth emphasizing that there are major transition and handoff issues that occur in community practice. One study tracked the information exchange between outpatient providers who cared for a patient following a hospital discharge, and discovered that information from the previous visit was available only 22% of the time.[38] This problem is magnified by the sheer volume of information that an outpatient provider needs to manage. In one large practice, the average primary care physician was responsible for following up on 800 chemistry/hematology tests, 40 radiographs, and 12 pathology specimens *in a typical week*.[39] Add to all that the need for consultation, and things look even grimmer. In another study, two-thirds of primary care physicians (and one-third of the specialists) were dissatisfied with the referral process, which isn't a surprise since the majority of specialists reported that they usually received no information from the primary care doctor, and one in four primary care doctors had not heard back from specialists within a month of their referral.[40]

While the solutions here would seem to rest with better information technology, this is proving harder than it looks. In one study, the VA system created an electronic alert for abnormal imaging results—alerts went to both the receiving physician and the radiologist. Despite what appeared to be a foolproof system, flawed follow-up remained distressingly common.[41] Similarly, computerized order entry has been held out as the savior for many errors in transitions and medication reconciliation. Researchers examined 4000 computer-generated prescriptions and found a 12% error rate.[42] Clearly, our efforts to solve transitional problems with information technology will need to be accompanied by equal efforts to apply human factors thinking, be alert for unanticipated consequences, and remain attuned to the challenges of trying to change care patterns in complex systems (Chapter 2).

The issues surrounding one distinctive and risky handoff—the end-of-year transition that occurs when residents graduate and turn their practices over to new interns[43]—will be discussed in Chapter 16.

PREVENTING READMISSIONS: BEST PRACTICES FOR HOSPITAL DISCHARGE

As discussed earlier, we have seen an abundance of evidence that the hospital discharge transition is one we manage exceptionally poorly. This was highlighted by the seminal study by Jencks et al., which found that 20% of Medicare patients are readmitted within a month of discharge and one-third return within 90 days.[12] The authors estimated the cost of preventable readmissions at $17 billion.

Other studies have chronicled a litany of additional postdischarge disasters:

- Nearly 20% of patients experience adverse events within 3 weeks of discharge.[4]
- Forty percent of patients are discharged with tests pending, and many of these balls are dropped.[5]
- Fifteen percent of discharged patients have a discrepancy in their medication lists.[44]
- Astonishingly few discharge summaries reach the primary care physician by the time the patient returns for his or her first postdischarge visit.[45]

Despite powerful literature that shows that relatively simple interventions—such as *postdischarge phone calls* or the use of a *transitions coach*—can lead to striking improvements in postdischarge care and decreased readmission rates,[46,47] only a small fraction of hospitals have implemented them. Moreover, few hospitals outside of integrated delivery systems have become electronically linked to their referring physicians' offices.

Recent policy changes such as readmission penalties[13] and value-based purchasing (Table 3-5) have turned improving the discharge transition into an imperative for hospitals, primary care doctors, and their respective systems. Luckily, a number of best practices have been identified, with proven beneficial effects on readmission rates and other meaningful outcomes.

In considering these best practices, several themes have emerged. First, hospitals will need to improve their discharge processes so that they can reliably: (a) get a discharge summary in the hands of an outpatient doctor on the day of discharge; (b) ensure that patients receive robust and understandable discharge instructions (not simply a check box on a form) (Figure 8-4 shows a discharge checklist, drawn from the Society of Hospital Medicine's Project BOOST[48]); and (c) keep in touch with patients via a follow-up phone call (or

Universal patient discharge checklist		Initials
1. GAP assessment (see below) completed with issues addressed................................YES □ NO □		_____
2. Medications reconciled with pre-admission list..YES □ NO □		_____
3. Medication use/side effects reviewed using Teach-Back with patient/caregiver(s).......................YES □ NO □		_____
4. Teach-Back used to confirm patient/caregiver understanding of disease, prognosis and self-care requirements..YES □ NO □		_____
5. Action plan for management of symptoms/side effects/complications requiring medical attention established and shared with patient/caregiver using Teach-Back................................YES □ NO □		_____
6. Discharge plan (including educational materials; medication list with reason for use and highlighted new/changed/discontinued drugs, follow-up plans) taught and provided to patient/caregiver at discharge................................YES □ NO □		_____
7. Discharge communication provided to principal care provider(s)................................YES □ NO □		_____
8. Documented receipt of discharge information from principal care provider(s)................YES □ NO □		_____
9. Arrangements made for outpatient follow-up with principal care provider(s)................YES □ NO □		_____
For increased risk patients, consider................................Not applicable □		_____
1. Face-to-face multidisciplinary rounds pnor to discharge................................YES □ NO □		_____
2. Direct communication with principal care provider *before* discharge................................YES □ NO □		_____
3. Phone contact with patient/caregiver arranged within 72 hours post-discharge to assess condition, discharge plan comprehension and adherence, and to reinforce follow-up..................YES □ NO □		_____
4. Follow-up appointment with principal care provider within 7 days of discharge.............YES □ NO □		_____
5. Direct contact information for hospital personnel familiar with patient's course provided to patient/caregiver to address questions/concerns *if unable to reach principal care provider* prior to first follow-up................................YES □ NO □		_____

Confirmed by: _____ _____ __/__/__
Signature Print name Date

Figure 8-4 ▪ An example of a discharge checklist, from Project BOOST®. (Copyright © Mark Williams et al. Project Boost Mentoring Program, Society of Hospital Medicine, 2010, http://www.hospitalmedicine.org/ResourceRoom Redesign/RR_CareTransitions/PDFs. Reproduced with permission.)

e-mail or Tweet—whatever gets the job done!). Second, high-risk patients will require something more: a postdischarge clinic visit, perhaps, or a discharge or transitions coach or a high-risk case manager. This isn't rocket science—all these interventions make sense, have manageable costs, and are challenging but not impossible to implement. They simply take institutional will, strong teamwork, and an appreciation of the principles of quality improvement and change management.

Of all of the discharge transition programs, perhaps the most creative has been *Project RED* ("Re-Engineered Discharge"), developed by a team at Boston University.[47] The RED protocol involves giving patients intensive predischarge counseling, a customized discharge document (Figure 8-5), an early postdischarge phone call, and a rapid follow-up appointment. The intervention resulted in a 30% decrease in readmissions and modest cost savings.

One of the most expensive parts of the intervention was the discharge counseling: an RN spent nearly 90 minutes with each patient and family, at significant cost. To address this issue, the BU investigators developed an animated conversational character, nicknamed "Louise." Louise is preprogrammed with individual patient information, which she combines with answers to disease-

** Bring this Plan to ALL Appointments**

After Hospital Care Plan for:

John Doe

Discharge Date: October 20, 2006

Question or Problem about this Packet? Call your Discharge Advocate: (617) 444-1111

Serious health problem? Call Dr. Brian Jack: (617) 444-2222

© Copyright 2006 by Boston Medical Center Corporation

EACH DAY follow this schedule:

MEDICINES

What time of day do I take this medicine?	Why am I taking this medicine?	Medication name Amount	How much do I take?	How do I take this medicine?
Morning	Blood pressure	PROCARDIA XL NIFEDIPINE 90 mg	1 pill	By mouth
	Blood pressure	HYDROCHLOROTHIAZIDE 25 mg	1 pill	By mouth
	Blood pressure	CLONIDINE HCI 0.1 mg	3 pills	By mouth
	cholesterol	LIPITOR ATORVASTATIN CALCIUM 20 mg	1 pill	By mouth
	stomach	PROTONIX PANTOPRAZOLE SODIUM 40 mg	1 pill	By mouth

© Copyright 2006 by Boston Medical Center Corporation

Figure 8-5 ▪ An example of a customized patient discharge care plan, from Project RED. (Courtesy of Boston University, Department of Family Medicine. Reproduced with permission.)

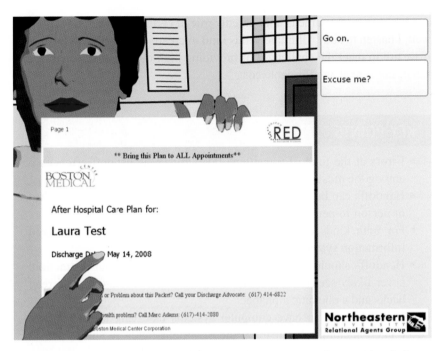

Figure 8-6 ▪ Louise, the "animated conversational character" who provides discharge instructions to patients. From Project RED. (Courtesy of Boston University, Department of Family Medicine. Reproduced with permission.)

specific and general questions. She—a pleasant-looking middle-aged woman of purposely ambiguous race and ethnicity—appears on a computer screen wheeled to the patient's bedside (Figure 8-6). Speaking to the patient in a relatively fluent but unmistakable computer voice (with synchronized animation), she might say: *The doctors tell me that your primary condition is atrial fibrillation… it usually causes a rapid heart beat. Do you have any questions about this condition?* Patients answer Louise's questions by picking choices off a touch-screen interface. She then responds according to her algorithm.

In a pilot study, Louise's performance was equivalent to that of the human discharge coach, while saving nearly $150 per encounter.[49] More interestingly, not only did most patients find Louise to be personable and responsive, but also three out of four preferred interacting with "her" to receiving discharge instructions from a live physician or nurse.

Let's be clear. While Louise can calmly walk a patient down an algorithmic path, answer simple questions, and test basic understanding, dealing with complex situations, managing ambiguity, and showing empathy are not her forte. Nevertheless, Louise's success indicates that certain functions that we call "nursing" can probably be accomplished by other people or technologies, at a lower cost (the same is undoubtedly true of certain doctoring functions as well, I hasten to add). Ultimately, this kind of creative thinking will be needed if we are to meet the challenges of providing high-quality, safe, reliable, and satisfying care at an affordable cost.

KEY POINTS

- Errors at the time of transitions (also known as handoff errors) are among the most common errors in healthcare.
- Handoffs can be site-to-site (e.g., hospital to skilled nursing faculty) or person-to-person (e.g., one physician signing out to another).
- For both kinds of handoffs, solutions will involve both improved information systems and standardized protocols.
- Handoffs should occur at designated times and without distraction, cover likely scenarios, include "if/then" statements, and utilize read backs and a phonetic alphabet.
- It will be vital to have computer systems that "talk to each other" ("interoperability"); creating these systems will require that we address legitimate concerns about patient privacy.
- Increasing pressure to improve transitions is coming from a variety of policies (public reporting and financial penalties for high rates of read-missions). Luckily, several comprehensive programs have resulted in markedly decreased readmission rates, and practices have been identified that appear to improve other transitions and handoffs as well.

REFERENCES

1. Vidyarthi AR. Triple handoff. *AHRQ WebM&M* (serial online); September 2006. Available at: http://www.webmm.ahrq.gov/case.aspx?caseID=134.
2. Patterson ES, Wears RL. Patient handoffs: standardized and reliable measurement tools remain elusive. *Jt Comm J Qual Patient Saf* 2010;36:52–61.
3. Cook RI, Render M, Woods DD. Gaps in the continuity of care and progress on patient safety. *BMJ* 2000;320:791–794.
4. Forster AJ, Murff HJ, Peterson JF, et al. The incidence and severity of adverse events affecting patients after discharge from the hospital. *Ann Intern Med* 2003;138: 161–167.
5. Roy CL, Poon EG, Karson AS, et al. Patient safety concerns arising from test results that return after hospital discharge. *Ann Intern Med* 2005;143:121–128.

6. Petersen LA, Brennan TA, O'Neil AC, et al. Does housestaff discontinuity of care increase the risk for preventable adverse events? *Ann Intern Med* 1994;121:866–872.

7. Petersen LA, Orav EJ, Teich JM, et al. Using a computerized sign-out program to improve continuity of inpatient care and prevent adverse events. *Jt Comm J Qual Improv* 1998;24:77–87.

8. Rogers AE, Hwang WT, Scott LD, et al. The working hours of hospital staff nurses and patient safety. *Health Aff (Millwood)* 2004;23:202–212.

9. Landrigan CP, Rothschild JM, Cronin JW, et al. Effect of reducing interns' work hours on serious medical errors in intensive care units. *N Engl J Med* 2004;351: 1838–1848.

10. Wachter RM, Goldman L. The emerging role of "hospitalists" in American health care. *N Engl J Med* 2006;335:514–517.

11. Vidyarthi AR, Arora V, Schnipper JL, et al. Managing discontinuity in academic medical centers: strategies for a safe and effective resident sign-out. *J Hosp Med* 2006;1:257–266.

12. Jencks SF, Williams MV, Coleman EA. Rehospitalizations among patients in the Medicare fee-for-service program. *N Engl J Med* 2009;360:1418–1428.

13. Epstein AM. Revisiting readmissions—changing the incentives for shared accountability. *N Engl J Med* 2009;360:1457–1459.

14. Naik G. A hospital races to learn lessons of Ferrari pit stop. *Wall Street Journal.* November 14, 2006:A1.

15. Catchpole KR, de Leval MR, McEwan A, et al. Patient handover from surgery to intensive care: using Formula 1 pit-stop and aviation models to improve safety and quality. *Paediatr Anaesth* 2007;17:470–478.

16. Catchpole K, Sellers R, Goldman A, et al. Patient handovers within the hospital: translating knowledge from motor racing to healthcare. *Qual Saf Health Care* 2010;19:318–322.

17. Anderson J, Shroff D, Curtis A, et al. The Veterans Affairs shift change physician-to-physician handoff project. *Jt Comm J Qual Patient Saf* 2010;36:62–71.

18. Van Eaton EG, Horvath KD, Lober WB, et al. A randomized, controlled trial evaluating the impact of a computerized rounding and sign-out system on continuity of care and resident work hours. *J Am Coll Surg* 2005;200:538–545.

19. Horwitz LI, Moin T, Krumholz HM, et al. What are covering doctors told about their patients? Analysis of sign-out among internal medicine house staff. *Qual Saf Health Care* 2009;18:248–255.

20. Wachter RM, Shojania KG. *Internal Bleeding: The Truth Behind America's Terrifying Epidemic of Medical Mistakes.* New York, NY: Rugged Land; 2004.

21. Barenfanger J, Sautter RL, Lang DL, et al. Improving patient safety by repeating (read-back) telephone reports of critical information. *Am J Clin Pathol* 2004;121:801–803.

22. Horwitz LI, Moin T, Krumholz HM, et al. Consequences of inadequate sign-out for patient care. *Arch Intern Med* 2008;168:1755–1760.

23. Arora VM, Manjarrez E, Dressler DD, et al. Hospitalist handoffs: a systematic review and task force recommendations. *J Hosp Med* 2009;4:433–440.

24. Australian Medical Association. *Safe Handover: Safe Patients.* Kingston, ACT, Australia: Australian Medical Association; 2006.

25. Thompson D, Holzmueller C, Hunt D, et al. A morning briefing: setting the stage for a clinically and operationally good day. *Jt Comm J Qual Patient Saf* 2005;31: 476–479.

26. Pronovost P, Berenholtz S, Dorman T, et al. Improving communication in the ICU using daily goals. *J Crit Care* 2003;18:71–75.

27. Sehgal NL, Green A, Vidyarthi AR, et al. Patient whiteboards as a communication tool in the hospital setting: a survey of practices and recommendations. *J Hosp Med* 2010;5:234–239.

28. Committee on Quality of Healthcare in America, Institute of Medicine. *Crossing the Quality Chasm: A New Health System for the 21st Century*. Washington, DC: National Academy Press; 2001.

29. Struijs JN, Baan CA. Integrating care through bundled payments—lessons from the Netherlands. *N Engl J Med* 2011;364:990–991.

30. McClellan M, McKethan AN, Lewis JL, et al. A national strategy to put accountable care into practice. *Health Aff (Millwood)* 2010;29:982–990.

31. Luft HS. Becoming accountable—opportunities and obstacles for ACOs. *N Engl J Med* 2010;363:1389–1391.

32. Blumenthal D, Tavenner M. The "meaningful use" regulation for electronic health records. *N Engl J Med* 2010;363:501–504.

33. Lo B, Dornbrand L, Dubler NN. HIPAA and patient care: the role for professional judgment. *JAMA* 2005;293:1766–1771.

34. Halamka J. Straight from the shoulder. *N Engl J Med* 2005;353:331–333.

35. Ong MS, Coiera E. A systematic review of failures in handoff communication during intrahospital transfers. *Jt Comm J Qual Patient Saf* 2011;37:274–284.

36. Schell H, Wachter RM. Moving pains. *AHRQ WebM&M* (serial online); July 2006. Available at: http://webmm.ahrq.gov/case.aspx?caseID=128.

37. Pesanka DA, Greenhouse PK, Rack LL, et al. Ticket to ride: reducing handoff risk during hospital patient transport. *J Nurs Care Qual* 2009;24:109–115.

38. van Walraven C, Taljaard M, Bell CM, et al. Information exchange among physicians caring for the same patient in the community. *CMAJ* 2008;179:1013–1018.

39. Poon EG, Wang SJ, Gandhi TK, et al. Design and implementation of a comprehensive outpatient Results Manager. *J Biomed Inform* 2003;36:80–91.

40. Gandhi TK, Sittig DF, Franklin M, et al. Communication breakdown in the outpatient referral process. *J Gen Intern Med* 2000;15:626–631.

41. Singh H, Thomas EJ, Mani S, et al. Timely follow-up of abnormal diagnostic imaging test results in an outpatient setting: are electronic medical records achieving their potential? *Arch Intern Med* 2009;169:1578–1586.

42. Nanji KC, Rothschild JM, Salzberg C, et al. Errors associated with outpatient computerized prescribing systems. *J Am Med Inform Assoc* 2011;18:767–773.

43. Young JQ, Wachter RM. Academic year-end transfers of outpatients from outgoing to incoming residents: an unaddressed patient safety issue. *JAMA* 2009;302: 1327–1329.

44. Coleman EA, Smith JD, Raha D, et al. Posthospital medication discrepancies: prevalence and contributing factors. *Arch Intern Med* 2005;165:1842–1847.

45. Kripalani S, LeFevre F, Phillips CO, et al. Deficits in communication and information transfer between hospital-based and primary care physicians: implications for patient safety and continuity of care. *JAMA* 2007;297:831–841.
46. Coleman EA, Parry C, Chalmers S, et al. The care transitions intervention: results of a randomized controlled trial. *Arch Intern Med* 2006;166:1822–1828.
47. Jack BW, Chetty VK, Anthony D, et al. A reengineered hospital discharge program to decrease rehospitalization: a randomized trial. *Ann Intern Med* 2009;150:178–187.
48. Society of Hospital Medicine. *BOOSTing Care Transitions Resource Room. Project BOOST (Better Outcomes for Older Adults Through Safe Transitions)*. Philadelphia, PA: Society of Hospital Medicine. Available at: http://www.hospitalmedicine.org/ResourceRoomRedesign/RR_CareTransitions/CT_Home.cfm.
49. Hendren R. Virtual discharge assistant cuts readmissions, costs. *HealthLeaders Media*. March 8, 2011. Available at: http://www.healthleadersmedia.com/page-1/NRS-263439/Virtual-Discharge-Assistant-Cuts-Readmissions-Costs.

ADDITIONAL READINGS

Arora V, Johnson J, Lovinger D, et al. Communication failures in patient sign-out and suggestions for improvement: a critical incident technique. *Qual Saf Health Care* 2005;14:401–407.

Care Transitions Program. Aurora, CO: The Division of Health Care Policy and Research, University of Colorado Health Sciences Center. Available at: http://www.caretransitions.org/.

Dalal AK, Poon EG, Karson AS, et al. Lessons learned from implementation of a computerized application for pending tests at hospital discharge. *J Hosp Med* 2011;6:16–21.

Gandhi TK. Fumbled hand-offs: one dropped ball after another. *Ann Intern Med* 2005;142:352–358.

Gandhi TK, Lee TH. Patient safety beyond the hospital. *N Engl J Med* 2010;363:1001–1003.

Hansen LO, Young RS, Hinami K, et al. Interventions to reduce 30-day rehospitalization: a systematic review. *Ann Intern Med* 2011;155:520–528.

Patterson ES, Roth EM, Woods DD, et al. Handoff strategies in settings with high consequences for failure: lessons for health care operations. *Int J Qual Health Care* 2004;16:125–132.

Project Red (Re-Engineered Discharge). Boston, MA: Boston University Medical Center. Available at: http://www.bu.edu/fammed/projectred/index.html.

Were MC, Li X, Kesterson J, et al. Adequacy of hospital discharge summaries in documenting tests with pending results and outpatient follow-up providers. *J Gen Intern Med* 2009;24:1002–1006.

TEAMWORK AND COMMUNICATION ERRORS 9

A "Code Blue" is called when a patient on a medical-surgical ward is discovered pulseless and not breathing. The code team rushes in and begins CPR. "Does anybody know this patient?" the team leader barks as the team continues its resuscitative efforts. A few moments later, a resident skids into the room, having pulled the patient's chart from the rack in the nurse's station. "This patient is a No Code!" he blurts, and all activity stops.

As the Code Blue team members collect their paraphernalia, the patient's young nurse wonders in silence. After all, she received sign-out on this patient only a couple of hours ago, and she was told that the patient was a "full code." She thinks briefly about questioning the physician, but reconsiders. One of the doctors must have changed the patient's code status to do not resuscitate (DNR) and forgotten to tell me, she decides. Happens all the time. So she keeps her concerns to herself.

Only later, after someone picks up the chart that the resident brought into the room, does it become clear that he had inadvertently pulled the wrong chart from the chart rack. The young nurse's suspicions were correct—the patient was a full code! A second Code Blue was called, but the patient could not be resuscitated.[1]

SOME BASIC CONCEPTS AND TERMS

All organizations need structure and hierarchies, lest there be chaos. Armies must have generals, large organizations must have CEOs, and children must have parents. This is not a bad thing, but taken to extremes, these hierarchies can become so rigid that frontline workers withhold critical information from leaders or reveal only the information they believe their leaders want to hear. This state can easily spiral out of control, leaving the leaders without the information they need to improve the system and the workers believing that the leaders are not listening, are not open to dissenting opinions, and are perhaps not even interested.

The psychological distance between a worker and a supervisor is sometimes called an *authority gradient,* and the overall steepness of this gradient is referred to as the *hierarchy* of an organization. Healthcare has traditionally been characterized by steep hierarchies and very large authority gradients, mostly between physicians and the rest of the staff. Errors like those in the wrong DNR case—in which a young nurse suspected that something was terribly wrong but did not feel comfortable raising her concerns in the face of a physician's forceful (but ultimately incorrect) proclamation—have alerted us to the safety consequences of this kind of a hierarchy.

THE ROLE OF TEAMWORK IN HEALTHCARE

Teamwork may have been less important in healthcare 50 years ago than it is today. The pace was slower, the technology less overwhelming, the medications less toxic (also less effective), and quality and safety appeared to be under the control of physicians; everyone else played a supporting role. But the last half century has brought a sea change in the provision of medical care, with massively increased complexity (think liver transplant or electrophysiology), huge numbers of new medications and procedures, and overwhelming evidence that the quality of teamwork often determines whether patients receive appropriate care promptly and safely. For example, the outcomes of trauma care, obstetrical care, care of the patient with an acute myocardial infarction or stroke, and care of the immunocompromised patient are likely to hinge more on the quality of teamwork than the brilliance of the supervising physician.

After recognizing the importance of teamwork to safety and quality, healthcare looked to the field of aviation for lessons. In the late 1970s and early 1980s, a cluster of deadly airplane crashes occurred in which a steep authority gradient appeared to be an important culprit. Probably the best known of these tragedies was the 1977 collision of two 747s on the runway at Tenerife in the Canary Islands.

On March 27, 1977, Captain Jacob Van Zanten, a copilot, and a flight engineer sat in the cockpit of their KLM 747 awaiting clearance to take off on a foggy morning in Tenerife. Van Zanten was revered among KLM employees: as director of safety for KLM's fleet, he was known as a superb pilot. In fact, with tragic irony, in each of the KLM's 300 seatback pockets that morning there was an article about him, including his picture. The crew of the KLM had spotted a Pan Am 747 on the tarmac earlier that morning, but it was taxiing toward a spur off the lone main runway and it was logical to believe that it was out of the way. The fog now hung thick, and there was no ground radar to signal to the cockpit crew whether the runway was clear—the crew relied on its own eyes, and those of the air traffic controllers.

A transmission came from the tower to the KLM cockpit radio, but it was garbled—although the crew did hear enough of it to tell that it had something to do with the Pan Am 747. Months later, a report from the Spanish Secretary of Civil Aviation described what happened next:

> On hearing this, the KLM flight engineer asked: "Is he not clear then?" The [KLM] captain didn't understand him and [the engineer] repeated, "Is he not clear, that Pan American?" The captain replied with an emphatic, "Yes" and, *perhaps, influenced by his great prestige, making it difficult to imagine an error of this magnitude on the part of such an expert pilot,* both the co-pilot and flight engineer made no further objections. [Italics added][2]

A few moments later, Van Zanten pulled the throttle and his KLM jumbo jet thundered down the runway. Emerging from the fog and now accelerating for takeoff, the pilot and his crew now witnessed a horrifying sight: the Pam Am plane was sitting squarely in front of them on the main runway. Although Van Zanten managed to get the nose of the KLM over the Pan Am, doing so required such a steep angle of ascent that his tail dragged along the ground, and then through the upper deck of the Pan Am's fuselage. Both planes exploded, causing the deaths of 583 people. Thirty-five years later, the Tenerife accident remains the worst air traffic collision of all time.

Tenerife and similar accidents taught aviation leaders the risks of a culture in which it was possible for individuals (such as the KLM flight engineer) to suspect that something was wrong yet not feel comfortable raising these concerns with the leader. Through many years of teamwork and communications training (called crew resource management [CRM], see Chapter 15), commercial airline crews have learned to speak up and raise concerns. Importantly, the programs have also taught pilots how to create an environment that makes it possible for those lower on the authority totem pole to raise issues. The result has been commercial aviation's remarkable safety record over the past 40 years (Figure 9-1), a record that many experts attribute largely to this "culture of safety"—particularly the dampening of the authority gradient.

How well do we do on this in healthcare? In a 2000 study, Sexton et al. asked members of operating room and aviation crews similar questions about culture, teamwork, and hierarchies.[3] While attending surgeons perceived that teamwork in their operating rooms was strong, the rest of the team members disagreed (see Figure 15-3), proving that one should ask the

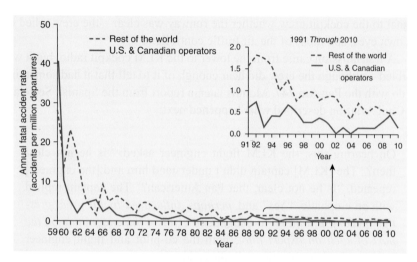

Figure 9-1 ▪ Commercial aviation's remarkable safety record. Graphs shows annual fatal accident rate in accidents per million departures, broken out for U.S. and Canadian operators (solid line) and the rest of the world's commercial jet fleet (hatched line). (Source: http://www.boeing.com/news/techissues/pdf/statsum.pdf, Slide 18. Used with permission from Boeing.)

followers, not the leader, about the quality of teamwork. Perhaps more germane to the patient safety question, while virtually all pilots would welcome being questioned by a coworker or subordinate, nearly 50% of surgeons would not (Figure 9-2). In a 2011 study, while these differences in perceptions among surgeons, anesthesiologists, and nurses had narrowed somewhat, they had not gone away.[4]

It is important to recognize that the attitudes now held by surgeons were common among pilots in the past, until pilots recognized that these attitudes (and the culture they represented) made crashes far more likely. As we consider strategies to improve teamwork and dampen down hierarchies in healthcare, it is also worth noting that pilots did not automatically jump for joy at the prospect of teamwork training when it was first introduced in the early 1980s (in fact, many pilots derisively referred to CRM training as "charm school"). Yet today it is difficult to find a pilot, or anyone else in commercial aviation, who questions the contribution of CRM training to airline safety. The adaptation of such training programs to medicine is further explored in Chapter 15, although it is worth foreshadowing now that studies have demonstrated that they improve both culture and outcomes in healthcare.[5-7]

While enthusiasm for teamwork training in healthcare is warranted, it is important to appreciate the complexity of this undertaking and the limitations

Figure 9-2 ▪ Percent of pilots and surgeons who would not welcome being questioned by a subordinate. (Reproduced with permission from Sexton JB, Thomas EJ, Helmreich RL. Error, stress, and teamwork in medicine and aviation: cross sectional surveys. *BMJ* 2000;320:745–749.)

of the aviation analogy. Changing the cockpit environment to prevent the next Tenerife involved improving teamwork between two or three individuals—captain, first officer, and perhaps flight engineer—who share similar training, expertise, social status, income, and confidence. In a busy operating room, it may be the high school–educated clerk or young nursing assistant who harbors a crucial concern that needs to be transmitted to the senior surgeon. Those interested in improving safety in healthcare need to recognize that transforming *this* culture is far more challenging than changing the culture of the cockpit.

FIXED VERSUS FLUID TEAMS

Some in healthcare point to our fluid teams—the fact that a surgeon is likely to work with a different set of nurses, technicians, and perfusionists every day—as an additional obstacle to better teamwork. Many do not realize that commercial aviation has precisely the same problem: when you fly a commercial airliner, the norm is that your pilot and copilot have never flown together previously. Because fluid teams are so common, it is critical to develop strategies and protocols that do not rely on individuals having worked together to ensure safety. In fact, some observers of both healthcare and aviation believe that fixed teams (in which the same groups of people work together repetitively) may be *more* dangerous, because they are more likely to get sloppy, make incorrect assumptions, regenerate fixed hierarchies, and suffer from "groupthink."[8]

That said, there are logistical challenges in trying to promote teamwork when team members don't work together with any regularity, and the desire to be surrounded by familiar faces at stressful times is understandable. Some surgeons feel so strongly about this issue that they insist on working with "their team" in the operating room. There are no data available to determine whether this makes a difference in safety, but it might.

On the medical ward, the concept of *geographic units* is increasingly popular—a unit in which the nurses and physicians are tied to a given locale. The hope is that this structure will lend itself to better team behaviors, both in the care of individual patients and in doing the hard work of improving systems of care. Recent studies have demonstrated that such units are associated with improved nurse–physician communication and, when combined with structured interdisciplinary rounds, fewer preventable adverse events.[9,10] The logistical and political complexity of guaranteeing fixed teams in the operating room and geographic units on the wards (particularly in hospitals that tend to run full) should not be underestimated.

TEAMWORK AND COMMUNICATION STRATEGIES

Data from the Joint Commission's sentinel event program have demonstrated that communication problems are the most common root cause of serious medical errors (Figure 9-3). Well-functioning teams employ a number of strategies (emphasized in CRM training programs, Chapter 15) to improve communication and teamwork. (In addition, many of the strategies to improve handoffs reviewed in Chapter 8 are relevant here as well.)

The first set of strategies focuses on ways to dampen authority gradients. These efforts can include very simple techniques, such as having the leader introduce himself or herself, learn the names of the other workers, admit his or her limitations, and explicitly welcome input from all the members of the team. These techniques can be incorporated into the surgical "time out" described in Chapter 5. But they shouldn't be limited to the presurgical or preprocedural pause: a medicine attending might employ them on the first day of a ward rotation, as might an obstetrician beginning a shift on the labor and delivery floor. For example, a surgeon might introduce himself (and have everyone else do the same) to all the members of his operating room crew, and then say, "You know, there will be times when I miss something, or when I'm going in the wrong direction in the middle of a complicated case. I really

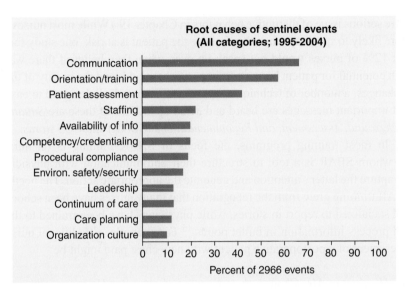

Figure 9-3 ▪ Frequency of communication problems among Joint Commission sentinel events. (Reproduced with permission from the Joint Commission. © The Joint Commission, 2011.)

depend on all of you to be my eyes and ears. If you see anything that you're not comfortable with—anything—including things that I'm doing, I really want you to bring them up. Together, we can be far safer than any of us can be individually." In his insightful book, *The Checklist Manifesto,* surgeon and patient safety expert Atul Gawande emphasizes the role of checklists in supporting such team behaviors—in contrast to the traditional view of checklists as tools to simply promote the completion of tasks (more on this in Chapter 15).[11]

There are also powerful opportunities to improve team performance after a procedure or a clinical encounter is over. Known in the military and aviation as a *debriefing,* all team members take a moment at the end of the procedure and explicitly, in a blame-free way, discuss what went wrong and right.[12] The lessons from these debriefings are often invaluable, and just as importantly, the sessions reinforce the value of team behaviors, the critical importance of speaking up, and the fact that everyone—even the leader—is fallible. Implementing standardized briefings and debriefings in the operating rooms of a regional medical center led to improved perceptions of teamwork and communication among the providers.[13]

It is one thing to tell nurses, clerks, or medical students to speak up, and another to give them the tools to do so productively. Many nurses recall having tried to raise concerns with physicians, only to be rebuffed. (I'll return to the more serious issue of disruptive behaviors in Chapter 19.) While most nurses are more likely to speak up when they believe the patient is at risk, one study found that 12% of nurses would not speak up even when they believed there was a high potential for patient harm.[14] To improve these odds and the quality of these exchanges, a number of techniques have been promoted, all designed to ensure that important messages are heard and acted upon. Two of these are *Situation, Background, Assessment, and Recommendations* (SBAR) and *CUS words.*

In most training programs, the focus of SBAR training is on nurses, for whom SBAR is a tool to structure their communication with physicians to capture the latter's attention and generate the appropriate action. The need for SBAR training grew from the recognition that many nurses have been schooled and socialized to report in stories, while physicians have been trained to think and process information in bullet points.[15] For example, a traditional nursing assessment of a postoperative patient with new chest pain might be:

> *Hi, doctor. Mr. Chow is having some chest pain. He was walking around the floor earlier, and he ate a good dinner. I don't really know what is going on, but I'm getting an electrocardiogram. He was a little sweaty when he had his pain, but I gave him the rest of his medicines, including his insulin and his antibiotic. He had surgery earlier today, and he's on a PCA pump right now.*

After SBAR training, the same nurse might call the physician and say:

> *This is Grace Jones. I'm a nurse on 7 North and I'm seeing your patient Edward Chow. He developed 8 out of 10 chest pain about 5 minutes ago, associated with shortness of breath, diaphoresis, and some palpitations (**Situation**). He is a 68-year-old man with no prior history of cardiac disease who had an uncomplicated abdominal-peritoneal resection yesterday (**Background**). I am obtaining an electrocardiogram, and my concern is that he might be having cardiac ischemia or a pulmonary embolism (**Assessment**). I'm giving him a nitroglycerin and would really appreciate it if you could be here in the next five minutes (**Recommendation**).*

Another technique to improve communication is the use of "CUS words." These involve escalating levels of concern, again usually on the part of a nurse, but they would be equally applicable to many other workers: medical students, respiratory therapists, pharmacists—anyone lower on a hierarchy who needs to get the attention of someone higher up. In escalating order, it begins with the use of the words, "I'm *concerned* about …," then "I'm *uncomfortable* …," and finally, "This is a *safety* issue!" It is important to teach those who might be receiving such messages (usually physicians) to appreciate their meaning and respond appropriately, and those who use CUS words to avoid overusing them to ensure that they have the intended impact.

Finally, strong teams depend on members—individually and collectively—responding appropriately to crises, particularly when the "fog of war" sets in. The concept of *situational awareness* refers to the degree to which one's perception of a situation matches reality.[16–18] Failure to maintain situational awareness during a crisis can result in various problems that compound the crisis. The classic examples come from certain airline crashes, where postcrash investigations revealed that the crew was focused, laser-like, on a trivial flashing light or gauge, as the plane ran out of fuel or crashed into a mountain.

We see similar problems in healthcare. For instance, during a resuscitation, an individual or entire team may focus on a particular task (such as a difficult central line insertion or administering a particular medication), while neglecting to address immediately life-threatening problems such as respiratory failure or a pulseless rhythm. In this context, maintaining situational awareness might be seen as equivalent to keeping the "big picture" in mind. Or, to cite one of the famous "Laws of the House of God" (the influential 1979 satire of the world of medical training), "at a cardiac arrest, the first procedure is to take your own pulse."[19]

KEY POINTS

- The provision of high-quality, safe healthcare is increasingly a team sport.
- Well-functioning teams are characterized by appropriate authority gradients and hierarchies that don't stifle the free flow of information.
- Healthcare has looked to the field of aviation for guidance regarding how best to dampen down hierarchies; the specific training model in aviation (which has been adapted to healthcare) is known as CRM.
- As long as effective teamwork and communication strategies are employed, the presence of fluid (rather than fixed) teams should not be a safety hazard.
- High functioning teams use strategies such as effective introductions and debriefings.
- Strategies to improve communications, particularly up the authority gradient, include the use of SBAR and CUS words.
- Strong teams manage to maintain "situational awareness" (focusing on the big picture) even during crises.

REFERENCES

1. Wachter RM, Shojania KG. *Internal Bleeding: The Truth Behind America's Terrifying Epidemic of Medical Mistakes.* New York, NY: Rugged Land; 2004.
2. Secretary of Aviation (Spain) Report on Tenerife Crash. Aircraft Accident Digest (ICAO Circular 153-AN/56); 1978:22–68.
3. Sexton JB, Thomas EJ, Helmreich RL. Error, stress, and teamwork in medicine and aviation: cross sectional surveys. *BMJ* 2000;320:745–749.
4. Wauben LS, Dekker-van Doorn CM, van Wijngaarden JD, et al. Discrepant perceptions of communication, teamwork and situation awareness among surgical team members. *Int J Qual Health Care* 2011;23:159–166.
5. Neily J, Mills PD, Young-Xu Y, et al. Association between implementation of a medical team training program and surgical mortality. *JAMA* 2010;304:1693–1700.
6. Wolf FA, Way LW, Stewart L. The efficacy of medical team training: improved team performance and decreased operating room delays: a detailed analysis of 4863 cases. *Ann Surg* 2010;252:477–485.
7. Morey JC, Simon R, Jay GD, et al. Error reduction and performance improvement in the emergency department through formal teamwork training: evaluation results of the MedTeams project. *Health Serv Res* 2002;37:1553–1581.
8. In conversation with … Jack Barker. *AHRQ WebM&M* (serial online); January 2006. Available at: http://webmm.ahrq.gov/perspective.aspx?perspectiveID=17.
9. Gordon MB, Melvin P, Graham D, et al. Unit-based care teams and the frequency and quality of physician–nurse communications. *Arch Pediatr Adolesc Med* 2011;165:424–428.
10. O'Leary KJ, Buck R, Fligiel HM, et al. Structured interdisciplinary rounds in a medical teaching unit: improving patient safety. *Arch Intern Med* 2011;171:678–684.
11. Gawande A. *The Checklist Manifesto: How to Get Things Right.* New York, NY: Metropolitan Books; 2009.
12. Makary MA, Holzmueller CG, Sexton JB, et al. Operating room debriefings. *Jt Comm J Qual Patient Saf* 2006;32:407–410, 357.
13. Berenholtz SM, Schumacher K, Hayanga AJ, et al. Implementing standardized operating room briefings and debriefings at a large regional medical center. *Jt Comm J Qual Patient Saf* 2009;35:391–397.
14. Lyndon A, Sexton JB, Simpson KR, et al. Predictors of likelihood of speaking up about safety concerns in labour and delivery. *BMJ Qual Saf* July 1, 2011 [Epub ahead of print].
15. Haig KM, Sutton S, Whittington J. SBAR: a shared mental model for improving communication between clinicians. *Jt Comm J Qual Patient Saf* 2006;32:167–175.
16. Weick KE. The collapse of sensemaking in organizations: the Mann Gulch disaster. *Adm Sci Q* 1993;38:628–652.
17. Weick KE, Sutcliffe KM. *Managing the Unexpected: Assuring High Performance in an Age of Complexity.* San Francisco, CA: Jossey-Bass; 2001.
18. Berwick DM. *Escape Fire: Lessons for the Future of Health Care.* New York, NY: The Commonwealth Fund; 2002.
19. Shem S. *The House of God.* New York, NY: Putnam; 1979.

ADDITIONAL READINGS

Connor M, Ponte PR, Conway J. Multidisciplinary approaches to reducing error and risk in a patient care setting. *Crit Care Nurs Clin North Am* 2002;14:359–367.

Donaldson L. *An Organisation with a Memory: Report of an Expert Group on Learning from Adverse Events in the NHS Chaired by the Chief Medical Officer.* London: The Stationery Office; 2000.

Helmreich RL. On error management: lessons from aviation. *BMJ* 2000;320:781–785.

Leape LL. Error in medicine. *JAMA* 1994;272:1851–1857.

Sachs BP. A 38-year-old woman with fetal loss and hysterectomy. *JAMA* 2005;294: 833–840.

Thomas EJ. Improving teamwork in healthcare: current approaches and the path forward. *BMJ Qual Saf* 2011;20:647–650.

Vincent C. *Patient Safety.* 2nd ed. London: Elsevier; 2010.

HEALTHCARE-ASSOCIATED INFECTIONS | 10

GENERAL CONCEPTS AND EPIDEMIOLOGY

Before the patient safety movement began, the prevention of hospital-acquired infections was seen as the job of the hospital epidemiologist and other infection control staff, who tried (often unsuccessfully) to engage clinicians in prevention efforts. Branding healthcare-associated infections (HAIs) as a patient safety problem (which by extension rendered failure to engage in appropriate infection control practices a form of medical error) has elevated the importance of these infections and propelled prevention into the mainstream.

Gratifyingly, evidence is accumulating that healthcare organizations can markedly decrease the frequency of HAIs. Some hospitals, having religiously implemented a variety of prevention strategies, are reporting intervals of months, even years, between previously commonplace infections such as ventilator-associated pneumonias (VAP), methicillin-resistant *Staphylococcus aureus* (MRSA), and central line–associated bloodstream infections (CLABSI) (Figure 10-1).

If we consider HAIs resulting from failure to adhere to evidence-based practices preventable adverse events (a position I endorse), then HAIs may well be the most common source of serious and preventable harm in healthcare. The Centers for Disease Control and Prevention (CDC) estimates that 1 in 10–20 hospitalized patients will develop an HAI, that HAIs are responsible for approximately 100,000 deaths per year in U.S. hospitals, and that these infections are responsible for $30 to 40 billion in attributable costs.[1,2] Beginning in 2008, Medicare began withholding payments to hospitals for the care of certain HAIs (CLABSI, healthcare-associated urinary tract infections, and *Clostridium difficile* infections) it considered largely preventable (Chapter 20 and Appendix VIII).[3]

For many HAIs (and other complications of healthcare, see Chapter 11), a variety of processes or structural changes appear to be correlated with improvement. In the past, infection control experts and regulators have underscored

Figure 10-1 ■ Marked decrease in catheter-related bloodstream infections after implementation of safety practices at Johns Hopkins Hospital. (Reproduced with permission from Berenholtz SM, Pronovost PJ, Lipsett PA, et al. Eliminating catheter-related bloodstream infections in the intensive care unit. *Crit Care Med* 2004;32:2014–2020.)

the need to increase adherence to individual prevention elements—for example, if there were five strategies thought to be effective in preventing a certain type of infection, a hospital might get "credit" for achieving 100% adherence on one of the five elements, 80% on another, and 50% on the other three. The Institute for Healthcare Improvement (IHI) has promoted a "*bundle*" approach, emphasizing that the chances of preventing complications seem to improve with complete adherence to a "bundle" of preventive strategies.[4] Under this model, institutions receive credit for their quality and safety efforts only for above-threshold adherence (i.e., >80%) on *all* of the preventive strategies, not just some. This approach rests on the theory that not only does better adherence to the individual elements increase the chances of prevention but also achieving high bundle adherence rates usually requires reengineering the entire clinical process of care. Changes born of this kind of reengineering may be more durable than those that result from short-term projects or cheerleading. This theory, though conceptually attractive and useful as a motivational tool, has not been empirically validated.

By this point in the book, you won't be surprised to learn that successfully eradicating HAIs is not as simple as creating and promoting the use of an evidence-based bundle of practices. In an insightful study, Saint et al. surveyed 86 people from a variety of disciplines (physicians, hospital executives, nurses, infection control preventionists, and others) to determine the barriers to successful implementation of evidence-based HAI prevention strategies.[5]

They identified two kinds of personnel—active resistors and "organizational constipators"—who impeded these efforts. To illustrate the resistor category, the authors quote one hospital chief of staff, who gave the following advice to those charged with getting surgeons to follow HAI guidelines:

> Surgeons are very tribal so if you, what you need to do, is you have something that you think is a best practice at your hospital... you need to get...either the chair of surgery or some reasonable surgeon...If you come in and you're an internist...into a group of surgeons...the first thing we're going to do is we're going to say, "Look, you're not one of us"...the way to get buy-in from surgeons is you got to have a surgeon on your team.

A quality manager who agreed to participate in a two-day quality collaborative was reprimanded by the chief nurse—who Saint et al. label as an organizational constipator—for her involvement:

> When [the chief nurse] found out I went to the first day, I was told I wasn't allowed to go to the second day...no one else could understand why...there was a control issue.

Table 10-1 chronicles some of the major themes from this study and best practices for overcoming both sources of resistance.

It is beyond the scope of this book to cover all aspects of HAIs in great detail; the interested reader is referred to other resources.[6–8] Instead, this chapter will highlight some of the patient safety principles involved in preventing the most common HAIs, ending with a discussion of what the patient safety movement can learn from the more established field of infection prevention. Table 10-2 summarizes some of the key evidence-based practices for the prevention of surgical site infections, VAP, CLABSI, and catheter-associated urinary tract infection.[6,9] (Note that hand hygiene is an essential practice for the prevention of *all* HAIs.)

SURGICAL SITE INFECTIONS

Surgical site infections are among the most common adverse events in hospitalized patients,[10] and they cause substantial increases in mortality, readmission rates, and costs. Approximately 1 in 30 "clean" surgeries will be complicated by a surgical site infection. The rate is significantly higher for "dirty" (i.e., after trauma), emergency, or prolonged surgeries, and for patients with medical comorbidities.

Table 10-1   **MAJOR UNIFYING AND RECURRENT THEMES SURROUNDING THE ROLES OF HOSPITAL PERSONNEL IN THWARTING HEALTHCARE-ASSOCIATED INFECTION PREVENTION EFFORTS, WITH IDEAS FOR OVERCOMING THESE BARRIERS**

1. ***Active resistance*** to a change in practice is pervasive, whether by attending physicians, resident physicians, or nurses. Successful efforts to overcome active resistance included the following:
   (a) Data feedback comparing local infection rates to national rates
   (b) Data feedback comparing rates of compliance with the practices to rates of others in the same area
   (c) Effective championing by an engaged and respected change agent who can speak the language of the staff he or she is guiding (e.g., a surgeon to motivate other surgeons)
   (d) Participation in collaborative efforts that generally align hospital leadership and clinicians in the goal of reducing healthcare-associated infection
2. ***Organizational constipators***: mid- to high-level executives who act as insidious barriers to change—they present added challenges to change in practice. Once leadership recognizes the problem and the negative effect on other staff, various techniques were used to overcome this barrier:
   (a) Include the organizational constipator early in group discussions in order to improve communication and obtain buy-in
   (b) Work around the individual, realizing that this is likely a shorter-term solution
   (c) Terminate the constipator's employment
   (d) Take advantage of turnover opportunities when the constipator leaves the organization by hiring a person who has a very high likelihood of being effective

Reproduced with permission from Saint S, Kowalski CP, Banaszak-Holl J, et al. How active resisters and organizational constipators affect health care–acquired infection prevention efforts. *Jt Comm J Qual Patient Saf* 2009;35:239–246.

Guidelines produced as recently as 2008[6,9] recommend the following strategies to prevent surgical site infections: appropriate use of prophylactic antibiotics (giving guideline-endorsed antibiotics within an hour of the incision, and stopping it/them within 24 hours after surgery), use of clippers (rather than razors) for hair removal prior to surgery, maintenance of postoperative normothermia,[11] and maintenance of relatively tight glucose control in the postoperative period.

That final recommendation was driven largely by a prominent 2001 study, which led to great enthusiasm for perioperative intensive insulin therapy.[12] Unfortunately, subsequent studies found no evidence of benefit and striking

Table 10-2 **SPECIFIC MEASURES FOR PREVENTION OF FOUR MAJOR HEALTHCARE-ASSOCIATED INFECTIONS**

Healthcare-Associated Infection	Preventive Measure	Definition or Comment
All healthcare-associated infections	Hand hygiene	Cleaning hands before and after each patient contact
Surgical site infection	Appropriate use of perioperative antibiotics	Administration of appropriate prophylactic antibiotic, generally begun within 1 hour of skin incision and discontinued within 24 hours
	Avoidance of shaving the operative site	Use clippers or other methods for hair removal in the area of incision(s)
	Perioperative normothermia	*Recommended by some guidelines but controversial*
	Glucose control	*Previous recommendation for tight glucose control has been relaxed after trials showed harm; aim for less than 180 mg/dL*
Ventilator-associated pneumonia	Semirecumbent positioning	Elevation of the head of the bed to more than 30° for all mechanically ventilated patients
	Daily assessment of readiness for weaning	Minimize duration of mechanical ventilation by limiting sedative administration and/or using protocolized weaning
	Regular antiseptic oral care	At least every shift
	Draining subglottic secretions/ silver-coated endotracheal tube	*Recommended by some guidelines but controversial*
Central line–associated bloodstream infection	Maximum barrier precautions	Use aseptic technique, including cap, mask, sterile gown, sterile gloves, and a large sterile sheet for the insertion of all central venous catheters
	Chlorhexidine skin antisepsis	Use 2% chlorhexidine gluconate solution for skin sterilization at the insertion site
	Appropriate insertion site selection	Subclavian vein is preferred site for nontunneled catheters; avoid femoral site for nonemergency insertions
	Prompt removal of unnecessary catheters	Remove when no longer essential for care
Catheter-associated urinary tract infection	Aseptic insertion and catheter care	Use of skin antisepsis at insertion and proper technique for maintenance of catheter and drainage bag; use of closed drainage system
	Prompt removal of unnecessary catheters	Remove catheter when no longer essential for care
	Silver- or antimicrobial-coated catheters	*Recommended by some guidelines but controversial*

Drawn from References 6, 9, and 31. Controversial or no longer recommended items in italics.

evidence of harm, mostly in the form of frequent hypoglycemic episodes.[13,14] As of 2012, therefore, tight glucose control to prevent surgical site infections (or for any perioperative indication) was no longer recommended. Most authorities now recommend keeping glucose levels at less than 180 mg/dL, but not to aim for tight control.[15]

VENTILATOR-ASSOCIATED PNEUMONIA

Of all HAIs, VAP is the leading cause of death, with far more fatal cases of VAP than of nosocomial urinary tract infections, CLABSI, or surgical site infections.[16] About 15% of patients receiving mechanical ventilation, particularly for long periods, will develop VAP, which in turn results in prolonged mechanical ventilation and longer hospital stays. Ventilated patients who develop VAP have a significantly higher mortality rate (46%) than those who don't (32%).

Many cases of VAP can be prevented by strict adherence to a variety of preventive strategies. The first is elevation of the head of the bed to semirecumbent (at least 30°) position, which in one trial resulted in an 18% decrease in VAP cases.[17] Head-of-bed (HOB) elevation decreases the risk of microaspiration of gastrointestinal tract and upper respiratory tract secretions into the lungs, which can serve as a nidus for infection. Although this intervention might seem like a relatively simple undertaking, experience has demonstrated that it can be a challenge, usually because of changes in patient position.[18] Several tactics have been recommended to increase adherence with HOB elevation, including enlisting the support of respiratory therapists and family members and placing a visual cue (such as a line on the wall) to help identify whether the bed is in the correct position. Some modern ICU beds come with a built-in tool to provide continuous monitoring of the angle of incline.[6]

A second effective strategy is daily interruption of sedation for ventilated patients.[19] Under one popular protocol, patients' sedative infusions are stopped each day, allowing patients to "lighten" to the point that they can answer simple questions. This strategy, when coupled with a program of systematic assessment (usually by trained respiratory therapists) regarding readiness for weaning, results in shorter duration of mechanical ventilation, presumably lowering the risk of VAP.[20]

Several other strategies have been included in various "VAP bundles." Regular antiseptic oral care has been proven to reduce the incidence of VAP.[21] Several systematic reviews have found that continuous drainage of subglottic secretions can lower VAP rates, but the procedure is technically difficult and relatively few institutions utilize it.[22,23] Finally, recent evidence has supported the use of silver-coated endotracheal tubes to prevent biofilm generation and ultimately VAP, although the cost-effectiveness of this strategy is still being debated and it is not standard practice as of this writing.[24]

VAP, like the other HAIs, has been considered for inclusion in a variety of public reporting and payment policies. One challenge, though, is that there are several VAP definitions, which means that the determination of whether an individual patient has VAP may be subject to interpretation. This, of course, opens the door to the possibility that hospitals that use conservative definitions or vigorously monitor their patients for infections may unfairly appear to be unsafe.[25,26]

The broader topic of hospital-acquired pneumonia will not be covered here. Interested readers are referred to recent reviews.[27,28]

CENTRAL LINE–ASSOCIATED BLOODSTREAM INFECTIONS

As catheter access to the central circulation has become ubiquitous in healthcare (to provide long-term antibiotics, nutrition, and vasoactive medications, as well as to permit central blood sampling), so too have infectious complications of these lines. The vast majority of CLABSI cases are associated with central venous catheters (CVCs).[29] Patients in ICUs, nearly half of whom have CVCs, are particularly vulnerable; it has been estimated that more than 20,000 people die each year from CLABSI in the United States alone.[30] The recommended bundle to prevent central line infections includes six practices (Table 10-2).[31]

The prevention of CLABSI has been one of the great success stories of the patient safety movement. Analyzing the history of this success is instructive, as it is built on a series of small-scale, and then increasingly ambitious, interventions—interventions that blended tools and recommended practices with change and measurement strategies.

First, of course, came the science: identifying a series of evidence-based practices that each reduced the incidence of CLABSI, and had an even more powerful effect when bundled together. Next, Berenholtz et al. demonstrated that high rates of adherence to these practices (Table 10-2) led to a near-zero rate of CLABSI in the ICUs at Johns Hopkins Hospital (Figure 10-1).[31] This was followed by the Keystone Project, in which widespread implementation of this bundle of practices in more than 100 ICUs in Michigan resulted in a breathtaking 66% reduction in CLABSIs over 18 months, a result that was subsequently sustained over 18 additional months.[32,33]

While the results in Michigan have famously been attributed to the use of a checklist that prompted the providers to adhere to the recommended practices,[34] the Hopkins-based investigators and colleagues have taken pains to highlight the importance of co-interventions aimed at improving teamwork

Figure 10-2 ■ The conceptual model for the Michigan study. (Reproduced with permission from Dixon-Woods M, Bosk CL, Aveling EL, et al. Explaining Michigan: developing an ex post theory of a quality improvement program. *Milbank Q* 2011;89: 167–205.)

and culture (Chapter 15).[35,36] A recent analysis of the Michigan experience led by the British sociologist Mary Dixon-Woods is a masterful guide to understanding the pathophysiology of change in complex organizations.[36] Dixon-Woods and her coworkers proposed a conceptual model (Figure 10-2) and six macrolevel key success factors to "explain Michigan" (Table 10-3). Anyone interested in promoting large-scale change in complex systems of care would do well to read this analysis.

Moving from the macro/sociopolitical to the bedside, the Michigan investigators did a number of things right here as well. Institutions that have made major gains in hand hygiene often empower nurses (and patients or families; Chapter 21) to question those entering patient rooms about whether they've cleaned their hands, and the Michigan team encouraged this kind of culture change.[37] The use of maximal sterile barrier precautions prior to line insertion, which has been strongly associated with lower infection rates,[38] was facilitated by the availability of a dedicated cart containing all the necessary equipment (a human factors intervention; Chapter 7). Importantly, although removal of central lines at the earliest possible date is a key preventive strategy (and should be encouraged by a daily team discussion of the risks and benefits of continued central access), routine line replacement (either by a

Table 10-3	**PROPOSED MECHANISMS BY WHICH THE MICHIGAN KEYSTONE PROJECT ACHIEVED ITS SUCCESSES**

1. It generated isomorphic pressures (the desire to conform to a group norm) for ICUs to join the program and conform to its requirements
2. It created a densely networked community with strong horizontal links that exerted normative pressure on its members
3. It reframed catheter-associated bloodstream infections as a social problem and addressed it through a professional movement that combined "grassroots" features and a vertically integrating program structure
4. It used several interventions that functioned in different ways to shape a culture of commitment to doing better in practice
5. It harnessed data on infection rates as a disciplinary force
6. It used "hard edges" (i.e., the leaders were not afraid to be tough at times, using "activist tactics" and threatening sanctions against laggards) when they were needed

From Dixon-Woods M, Bosk CL, Aveling EL, et al. Explaining Michigan: developing an ex post theory of a quality improvement program. *Milbank Q* 2011;89:167–205.

new line at a fresh site or by a line placed over a guidewire at the same site) does not result in fewer catheter-related infections, and was not part of the intervention.[39]

The Keystone Project is an important model for successfully implementing patient safety practices on a broad scale, accompanied by rigorous measures of effectiveness. One of the key questions for the safety field going forward is whether the factors that led to Michigan's success can be replicated in other venues, under different circumstances, and for other safety targets. I offer my own assessment of this provocative issue in Table 10-4.

CATHETER-ASSOCIATED URINARY TRACT INFECTIONS

Urinary tract infections are the most common HAIs, accounting for about 40% of HAIs in the United States. The vast majority are associated with indwelling urinary catheters, and risk factors include the duration of catheterization, patient age, and history of malignancy.[40] Although more common than VAP and CLABSI, urinary tract infections are less often fatal, and thus have received less attention in the patient safety and infection control literatures. But they have received more notice of late, particularly after they were included on Medicare's "no pay" list in 2008 (Appendix VIII) and, in 2012, became the subject of a Joint Commission National Patient Safety Goal (Appendix IV).

responsibility for infection control. Fourteen percent of patients were found to be colonized or infected at the time of admission. (Importantly, there were no recommendations to try to decolonize patients who tested positive, with either topical mupirocin or chlorhexidine baths; there is no good evidence that either strategy improves outcomes.[53,54]) Over two years, the VA's ICU MRSA infection rate fell by 62% (from 1.64 infections per 1000 patient-days to 0.62), and the non-ICU rate fell by 45% (0.47 per 1000 patient-days to 0.26).

Before we get too excited about having identified the magic bullet—or bundle—it is worth noting, with frustration, that another large MRSA prevention trial, reported in the same issue of the *New England Journal of Medicine,* found no impact on infection rates,[55] despite employing a similar array of activities. For now, the optimal approach to surveillance remains up in the air, pending additional research.[56] Many institutions favor a strategy of selective active surveillance, focusing on high-risk patients such as those admitted to the ICU or receiving chronic hemodialysis.

C. DIFFICILE INFECTION

C. difficile is the most common cause of infectious diarrhea in hospitalized patients, and both its incidence and severity have increased in recent years.[57] It is associated with substantial morbidity and mortality; a 2010 study found that 1 in 100 hospitalized patients is diagnosed with the infection, and patients with *C. difficile* had a threefold increased risk of death during the hospitalization.[58] Patients over age 65 are at particularly high risk.

The mainstays of prevention are strict contact precautions, hand hygiene (most authorities recommend the use of traditional hand washing with soap and water, rather than alcohol hand gels, which do not kill the organism), cleaning and disinfecting rooms and equipment, and *antibiotic stewardship.* The latter is vital since the main risk factor for *C. difficile* is prior antibiotic use, and decreasing unnecessary use will not only prevent this infection but also decrease antibiotic resistance. The mainstays of antibiotic stewardship are: avoid prolonged use of empiric antibiotics, narrow the spectrum of antibiotics whenever possible, and discontinue antibiotics promptly when appropriate.[59] Boston's Brigham and Women's Hospital combined an educational campaign, a prevention bundle (including newly designed "Contact Precautions Plus" signs for the doors of patients with *C. difficile,* Figure 10-3), and a treatment bundle (which guides the use of metronidazole or oral vancomycin, as well as the need for abdominal imaging and consultation), and saw a 40% decrease in the incidence of *C. difficile.*[60]

Figure 10-3 ▪ The Contact Precautions Plus sign, developed by Brigham and Women's Hospital, to be displayed outside the room of patients with *C. difficile* infection. (Reproduced with permission from Abbett SK, Yokoe DS, Lipsitz SR, et al. Proposed checklist of hospital interventions to decrease the incidence of healthcare-associated *Clostridium difficile* infection. *Infect Control Hosp Epidemiol* 2009;30:1062–1069.)

WHAT CAN PATIENT SAFETY LEARN FROM THE APPROACH TO HOSPITAL-ASSOCIATED INFECTIONS?

As a relatively new field, patient safety has looked outside of healthcare—to fields such as commercial aviation, clinical psychology, informatics, and engineering—for many of its lessons and guiding principles (Chapter 1). However, the patient safety movement can also learn from the much older fields of infection control and hospital epidemiology. Former CDC director Julie Gerberding made this important point in 2002, in the early years of the patient safety movement:

> Precise and valid definitions of infection-related adverse events, standardized methods for detecting and reporting events, confidentiality protections, appropriate rate adjustments for institutional and case-mix differences, and evidence-based intervention programs come to mind. Perhaps most important, reliance on skilled professionals to promote ongoing improvements in care has contributed to the 30-year track record of success in infection prevention and control.

Analogously, in approaching patient safety, standard definitions should be used as much as possible when discussing adverse events and preventability. Health care organizations should be encouraged to pool data on adverse events in a central repository to permit benchmarking, and such data should be appropriately adjusted and reported. Finally, institutions should consider hiring dedicated, trained patient safety officers (comparable to infection control practitioners) ....[61]

KEY POINTS

- Since the start of the patient safety movement, infection control activities have been considered a subset of patient safety, implying that many HAIs are best seen as preventable adverse events caused by medical errors (failure to adhere to evidence-based prevention strategies).
- Many surgical site infections can be prevented by appropriate use of prophylactic antibiotics, clipping rather than shaving the surgical site, and reasonable postoperative glucose control. However, enthusiasm for tight glucose control waned after the publication of studies demonstrating high rates of hypoglycemia.
- Many cases of VAP can be prevented by elevating the head of the bed and by strategies designed to minimize the duration of mechanical ventilation (particularly daily interruption of sedation).
- Many cases of CLABSI and healthcare-associated urinary tract infections can be prevented by rigorous hand hygiene, strict infection control procedures at the time of insertion, and removal of the foreign bodies at the earliest possible time. The Keystone Project, which demonstrated major reductions in CLABSI rates in 100 Michigan ICUs, is one of the striking successes of the young field of patient safety.
- Recently, MRSA and *C. difficile* infection have been added to the list of HAIs considered largely preventable, and thus fair game for the kinds of policy pressures that we've seen with the other HAIs.
- The new field of patient safety can learn much from the older fields of hospital epidemiology and infection control, particularly the use of standardized definitions, the importance of data collection and analysis, and the key role of professionals to monitor safety problems and implement safe practices.

REFERENCES

1. Centers for Disease Control and Prevention. *Estimates of Healthcare-Associated Infections*; May 30, 2007. Atlanta, GA: Centers for Disease Control and Prevention. Available at: http://www.cdc.gov/HAI/burden.html.

2. Scott RD. The direct medical costs of healthcare-associated infections in U.S. hospitals and the benefits of prevention. Atlanta, GA: Centers for Disease Control and Prevention; March 2009. Available at: http://www.cdc.gov/ncidod/dhqp/pdf/Scott_CostPaper.pdf.

3. Wachter RM, Foster NE, Dudley RA. Medicare's decision to withhold payment for hospital errors: the devil is in the details. *Jt Comm J Qual Patient Saf* 2008;34:116–123.

4. Nolan T, Berwick DM. All-or-none measurement raises the bar on performance. *JAMA* 2006;295:1168–1170.

5. Saint S, Kowalski CP, Banaszak-Holl J, et al. How active resisters and organizational constipators affect health care–acquired infection prevention efforts. *Jt Comm J Qual Patient Saf* 2009;35:239–246.

6. Yokoe DS, Mermel LA, Anderson DJ, et al. A compendium of strategies to prevent healthcare-associated infections in acute care hospitals. *Infect Control Hosp Epidemiol* 2008;29:901–994.

7. Lautenbach E, Woeltje KF, Malani PN. *Practical Healthcare Epidemiology.* 3rd ed. Chicago: University of Chicago Press; 2010.

8. Jarvis WR. *Bennett & Brachman's Hospital Infections.* 5th ed. Philadelphia: Lippincott Williams & Wilkins; 2007.

9. Ranji SR, Shetty K, Posley KA. *Closing the Quality Gap: A Critical Analysis of Quality Improvement Strategies (Vol. 6: Prevention of Healthcare–Associated Infections).* Technical Review 9. Rockville, MD: Agency for Healthcare Research and Quality; 2007. AHRQ Publication No. 04-0051-6.

10. Brennan TA, Leape LL, Laird NM, et al. Incidence of adverse events and negligence in hospitalized patients. Results of the Harvard Medical Practice Study I. *N Engl J Med* 1991;324:370–376.

11. Melling AC, Ali B, Scott EM, et al. Effects of preoperative warming on the incidence of wound infection after clean surgery: a randomised controlled trial. *Lancet* 2001;358:876–880.

12. Van den Berghe G, Wouters P, Weekers F, et al. Intensive insulin therapy in the critically ill patients. *N Engl J Med* 2001;345:1359–1367.

13. NICE-SUGAR Study Investigators, Finfer S, Chittock DR, Su SY, et al. Intensive versus conventional glucose control in critically ill patients. *N Engl J Med* 2009;360:1283–1297.

14. Kansagara D, Fu R, Freeman M. Intensive insulin therapy in hospitalized patients: a systematic review. *Ann Intern Med* 2011;154:268–282.

15. Wesley AJ, Solomkin JS, Edwards MJ. Updated recommendations for control of surgical site infections. *Ann Surg* 2011;253:1082–1093.

16. Ibrahim EH, Tracy L, Hill C, et al. The occurrence of ventilator-associated pneumonia in a community hospital: risk factors and clinical outcomes. *Chest* 2001;120:555–561.

17. Drakulovic MB, Torres A, Bauer TT, et al. Supine body position as a risk factor for nosocomial pneumonia in mechanically ventilated patients: a randomized trial. *Lancet* 1999;354:1851–1858.

18. van Nieuwenhoven CA, Vandenbroucke-Grauls C, van Tiel FH, et al. Feasibility and effects of the semirecumbent position to prevent ventilator-associated pneumonia: a randomized study. *Crit Care Med* 2006;34:396–402.

19. Kress JP, Pohlman AS, O'Connor MF, et al. Daily interruption of sedative infusions in critically ill patients undergoing mechanical ventilation. *N Engl J Med* 2000;342: 1471–1477.

20. Esteban A, Frutos F, Tobin MJ, et al. A comparison of four methods of weaning patients from mechanical ventilation. Spanish Lung Failure Collaborative Group. *N Engl J Med* 1995;332:345–350.

21. Labeau SO, Vyver VD, Brusselaers N, et al. Prevention of ventilator-associated pneumonia with oral antiseptics: a systematic review and meta-analysis. *Lancet Infect Dis* 2011;11:845–854.

22. Muscedere J, Rewa O, McKechnie K, et al. Subglottic secretion drainage for the prevention of ventilator-associated pneumonia: a systematic review and meta-analysis. *Crit Care Med* 2011;39:1985–1991.

23. Dezfulian C, Shojania K, Collard HR, et al. Subglottic secretion drainage for preventing ventilator-associated pneumonia: a meta-analysis. *Am J Med* 2005;118:11–18.

24. Afessa B, Shorr AF, Anzueto A, et al. Association between a silver-coated endotracheal tube and reduced mortality in patients with ventilator-associated pneumonia. *Chest* 2010;137:1015–1021.

25. Klompas M, Platt R. Ventilator-associated pneumonia—the wrong quality measure for benchmarking. *Ann Intern Med* 2007;147:803–805.

26. Pronovost PJ, Miller M, Wachter RM. The GAAP in quality measurement and reporting. *JAMA* 2007;298:1800–1802.

27. Amin A, Kollef MH. Health care-associated pneumonia. *Hosp Pract (Minneap)* 2010;38:63–74.

28. Dallas J, Kollef M. Severe hospital-acquired pneumonia: a review for clinicians. *Curr Infect Dis Rep* 2009;11:349–356.

29. Mermel LA. Prevention of intravascular catheter-related infections. *Ann Intern Med* 2000;132:391–402.

30. Pittet D, Tarara D, Wenzel RP. Nosocomial bloodstream infection in critically ill patients. Excess length of stay, extra costs, and attributable mortality. *JAMA* 1994;271:1598–1601.

31. Berenholtz SM, Pronovost PJ, Lipsett PA, et al. Eliminating catheter-related bloodstream infections in the intensive care unit. *Crit Care Med* 2004;32:2014–2020.

32. Pronovost P, Needham D, Berenholtz S, et al. An intervention to decrease catheter-related bloodstream infections in the ICU. *N Engl J Med* 2006;355:2725–2732.

33. Pronovost PJ, Goeschel CA, Colantuoni E, et al. Sustaining reductions in catheter related bloodstream infections in Michigan intensive care units: observational study. *BMJ* 2010;340:c309.

34. Gawande A. *The Checklist Manifesto: How to Get Things Right.* New York, NY: Metropolitan Books; 2009.

35. Bosk CL, Dixon-Woods M, Goeschel CA, et al. Reality check for checklists. *Lancet* 2009;374:444–445.

36. Dixon-Woods M, Bosk CL, Aveling EL, et al. Explaining Michigan: developing an ex post theory of a quality improvement program. *Milbank Q* 2011;89:167–205.

37. Gawande A. *Better: A Surgeon's Notes on Performance.* New York, NY: Metropolitan Books; 2007.

38. Raad II, Hohn DC, Gilbreath BJ, et al. Prevention of central venous catheter-related infections by using maximal sterile barrier precautions during insertion. *Infect Control Hosp Epidemiol* 1994;15(4 pt 1):231–238.

39. Cook D, Randolph A, Kernerman P, et al. Central venous catheter replacement strategies: a systematic review of the literature. *Crit Care Med* 1997;25:1417–1424.

40. Nicolle LE. Catheter-related urinary tract infection. *Drugs Aging* 2005;22:627–639.

41. Rebmann T, Greene LR. Preventing catheter-associated urinary tract infections: an executive summary of the Association for Professionals in Infection Control and Epidemiology, Inc, Elimination Guide. *Am J Infect Control* 2010;38:644–646.

42. Saint S, Wiese J, Amory JK, et al. Are physicians aware of which of their patients have indwelling urinary catheters? *Am J Med* 2000;109:476–480.

43. Saint S, Lipsky BA, Goold SD. Indwelling urinary catheters: a one-point restraint? *Ann Intern Med* 2002;137:125–127.

44. Saint S, Kaufman SR, Thompson M, et al. A reminder reduces urinary catheterization in hospitalized patients. *Jt Comm J Qual Patient Saf* 2005;31:455–462.

45. Saint S, Veenstra DL, Sullivan SD, et al. The potential clinical and economic benefits of silver alloy urinary catheters in preventing urinary tract infection. *Arch Intern Med* 2000;160:2670–2675.

46. Johnson JR, Kuskowski MA, Wilt TJ. Systematic review: antimicrobial urinary catheters to prevent catheter-associated urinary tract infection in hospitalized patients. *Ann Intern Med* 2006;144:116–126.

47. Saint S, Kaufman SR, Rogers MA, et al. Condom versus indwelling urinary catheters: a randomized trial. *J Am Geriatr Soc* 2006;54:1055–1061.

48. Cosgrove SE, Sakoulas G, Perencevich EN, et al. Comparison of mortality associated with methicillin-resistant and methicillin-susceptible *Staphylococcus aureus* bacteremia: a meta-analysis. *Clin Infect Dis* 2003;36:53–59.

49. Harbarth S, Fankhauser C, Screnzel J, et al. Universal screening for methicillin-resistant *Staphylococcus aureus* at hospital admission and nosocomial infection in surgical patients. *JAMA* 2008;229:1149–1157.

50. Robicsek A, Beaumont JL, Paule SM, et al. Universal surveillance for methicillin-resistant *Staphylococcus aureus* in 3 affiliated hospitals. *Ann Intern Med* 2008;148:409–418.

51. Cohen Al, Calfee D, Fridkin SK, et al. Recommendations for metrics for multidrug-resistant organisms in healthcare settings: SHEA/HICPAC position paper. *Infect Control Hosp Epidemiol* 2008; 29:901–913.

52. Jain R, Kralovic SM, Evans ME, et al. Veterans Affairs initiative to prevent methicillin-resistant *Staphylococcus aureus* infections. *N Engl J Med* 2011;364:1419–1430.

53. Hebert C, Robicsek A. Decolonization therapy in infection control. *Curr Opin Infect Dis* 2010;23:340–345.

54. Robicsek A, Beaumont JL, Thomson RB Jr, et al. Topical therapy for methicillin-resistant *Staphylococcus aureus* colonization: impact on infection risk. *Infect Control Hosp Epidemiol* 2009;30:623–632.

55. Huskins WC, Huckabee CM, O'Grady NP, et al.; STAR*ICU Trial Investigators. Intervention to reduce transmission of resistant bacteria in intensive care. *N Engl J Med* 2011;364:1407–1418.

56. Platt R. Time for a culture change? *N Engl J Med* 2011;364:1464–1465.

57. Zilberberg MD, Shorr AF, Kollef MH. Increase in adult *Clostridium difficile* related hospitalizations and case-fatality rate, United States, 2000–2005. *Emerg Infect Dis* 2008;14:929–931.

58. Oake N, Taljaard M, van Walraven C, et al. The effect of hospital-acquired *Clostridium difficile* infection on in-hospital mortality. *Arch Intern Med* 2010;170:1804–1810.

59. Rebmann T, Carrico RM, Association for Professionals in Infection Control and Epidemiology. Preventing *Clostridium difficile* infections: an executive summary of the Association for Professionals in Infection Control and Epidemiology's elimination guide. *Am J Infect Control* 2011;39:239–242.

60. Abbett SK, Yokoe DS, Lipsitz SR, et al. Proposed checklist of hospital interventions to decrease the incidence of healthcare-associated *Clostridium difficile* infection. *Infect Control Hosp Epidemiol* 2009;30:1062–1069.

61. Gerberding JL. Hospital-onset infections: a patient safety issue. *Ann Intern Med* 2002;137:665–670.

ADDITIONAL READINGS

Collard HR, Saint S, Matthay MA. Prevention of ventilator-associated pneumonia: an evidence-based systematic review. *Ann Intern Med* 2003;138:494–501.

Hugonnet S, Chevrolet JC, Pittet D. The effect of workload on infection risk in critically ill patients. *Crit Care Med* 2007;35:76–81.

Lin MY, Hota B, Khan YM, et al.; CDC Prevention Epicenter Program. Quality of traditional surveillance for public reporting of nosocomial bloodstream infection rates. *JAMA* 2010;304:2035–2041.

Pittet D, Donaldson L. Challenging the world: patient safety and health care-associated infection. *Int J Qual Health Care* 2006;18:4–8.

Stelfox HT, Bates DW, Redelmeier DA. Safety of patients isolated for infection control. *JAMA* 2003;290:1899–1905.

Stulberg JJ, Delaney CP, Neuhauser DV, et al. Adherence to Surgical Care Improvement Project measures and the association with postoperative infections. *JAMA* 2010;303:2479–2485.

Umscheid CA, Mitchell MD, Doshi JA, et al. Estimating the proportion of healthcare-associated infections that are reasonably preventable and the related mortality and costs. *Infect Control Hosp Epidemiol* 2011;32:101–114.

Waters HR, Korn R Jr, Colantuoni E, et al. The business case for quality: economic analysis of the Michigan Keystone Patient Safety Program in ICUs. *Am J Med Qual* 2011;26:333–339.

OTHER COMPLICATIONS OF HEALTHCARE $\Big|$ 11

GENERAL CONCEPTS

As with healthcare-associated infections (Chapter 10), the patient safety movement has broadened the concept of "adverse event" to include such outcomes as patient falls, delirium, pressure ulcers, and venous thromboembolism (VTE) occurring in healthcare facilities. The rationale for this inclusion is that the strategies to prevent these complications of medical care are similar to those used to prevent other errors. Such strategies include education, culture change, audit and feedback, improved teamwork, and the use of checklists and bundles.

Moreover, as a practical matter, inclusion of these complications under the broad umbrella of patient safety has increased their visibility, thus making available more resources to combat them. It has also facilitated their inclusion within policy initiatives being used to promote safety. For example, postoperative VTE is on the Agency for Healthcare Research and Quality (AHRQ) Patient Safety Indicators list (Appendix V), and is included among the preventable adverse events that are no longer reimbursed by Medicare (Appendix VIII).[1]

This chapter will highlight a few key complications of healthcare and the strategies that can help prevent them. Strategies to prevent readmissions and other handoff-related adverse events are covered in Chapter 8.

VENOUS THROMBOEMBOLISM PROPHYLAXIS

Hospitalized or institutionalized patients often have conditions that place them at high risk for VTE, including inactivity, comorbid diseases that increase the risk for clotting (e.g., cancer, nephrotic syndrome, heart failure), and indwelling catheters. Moreover, because such patients often have limited cardiopulmonary reserve, a pulmonary embolism (PE) can be quite consequential, even fatal. In fact, autopsy studies have shown approximately half the patients who die in hospitals have had a PE, with most of these cases unrecognized antemortem.[2]

The risk of VTE in a hospitalized patient is hard to determine with certainty, because it varies widely depending on the ascertainment method. Studies relying on clinical diagnosis have found rates of 20% for deep venous thrombosis and 1% to 2% for PE after major surgical procedures in the absence of prophylaxis. Rates after certain orthopedic procedures are even higher. Studies using more aggressive observational methods (i.e., Doppler ultrasounds on every postoperative patient) have found much higher rates. It is not known how many of these asymptomatic clots would have caused clinical problems, but surely some would have.

A detailed review of strategies to prevent VTE is beyond the scope of this chapter; the interested reader is referred to a number of excellent reviews, particularly the regularly updated guidelines published by the American College of Chest Physicians (ACCP).[3] Instead, in keeping with the patient safety focus on systems, our emphasis will be on creating systems that ensure that every eligible patient receives appropriate, evidence-based prophylaxis.

Given the complexity of the VTE prophylaxis decision (which varies by patient group and clinical situation, and changes rapidly with new research and pharmacologic agents), it seems unlikely that physician education, the traditional approach, is the best strategy to ensure that research is translated into practice. Rather, the emphasis should be on developing standardized protocols, through order sets and similar mechanisms and, when possible, building these protocols into clinical decision support systems (Chapter 13). In fact, the most recent ACCP guidelines strongly recommend that "every hospital develop a formal strategy that addresses the prevention of VTE."[3]

In a study of 2500 hospitalized patients, half the patients received standard care, while the other half's physicians received a computerized notice of their patient's own risk of thromboembolism. The latter group was required to acknowledge the notice and then explicitly choose to withhold prophylaxis or order it (graduated compression stockings, pneumatic boots, unfractionated or low-molecular-weight heparin, or warfarin). Physicians receiving the alerts were far more likely to order appropriate prophylaxis, and the rates of clinically diagnosed deep venous thrombosis or PE fell by 41% in their patients.[4] Two ICU-based studies reported on the adoption of a series of tools that promoted team communication, prompted clinicians with evidence-based recommendations for ICU prophylaxis (for VTE and other targets including ventilator-associated pneumonia and stress ulcers), and gave them real-time feedback on their performance. Both studies found significant improvements in the use of evidence-based prophylaxis.[5,6] In a comprehensive review of patient safety practices that several colleagues and I conducted for AHRQ, promoting the appropriate use of VTE prophylaxis was the most highly rated practice on the strength of evidence regarding impact and effectiveness.[7]

As with many patient safety targets, moving from local improvement strategies to national reporting and payment changes comes with some complexity. Many national programs determine whether VTE was present based on hospital administrative records, largely created for billing purposes. Several studies have shown that such data lack specificity for hospital-acquired VTE, because either the thrombosis was present on admission or the coding was inaccurate.[8–11]

In addition to accuracy of coding, the issue of preventability arises when hospitals are no longer reimbursed for certain cases of VTE.[1] Streiff and Haut have argued for a reimbursement strategy in which the presence of the adverse event—VTE in this case—would lead to a chart review to determine whether the evidence-based processes were carried out; reimbursement would be withheld only if they were not.[11] Although unwieldy and expensive, such a strategy seems fairer than penalizing hospitals when they did everything right.[12] A similar argument, of course, can be made for the other events on Medicare's "no pay" list that are only partly preventable (Appendix VIII).

PREVENTING PRESSURE ULCERS

Pressure ulcers—damage to skin or underlying structures caused by unrelieved pressure—cause pain, delay functional recovery, and predispose patients to local and systemic infections. It is estimated that about one in seven hospitalized patients in the United States has or develops a pressure ulcer, that 2.5 million patients are treated for pressure ulcers each year, and that more than 50,000 patients die each year from complications.[13,14]

Similar to patient falls (see Section "Preventing Falls"), the first step in preventing pressure ulcers is identifying at-risk patients with a validated risk assessment tool. A variety of such tools are available—most assess nutritional status, mobility, incontinence, and sensory deficiencies. In the United States, the most commonly used tool is the Braden Scale.[15,16] Risk should be assessed on admission (to the hospital or skilled nursing facility), then subsequently (daily, in the case of hospitalized patients). The goals of risk assessment are both overall prevention and preventing early stage pressure ulcers from becoming more severe (i.e., Stages III and IV) with deep tissue injury (Table 11-1).

These risk assessments are followed by a variety of preventive activities focused on at-risk patients. The Institute for Healthcare Improvement's (IHI) bundle includes the following strategies: daily inspection of skin from head to toe (with a special focus on high-risk locations such as sacrum, buttocks, and heels), keeping the patient dry and treating overly dry skin with moisturizers,

Table 11-1   **PRESSURE ULCER STAGING SYSTEM**

Suspected deep tissue injury

Purple or maroon localized area of discolored intact skin or blood-filled blister due to damage of underlying soft tissue from pressure and/or shear. The area may be preceded by tissue that is painful, firm, mushy, boggy, warmer, or cooler as compared to adjacent tissue

Stage I

Intact skin with nonblanchable redness of a localized area usually over a bony prominence. Darkly pigmented skin may not have visible blanching; its color may differ from the surrounding area

Stage II

Partial thickness loss of dermis presenting as a shallow open ulcer with a red pink wound bed, without slough. May also present as an intact or open/ruptured serum-filled blister

Stage III

Full thickness tissue loss. Subcutaneous fat may be visible but bone, tendon, or muscle is not exposed. Slough may be present but does not obscure the depth of tissue loss. May include undermining and tunneling

Stage IV

Full thickness tissue loss with exposed bone, tendon, or muscle. Slough or eschar may be present on some parts of the wound bed. Often includes undermining and tunneling

Unstageable

Full thickness tissue loss in which the base of the ulcer is covered by slough (yellow, tan, gray, green, or brown) and/or eschar (tan, brown, or black) in the wound bed.

Reproduced with permission from National Pressure Ulcer Advisory Panel and European Pressure Ulcer Advisory Panel. Pressure Ulcer Prevention and Treatment: Clinical Practice Guideline. Washington, DC: National Pressure Ulcer Advisory Panel, 2009.

optimizing nutrition and hydration, and minimizing pressure through frequent repositioning and the use of pressure relieving surfaces such as special beds. While several institutions have reported anecdotal success in decreasing pressure ulcer rates through the systematic implementation of these risk assessment and mitigation strategies,[17,18] to date, no large-scale, methodologically strong clinical trial has defined evidence-based best practices or the degree to which pressure ulcers are truly preventable.[19]

PREVENTING FALLS

Patient falls are common—each year, more than one-third of community-dwelling elders fall—and frequently morbid. As older patients are hospitalized or institutionalized, placed on multiple medications, and often immobilized, the risk of falls grows, with some studies suggesting that more than 50% of nursing home residents fall each year.[20] Approximately 20% of falls in institutionalized patients result in serious injury.[21] Interestingly, when asked about what they fear during a hospitalization, adult patients rate "falling and getting hurt" as a greater concern than "being misdiagnosed," "having the wrong test or procedure done," or "being mistaken for another patient," and only a bit below "errors with your medications" and "mistakes by nurses."[22] Patients who suffer serious fall-related injuries while hospitalized cost $14,000 more and stay seven days longer than age- and disease-matched controls.[23] This cost includes only the hospital stay, not the cost of rehabilitation or of any liability payments.[24]

All institutionalized patients should be assessed for fall risk with a validated instrument, such as the St. Thomas Risk Assessment Tool In Falling elderlY inpatients (*STRATIFY*) tool[25] (Figure 11-1). In a validation study, patients with two or more risk factors on the STRATIFY tool had approximately a 50% chance of

STRATIFY risk assessment tool

1 Did the patient present to hospital with a fall or has he or she fallen in the ward since admission?

(Yes = 1, No = 0)

Do you think the patient is (questions 2–5)

2 Agitated?

(Yes = 1, No = 0)

3 Visually impaired to the extent that everyday function is affected?

(Yes = 1, No = 0)

4 In need of especially frequent toileting?

(Yes = 1, No = 0)

5 Transfer and mobility score of 3 or 4?

(Yes = 1, No = 0)

Total score = [   ]

Figure 11-1 ▪ The STRATIFY risk assessment tool for falls.
Transfer and mobility score is a combination of transfer score (0, unable; 1, major help needed; 2, minor help; 3, independent) and mobility score (0, immobile; 1, independent with aid of wheelchair; 2, walks with help of one person; 3, independent). Patients with two or more fall risk factors have a 50% chance of falling in the next week. (Reproduced with permission from Oliver D, Britton M, Seed P, et al. Development and evaluation of evidence based risk assessment tool (STRATIFY) to predict which elderly inpatients will fall: case–control and cohort studies. *BMJ* 1997;315:1049–1053.)

Table 11-2   **RISK FACTORS FOR PATIENT FALLS IN THE HOSPITAL**
■ Fall as presenting complaint or history of falls
■ Mobility impairment or unstable gait
■ Muscle weakness
■ Use of assistive devices
■ Postural hypotension
■ Visual deficits
■ Cognitive impairment
■ Agitation
■ Urinary frequency
■ Medications (e.g., psychotropics, class IA antiarrhythmics, digoxin, and diuretics)
■ Environmental factors (e.g., poor lighting, loose carpets)
■ Arthritis
■ Depression
■ Age >80 years

Reproduced with permission from Bogardus ST. Another fall. *AHRQ WebM&M* (serial online); April 2003. Available at: http://www. webmm.ahrq.gov/case.aspx?caseID=6.

falling in the next week. In addition to the patient-centered risk factors captured in this tool, environmental (such as poor lighting and loose carpets) and extrinsic (such as polypharmacy) risk factors need to be considered (Table 11-2).[20] A systematic review found that the best predictors of future falls were a history of falls in the past year and the presence of active gait or balance problems.[26]

Particularly in patients found to be at risk for falls, active prevention efforts should be undertaken. Although the use of restraints (such as vests, bed rails, and wrist restraints) might appear to be a fall prevention strategy, evidence suggests just the opposite.[27] For this reason (as well as on ethical grounds), restraints should be used as a fall prevention strategy only as a last resort. Other important strategies include early mobilization and efforts to preserve patient strength. Using hip protectors to prevent hip fractures in high-risk patients who do fall has shown benefit in some studies but not others; their use remains controversial.[28,29] A number of other commonsensical practices have also not been convincingly demonstrated to help, including the use of bed alarms to signal patient egress and the use of specially padded floors (which appear to decrease harm from falls but may increase fall risk from tripping). Although unstudied and challenging to implement, moving the mattress to the floor does help prevent harm from falls, particularly for confused patients who are apt to leave their bed.[20]

Recently, two rigorous studies have demonstrated that fall prevention strategies truly work. In one, conducted at two Australian hospitals, patients received a comprehensive educational program, which included both written

Figure 11-2 ▪ Fall prevention tool kit user interface, used in Reference 31 (Reproduced with permission from Partners HealthCare System and Dykes PC, Carroll DL, Hurley A, et al. Fall prevention in acute care hospitals. A randomized trial. *JAMA* 2010;304:1912–1918. Copyright © 2010 American Medical Association. All rights reserved.)

and video-based materials and follow-up by a physical therapist.[30] Fall risk was reduced by approximately 50% among cognitively intact patients. Importantly, simply providing the educational materials without the physical therapist follow-up carried no benefit.

The second study tested the value of a fall prevention tool kit in four teaching hospitals.[31] The tool kit, which was implemented through a sophisticated hospital information technology system, included a risk assessment, tailored fall prevention interventions aimed at both patients and different providers (Figure 11-2), and a tailored educational intervention. The results were impressive: falls in older patients were reduced by about half. The study was not sufficiently powered to detect a change in fall-related injuries. Together, these studies tell us that fall rates can be cut through thoughtful implementation of programs that include risk assessment, comprehensive multidisciplinary prevention strategies, patient education, and use of information technology. These early successes are likely to become a model for other patient safety interventions.

PREVENTING DELIRIUM

Healthcare-acquired delirium is a relatively new planet to enter the patient safety universe. But its attributes largely follow those of the other noninfectious topics covered earlier: there are clear risk factors for its occurrence, many cases do relate to errors in management and/or can be prevented with

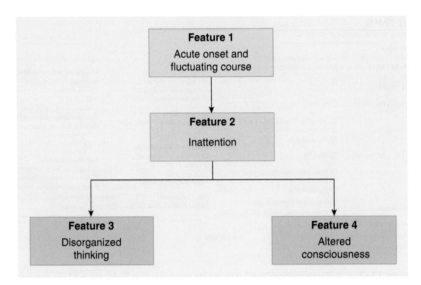

Figure 11-3 ▪ The Confusion Assessment Method (CAM) for the diagnosis of delirium. Diagnosis of delirium using the CAM requires the presence of both features 1 and 2, and either feature 3 or 4. (Reproduced with permission from Rudolph JL. Delirium or dementia? *AHRQ WebM&M* (serial online); May 2009. Available at: http://webmm.ahrq .gov/case.aspx?caseid=200.)

evidence-based interventions, and policymakers are increasingly scrutinizing the adverse events for possible public reporting requirements and payment changes.

One difference from VTE, falls, and even pressure ulcers, though, is that the diagnosis of delirium is often challenging to make, since there are many underlying causes and not all changes in mental status in hospitalized patients relate to delirium. That said, because delirium is so common and morbid in institutionalized patients, one should *assume that altered mental status in a patient in the hospital or long-term care facility is delirium* until proven otherwise.[32] The *Confusion Assessment Method* (CAM), a diagnostic algorithm based on this history and physical examination, is the most useful tool in diagnosing delirium (Figure 11-3).[33] It is noteworthy that published guidelines preclude making the diagnosis of dementia in the inpatient setting; many such diagnoses prove incorrect, the true cause being delirium.[32]

Delirium is common: one in four older patients on a general medical ward and as many as 80% of ICU patients will experience at least one episode of delirium during their hospitalization.[34] Certain patients are at higher risk than others, and a risk assessment using a validated tool should be performed at the time of admission to a hospital, ICU, and long-term care facility. One such tool, for use in medical patients, is shown in Table 11-3.[35]

Table 11-3	DELIRIUM PREDICTION RULE FOR HOSPITALIZED PATIENTS BASED ON ADMISSION CHARACTERISTICS	
Feature	**Measurement**	**Points Awarded**
Cognitive impairment	Mini-Mental State Examination (MMSE) score <24	1
Acute illness	Acute Physiology Age and Chronic Health Evaluation (APACHE) score >16	1
Visual impairment	Corrected >20/70	1
Evidence of dehydration	Blood urea nitrogen (BUN):creatinine ratio ≥18	1

The points are added. The incidence of delirium in patients scoring 0 points is 3% to 9%, 1 to 2 points is 16% to 23%, and ≥3 points is 32% to 83%. (From Inouye SK et al. A predictive model for delirium in hospitalized elderly medical patients based on admission characteristics. *Ann Intern Med* 1993;119:474–481.)

Delirium poses several risks. Making the correct diagnosis of the delirious patient's primary illness is often delayed, both because patients are unable to provide accurate histories and because providers become consumed with managing the delirium itself. Patients, particularly those who are agitated, are at risk for adverse events from the medications or restraints that are often administered. The general risks of hospitalization in older patients, including malnutrition, loss of muscle mass, aspiration, and line infections, are magnified. Remarkably, when taken together, the mortality risk associated with the onset of delirium in a hospitalized patient is comparable to that of patients with sepsis or myocardial infarction.[36]

A detailed description of delirium diagnosis and management is beyond our scope; interested readers would do well to read Rudolph's discussion of a misdiagnosed case of delirium in *AHRQ WebM&M*.[32] For our purposes, suffice it to say that many cases of delirium can be prevented through a program that includes risk assessment, careful medication management[37] and attention to psychosocial aspects of care (reorientation by caregivers and family, appropriate cognitive stimulation, preventing sleep deprivation), and rapid diagnosis and management of underlying precipitants, which are often infections, electrolyte disorders, medication effects, and even constipation. Studies in hospitalized older patients and in patients after hip fracture have demonstrated that these types of multicomponent interventions can prevent many cases of this highly morbid and, until recently, underemphasized adverse event.[38,39]

KEY POINTS

- Like healthcare-associated infections, several other complications of healthcare have been included under the patient safety umbrella. These include VTE, pressure ulcers, patient falls, and, more recently, delirium.
- VTE guidelines are complex and rapidly changing. Improving adherence to appropriate prophylactic strategies depends on building systems (including checklists and computerized decision support) to prompt their use.
- Many cases of pressure ulcers can be prevented with systematic risk assessment using validated tools, followed (particularly in at-risk patients) by extra attention to skin hygiene, nutrition and hydration, and avoiding undue pressure.
- Similarly, the approach to preventing falls begins with risk assessment, followed by strategies such as early mobilization, strength training, and lowering the mattress for at-risk patients.
- Delirium is a common complication of healthcare and is associated with considerable morbidity and mortality. All hospitalized patients with altered mental status should be assumed to have delirium until proven otherwise. Multimodal prevention efforts, targeted to high-risk patients, can decrease the frequency of this adverse event.

REFERENCES

1. Wachter RM, Foster NE, Dudley RA. Medicare's decision to withhold payment for hospital errors: the devil is in the details. *Jt Comm J Qual Patient Saf* 2008;34:116–123.
2. Shojania KG, Burton ED, McDonald KM, et al. Changes in rates of autopsy-detected diagnostic errors over time: a systematic review. *JAMA* 2003;289:2849–2856.
3. Gould MK, Garcia DA, Wren SM, et al. Prevention of VTE in nonorthopedic surgical patients: antithrombotic therapy and prevention of thrombosis. 9th ed. American College of Chest Physicians evidence-based clinical practice guidelines. *Chest* 2012;141:e227S–e277S.
4. Kucher N, Koo S, Quiroz R, et al. Electronic alerts to prevent venous thromboembolism among hospitalized patients. *N Engl J Med* 2005;352:969–977.
5. Byrnes MC, Schuerer DJ, Schallom ME, et al. Implementation of a mandatory checklist of protocols and objectives improves compliance with a wide range of evidence-based intensive care unit practices. *Crit Care Med* 2009;37:2775–2781.
6. Krimsky WS, Mroz IB, McIlwaine JK, et al. A model for increasing patient safety in the intensive care unit: increasing the implementation rates of proven safety measures. *Qual Saf Health Care* 2009;18:74–80.

7. Shojania KG, Duncan BW, McDonald KM, et al. Practices rated by strength of evidence. In: Shojania KG, Duncan BW, McDonald KM, et al., eds. *Making Health Care Safer: A Critical Analysis of Patient Safety Practices.* Evidence Report/Technology Assessment No. 43, AHRQ Publication No. 01-E058. Rockville, MD: Agency for Healthcare Research and Quality; 2001.

8. Bahl V, Thompson MA, Kau T-Y, et al. Do the AHRQ Patient Safety Indicators flag conditions that are present at the time of hospital admission? *Med Care* 2008;46:516–522.

9. White RH, Sadeghi B, Tancredi DJ, et al. How valid is the ICD-9-CM based AHRQ Patient Safety Indicator for postoperative venous thromboembolism? *Med Care* 2009;47:1237–1243.

10. Henderson KE, Recktenwald AJ, Reichley RM, et al. Clinical validation of the AHRQ postoperative venous thromboembolism patient safety indicator. *Jt Comm J Qual Patient Saf* 2009;35:370–376.

11. Streiff MB, Haut ER. The CMS ruling on venous thromboembolism after total knee or hip arthroplasty: weighing risks and benefits. *JAMA* 2009;301:1063–1065.

12. Pronovost PJ, Goeschel CA, Wachter RM. The wisdom and justice of not paying for "preventable complications." *JAMA* 2008;299:2197–2199.

13. Lyder CH. Pressure ulcer prevention and management. *JAMA* 2003;289:223–226.

14. Reddy M, Gill SS, Rochon PA. Preventing pressure ulcers: a systematic review. *JAMA* 2006;296:974–984.

15. Ayello EA, Braden B. How and why to do pressure ulcer risk assessment. *Adv Skin Wound Care* 2002;15:125–131 [quiz 132–133].

16. Prevention Plus. Home of the Braden Scale. Available at: http://www.bradenscale.com/.

17. Courtney BA, Ruppman JB, Cooper HM. Save our skin: initiative cuts pressure ulcer incidence in half. *Nurs Manage* 2006;37:36, 38, 40 passim.

18. Gibbons W, Shanks HT, Kleinhelter P, et al. Eliminating facility-acquired pressure ulcers at Ascension Health. *Jt Comm J Qual Patient Saf* 2006;32:488–496.

19. Soban LM, Hempel S, Munjas BA, et al. Preventing pressure ulcers in hospitals: a systematic review of nurse-focused quality improvement interventions. *Jt Comm J Qual Patient Saf* 2011;37:245–252.

20. Bogardus ST. Another fall. *AHRQ WebM&M* (serial online); April 2003. Available at: http://www.webmm.ahrq.gov/case.aspx?caseID=6.

21. Rubenstein LZ, Josephson KR. Falls and their prevention in elderly people: what does the evidence show? *Med Clin North Am* 2006;90:807–824.

22. Burroughs TE, Waterman BM, Gallagher TH, et al. Patients' concerns about medical errors during hospitalization. *Jt Comm J Qual Improv* 2007;33:5–14.

23. Wong CA, Recktenwald AJ, Jones ML, et al. The cost of serious fall-related injuries at three midwestern hospitals. *Jt Comm J Qual Patient Saf* 2011;37:81–87.

24. Oliver D, Killick S, Even T, et al. Do falls and falls-injuries in hospital indicate negligent care—and how big is the risk? A retrospective analysis of the NHS Litigation Authority Database of clinical negligence claims, resulting from falls in hospitals in England 1995 to 2006. *Qual Saf Health Care* 2008;17:431–436.

25. Oliver D, Britton M, Seed P, et al. Development and evaluation of evidence based risk assessment tool (STRATIFY) to predict which elderly inpatients will fall: case–control and cohort studies. *BMJ* 1997;315:1049–1053.

26. Ganz DA, Bao Y, Shekelle PG, et al. Will my patient fall? *JAMA* 2007;297:77–86.
27. Ejaz FK, Jones JA, Rose MS. Falls among nursing home residents: an examination of incident reports before and after restraint reduction programs. *J Am Geriatr Soc* 1994;42:960–964.
28. Agostini JV, Baker DI, Bogardus ST. Prevention of falls in hospitalized and institutionalized older people. In: Shojania KG, Duncan BW, McDonald KM, et al., eds. *Making Health Care Safer: A Critical Analysis of Patient Safety Practices.* Evidence Report/Technology Assessment No. 43, AHRQ Publication No. 01-E058. Rockville, MD: Agency for Healthcare Research and Quality; 2001.
29. Kiel DP, Magaziner J, Zimmerman S, et al. Efficacy of a hip protector to prevent hip fracture in nursing home residents: the HIP PRO randomized controlled trial. *JAMA* 2007;298:413–422.
30. Haines TP, Hill A-M, Hill KD, et al. Patient education to prevent falls among older hospital inpatients: a randomized controlled trial. *Arch Intern Med* 2011;171:516–524.
31. Dykes PC, Carroll DL, Hurley A, et al. Fall prevention in acute care hospitals. A randomized trial. *JAMA* 2010;304:1912–1918.
32. Rudolph JL. Delirium or dementia? *AHRQ WebM&M* (serial online); May 2009. Available at: http://webmm.ahrq.gov/case.aspx?caseid=200.
33. Inouye SK, van Dyck CH, Alessi CA, et al. Clarifying confusion: the confusion assessment method. A new method for detection of delirium. *Ann Intern Med* 1990;113:941–948.
34. McNicoll L, Pisani MA, Zhang Y, et al. Delirium in the intensive care unit: occurrence and clinical course in older patients. *J Am Geriatr Soc* 2003;51:591–598.
35. Inouye SK, Viscoli CM, Horwitz RI, et al. A predictive model for delirium in hospitalized elderly medical patients based on admission characteristics. *Ann Intern Med* 1993;119:474–481.
36. Inouye SK, Rushing JT, Foreman MD, et al. Does delirium contribute to poor hospital outcomes? A three-site epidemiologic study. *J Gen Intern Med* 1998;13:234–242.
37. Hamilton H, Gallagher P, Ryan C, Byrne S, O'Mahony D. Potentially inappropriate medications defined by STOPP criteria and the risk of adverse drug events in older hospitalized patients. *Arch Intern Med* 2011;171:1013–1019.
38. Inouye SK, Bogardus ST, Charpentier PA, et al. A multicomponent intervention to prevent delirium in hospitalized older patients. *N Engl J Med* 1999;340:669–676.
39. Marcantonio ER, Flacker JM, Wright JR, et al. Reducing delirium after hip fracture: a randomized trial. *J Am Geriatr Soc* 2001;49:516–522.

ADDITIONAL READINGS

Armstrong DG, Ayello EA, Capitulo KL, et al. New opportunities to improve pressure ulcer prevention and treatment: implications of the CMS inpatient hospital care present on admission indicators/hospital-acquired conditions policy: a consensus paper from the International Expert Wound Care Advisory Panel. *Adv Skin Wound Care* 2008;21:469–478.

Coussement J, De Paepe L, Schwendimann R, et al. Interventions for preventing falls in acute- and chronic-care hospitals: a systematic review and meta-analysis. *J Am Geriatr Soc* 2008;56:29–36.

Duncan KD. Preventing pressure ulcers: the goal is zero. *Jt Comm J Qual Improv* 2007;33:605–610.

Eikelboom JW, Karthikeyan G, Fagel N, et al. American Association of Orthopedic Surgeons and American College of Chest Physicians guidelines for venous thromboembolism prevention in hip and knee arthroplasty differ: what are the implications for clinicians and patients? *Chest* 2009;135:513–520.

Inouye SK. Current concepts: delirium in older persons. *New Engl J Med* 2006;354: 1157–1165.

Lederle FA, Zylla D, Macdonald R, et al. Venous thromboembolism prophylaxis in hospitalized medical patients and those with stroke: a background review for an American College of Physicians clinical practice guideline. *Ann Intern Med* 2011;155:602–615.

McInnes E, Jammali-Blasi A, Bell-Syer SE, et al. Support surfaces for pressure ulcer prevention. *Cochrane Database Syst Rev* 2011;(4):CD001735.

PATIENT SAFETY IN THE AMBULATORY SETTING

12

GENERAL CONCEPTS AND EPIDEMIOLOGY

The point has been well made that while most of the patient safety literature focuses on hospital errors, most healthcare is delivered in office settings. Consider this: for every one hospitalized patient, 28 people visit a physician's office.[1] Nevertheless, the early emphasis on patient safety in the hospital was natural: the stakes are higher, errors are more visible, and the resources to research safety problems and implement solutions are all greater there.

The scope of potential errors is also broader in the hospital. Although both settings are beset by medication and laboratory errors, and both inpatient and outpatient errors center on transitions of care and communication problems, the ambulatory setting will see fewer surgical errors (although the rapid increase in outpatient surgery makes these a growing problem) and healthcare-associated infections, pressure ulcers, and blood clots are lesser concerns. Moreover, the research focus on hospital safety also reflects the disproportionate emphasis by academic health centers on hospital care.

But interest in ambulatory safety is growing rapidly, accompanied by a number of new research and practice initiatives. Recent studies have shown that nearly 10% of adverse events occur in physician offices;[2] adverse drug events and diagnostic errors are particularly common.[3,4] Growing experience from outpatient-based patient safety networks indicates that ambulatory practices should focus on two main risky areas: prescription medications and the processing of lab, x-ray, and diagnostic tests.[5,6] Both areas will likely be transformed by the implementation of ambulatory electronic health records and computerized prescribing, presently being driven in the United States by incentive payments to office practitioners who implement information technology (IT) systems that meet certain standards of functionality and interoperability.[7,8]

Sarkar et al. have proposed a model for ambulatory safety[9] modified from the Chronic Care Model described by Wagner et al.[10] It encompasses cheese–related (Chapter 2) problems, along with the many opportunities for improvement in ambulatory test follow-up (Table 12-1).[12]

Note that a robust electronic backbone is only one component of an improved system. As with IT in all healthcare settings, it is relatively easy—natural, even—to think of IT as the Holy Grail: "if we just had a good IT system" is a common refrain. And there is no question that the need for such systems exists—just consider these sobering statistics:

- In a typical week, the average primary care physician is responsible for following up on 800 chemistry/hematology tests, 40 radiographs, and 12 pathology specimens.[13]
- Forty percent of patients have hospital test results that return after hospital discharge, with both hospital and primary care physicians often unaware of the (sometimes crucial) results.[14]
- Fewer than half of primary care physicians are satisfied with their system for managing test results, more than four in five reports having had at least one test result "they wished they had known about earlier" in the prior two months.[15]
- More often than not, some crucial piece of information (lab and radiology results, consultant and pathology reports, procedure notes, and more) is missing in primary care visits.[16] Another study showed that information from one outpatient visit was available at the next visit less than one-quarter of the time.[17]

Unfortunately, early evidence from ambulatory IT implementations demonstrates that IT is not a panacea. One primary care group nearly broke up over the challenges that accompanied implementing a new system (after the dust settled, none of the physicians could imagine going back to paper, though).[18] More sobering, several recent studies have found persistently high rates of errors in both medication and radiology information flow even after IT implementations,[19–21] and thus far there is no evidence that the presence of an ambulatory health record is associated with improved quality.[22]

At the same time, it is inconceivable that we can achieve highly reliable ambulatory care without effective IT. These sobering results simply illustrate, as always, that building and implementing IT is harder than it looks, that systems need to evolve based on provider and patient feedback, and that human factors need to be considered in the development and implementation of these systems (Chapters 7 and 13). Given both the limitations of IT systems and the fact that most ambulatory practices will not have them for the next few years, Nancy Elder's commonsensical steps that can be taken to improve ambulatory medication and test management safety are worth reviewing (Tables 12-2 and 12-3).[5]

Table 12-1	**BUILDING A SYSTEM FOR MORE RELIABLE TEST FOLLOW-UP IN THE AMBULATORY ENVIRONMENT***	
Redesign Recommendation	**Logic**	**Specifications**
Tests need to be tracked from order to completion, receipt, and action.	Failures need to be visible, rather than invisibly falling through cracks.	Each step needs to be acknowledged and documented. Critical tests ordered but not performed and results lacking acknowledgment or expected action need to be tracked.
Develop standardized approach for every test and test-generating area to define and flag clinically significant abnormal results.	"Panic values" were a major advance in the 1970s, but nonurgent, action-requiring abnormal results are now the biggest problem. Lack of standardized, coded system is difficult for clinicians and for systematic tracking.	Each testing area should delineate criteria for abnormal results using three levels of urgency—immediate/life threatening, urgent, and nonurgent but critical to follow up—defining time frames for receipt and action for each level of urgency and tagging results meeting criteria.
Eliminate ambiguities regarding whom to contact for critical abnormal results, and delineate their responsibilities.	Confusion leads to errors, particularly related to responsibilities of ordering specialists and cross-covering physicians versus primary caregivers. Redesign is needed to overcome fragmented outpatient services and increasing inpatient "shift work."	Emerging consensus that initial responsibility belongs to the *ordering* clinician to receive, act on, and/or relay critical results, backed up by the *covering* clinician when ordering clinician is unavailable, for more urgent results.
Outpatients should be informed about all test results, even normal results.	Creating expectation that they will hear about all results allows patients to serve as reliability backstop for unreported results.	Multiple ways to communicate with patients depending on the result, the patient, and available technology. Web-based secure patient "portals" are increasingly useful as ways to post results.
Tracking and system oversight monitoring	Just as someone needs to "own" each critical result, someone needs to be responsible for tracking outstanding results and identifying problems and system improvement opportunities.	Create test result quality office/person to track abnormal results unaddressed after predefined intervals, to troubleshoot/investigate when clinicians are not reachable or results are sent to wrong physician, and to monitor and improve performance based on incidents and aggregated data.

(continued)

Table 12-1	BUILDING A SYSTEM FOR MORE RELIABLE TEST FOLLOW-UP IN THE AMBULATORY ENVIRONMENT* (continued)	
Redesign Recommendation	**Logic**	**Specifications**
Advanced systems to support clinicians in test results management	Further overloading busy clinicians with more tests to follow up without supporting ability to do so is not effective system redesign. Need automation, delegation, and cognitive support tools.	Results management system redesign and tools featuring interoperability with all testing areas (e.g., cardiology, endoscopy), linking to contextual information (past results, problems, drugs), and electronic decision support to identify and streamline carrying out next actions.

Reproduced with permission from Schiff GD. A 60-year-old man with delayed care for a renal mass. *JAMA* 2011;305:1890–1898. Copyright © 2011 American Medical Association. All rights reserved.

*Adapted from multiple consensus guidelines and recommendations, including the Massachusetts Coalition for the Prevention of Medical Errors Communicating Critical Test Results Collaborative; the Partners Communicating Clinically Significant Test Results Task Force; the Alert Notification of Critical Radiology Results collaboration project of the Brigham and Women's Hospital, Beth Israel Deaconess Medical Center, and the University of Chicago; and the CRICO Risk Management Foundation's Office Practice: What Works.

Table 12-2	PRACTICES THAT MAY LEAD TO IMPROVED AMBULATORY MEDICATION SAFETY

Write understandable, legible prescriptions, and include the indication on the prescription. Use English instead of Latin abbreviations (i.e., writing "four times daily" or "once daily" instead of "qid" and "qd," respectively), and write the indication on the prescription (e.g., "for high blood pressure").

Use sample medications with care, if at all. Pharmacists serve as an important safety check when prescribing medications, often catching interactions and allergies that physicians miss.

Maintain accurate and usable medication lists and reconcile medications regularly. Use the "brown bag checkup" (i.e., ask patients to bring all the medicines in their medicine cabinet to a visit). Physicians and their staff need to confirm the medications at every visit. When discrepancies are found, it is the physician's task to resolve these.

Empower patients to serve as safety double checkers. Most patients can assume significant responsibility for discovering—and preventing—many medical errors from becoming harmful events.

Consider using an electronic prescribing system. An electronic prescribing system, especially when interfaced with an electronic health record, has the potential to decrease errors from illegibility and interactions. Direct electronic transmission to pharmacies may decrease errors even further.

Reproduced with permission from Elder NC. Patient safety in the physician office setting. *AHRQ WebM&M* (serial online); May 2006. Available at: http://webmm.ahrq.gov/perspective.aspx?perspectiveID=24.

Table 12-3 **PRACTICES THAT MAY LEAD TO IMPROVED AMBULATORY MANAGEMENT OF TEST RESULTS**

Implement a formal test-tracking system. A tracking system assures that all tests ordered are returned, ideally to the physician but at least to the practice. Although a formal tracking system can be incorporated within an electronic health record, this is not a requirement for having a working system. A system needs to be simple, have some built-in redundancies (to account for human error in entering data), and be accessible and accountable to multiple people (not just "Mary in the laboratory"). An electronic results manager can track results and provide reminders.

Make a policy of notifying every patient of every result. "No news is good news" should be a policy relegated to history. Practices should decide on a standardized system for notifying patients of both normal and abnormal results.

Empower patients to serve as safety double checkers. Patients should be educated as to what tests are being ordered, their purpose, and when (and how) results will be relayed. If patients do not receive their results within a specified time, they should be instructed to contact the office for the results.

Only file signed reports, letters, dictations, and results. Whereas many offices have a policy that nothing enters a chart (electronic or paper) without being signed first, too often, unsigned or inappropriately signed reports get filed. The response to the report (normal, abnormal) also needs to be noted by the physician.

Reproduced with permission from Elder NC. Patient safety in the physician office setting. *AHRQ WebM&M* (serial online); May 2006. Available at: http://webmm.ahrq.gov/perspective.aspx?perspectiveID=24.

The role of the patient is crucial in ambulatory safety, particularly since patients spend so little time with their providers. Strong emphasis should be placed on patient education (using proven methods such as the "teach back"[23]) and empowerment, with particular attention paid to the issues of health literacy and cultural differences. We will discuss these in more detail in Chapter 21.

Overall, improving safety in the ambulatory setting will not necessarily be harder or easier than in the hospital, just different.[11] As with much of the patient safety field, which often involves extrapolating experiences (Table P-1) from other settings (i.e., *Will crew resource management, which worked so well in commercial aviation, work in the labor and delivery suite? Will bar coding, which works so well in the supermarket, actually decrease medication errors?*), it will be important to remain sensitive to the differences in structure and culture as we try to translate what we know about safety from the hospital to the office setting.

While ambulatory safety was all-but-ignored during the first few years of the safety movement, research funders, accreditors, regulators, and specialty societies have come to appreciate its importance, as have patients and their advocates. All these stakeholders are beginning to exert their influence in this setting, so the next few years will see far more patient safety activity in the ambulatory arena, and far more pressure to improve.

KEY POINTS

- Until recently, the patient safety field's focus has been on hospital safety. Attention is now shifting to the ambulatory setting.
- Efforts to improve ambulatory safety should initially focus on decreasing medication errors and improving the management of test results.
- In approaching ambulatory safety, it will be important to appreciate major clinical, structural, and organizational differences between the hospital and the office. These include the inability to support specialized experts in many safety-related areas, and the employer–employee relationship between physicians and many nurses and other staff found in most U.S. office practices.
- The development and implementation of effective IT tools is essential to improving ambulatory safety, particularly in the areas of medication management and test results handling. Early experience with ambulatory IT has been sobering, with unexpectedly high rates of errors. Effective systems will need to integrate provider and patient feedback and take better account of human factors.

REFERENCES

1. Green LA, Fryer GE, Yawn BP, et al. The ecology of medical care revisited. *N Engl J Med* 2001;344:2021–2025.
2. Weingart SN, Wilson RM, Gibberd RW, et al. Epidemiology of medical error. *BMJ* 2000;320:774–777.
3. Gandhi TK, Weingart SN, Borus J, et al. Adverse drug events in ambulatory care. *N Engl J Med* 2003;348:1556–1564.
4. Gandhi TK, Kachalia A, Thomas EJ, et al. Missed and delayed diagnoses in the ambulatory setting: a study of closed malpractice claims. *Ann Intern Med* 2006;145:488–496.
5. Elder NC. Patient safety in the physician office setting. *AHRQ WebM&M* (serial online); May 2006. Available at: http://webmm.ahrq.gov/perspective.aspx?perspectiveID=24.
6. West D, Westfall JM, Araya-Guerra R, et al. Using reported primary care errors to develop and implement patient safety interventions: a report from the ASIPS Collaborative. In: *Advances in Patient Safety: From Research to Implementation.* Rockville, MD: Agency for Healthcare Research and Quality; 2005. AHRQ Publication No. 050021.
7. DesRoches CM, Campbell EG, Rao SR, et al. Electronic health records in ambulatory care—a national survey of physicians. *N Engl J Med* 2008;359:50–60.
8. Bruen BK, Ku L, Burke MF, Buntin MB. More than four in five office-based physicians could qualify for federal electronic health record incentives. *Health Aff (Millwood)* 2011;30:472–480.

9. Sarkar U, Wachter RM, Schroeder SA, et al. Refocusing the lens: patient safety in ambulatory chronic disease care. *Jt Comm J Qual Patient Saf* 2009;35:377–383.

10. Wagner EH, Austin BT, Von Korff M. Organizing care for patients with chronic illness. *Milbank Q* 1996;74:511–544.

11. Wachter RM. Is ambulatory patient safety just like hospital safety, only without the "stat?" *Ann Intern Med* 2006;145:547–549.

12. Schiff GD. A 60-year-old man with delayed care for a renal mass. *JAMA* 2011;305:1890–1898.

13. Poon EG, Wang SJ, Gandhi TK, et al. Design and implementation of a comprehensive outpatient results manager. *J Biomed Inform* 2003;36:80–91.

14. Roy CL, Poon EG, Karson AS, et al. Patient safety concerns arising from test results that return after hospital discharge. *Ann Intern Med* 2005;143:121–128.

15. Poon EG, Gandhi TK, Sequist TD, et al. "I wish I had seen this test result earlier!": dissatisfaction with test result management systems in primary care. *Arch Intern Med* 2004;164:2223–2228.

16. Smith PC, Araya-Guerra R, Bublitz C, et al. Missing clinical information during primary care visits. *JAMA* 2005;293:565–571.

17. van Walraven C, Taljaard M, Bell CM, et al. Information exchange among physicians caring for the same patient in the community. *CMAJ* 2008;179:1013–1018.

18. Baron RJ, Fabens EL, Schiffman M, et al. Electronic health records: just around the corner? Or over the cliff? *Ann Intern Med* 2005;143:222–226.

19. Abramson EL, Malhotra S, Fischer K, et al. Transitioning between electronic health records: effects on ambulatory prescribing safety. *J Gen Intern Med* 2011;26:868–874.

20. Nanji KC, Rothschild JM, Salzberg C, et al. Errors associated with outpatient computerized prescribing systems. *J Am Med Inform Assoc* 2011;18:767–773.

21. Singh H, Thomas EJ, Mani S, et al. Timely follow-up of abnormal diagnostic imaging test results in an outpatient setting: are electronic medical records achieving their potential? *Arch Intern Med* 2009;169:1578–1586.

22. Romano MJ, Stafford RS. Electronic health records and clinical decision support systems: impact on national ambulatory care quality. *Arch Intern Med* 2011;171:897–903.

23. Bertakis KD. The communication of information from physician to patient: a method for increasing patient retention and satisfaction. *J Fam Pract* 1977;5:217–222.

ADDITIONAL READINGS

Gandhi TK, Lee TH. Patient safety beyond the hospital. *N Engl J Med* 2010;363:1001–1003.

Gandhi TK, Weingart SN, Seger AC, et al. Outpatient prescribing errors and the impact of computerized prescribing. *J Gen Intern Med* 2005;20:837–841.

Gurwitz JH, Field TS, Harrold LR, et al. Incidence and preventability of adverse drug events among older persons in the ambulatory setting. *JAMA* 2003;289:1107–1116.

Modak I, Sexton JB, Lux TR, et al. Measuring safety culture in the ambulatory setting: the Safety Attitudes Questionnaire—ambulatory version. *J Gen Intern Med* 2007; 22:1–5.

Nassaralla CL, Naessens JM, Chaudhry R, et al. Implementation of a medication reconciliation process in an ambulatory internal medicine clinic. *Qual Saf Health Care* 2007;16:90–94.

Schauberger CW, Larson P. Implementing patient safety practices in small ambulatory care settings. *Jt Comm J Qual Patient Saf* 2006;32:419–425.

Taché SV, Sönnichsen A, Ashcroft DM. Prevalence of adverse drug events in ambulatory care: a systematic review. *Ann Pharmacother* 2011;45:977–989.

SECTION

III

SOLUTIONS

INFORMATION TECHNOLOGY | 13

HEALTHCARE'S INFORMATION PROBLEM

The provision of healthcare is remarkably information intensive. A large integrated healthcare system processes twice as many computerized transactions each day (approximately 10 million) as the NASDAQ stock exchange (5 million) processes.

But high volume is just the beginning. Consider the task of tracking a single patient's current diseases, past medical history, medications, allergies, test results, risk factors, and personal preferences (such as for cardiopulmonary resuscitation). Tricky? Sure, but now do it over months or years, and then add in the fact that the patient is seen by many different providers, scattered across a region.

Want more? To make payment decisions, the insurer needs access to some of this information, as does the source of the insurance, which in the United States is often the patient's employer. But, because of privacy concerns, both should receive only essential information; to tell them of the patient's HIV status, or her psychiatric or sexual history, would be highly inappropriate, damaging, and possibly illegal.

Now let's make it really hard. Assume that the patient is in a car accident and taken to an emergency department (ED) in a nearby state, where she is stabilized and admitted to the hospital. Ideally, the doctors and nurses would see the relevant clinical details of her past history, preferably in a format that highlighted the information they needed without overwhelming them with extraneous data. Orders must be processed instantaneously (none of "the system is down for planned maintenance" or "orders are processed on the next business day" so familiar from commercial transactions). During the patient's hospital stay, not only would there be seamless links among all of the new observations (the neurosurgeon can easily view the ED doctor's notes; the resident can quickly find the patient's vital signs and laboratory studies), but also the various components would weave together seamlessly. For example:

- The system would prompt the doctor with information regarding the appropriate therapy or test for a given condition (along with links to the evidence supporting any recommendations).
- The system would warn the nurse that the patient is allergic to a medicine before she administers it.
- The system would tell the doctor or pharmacist which medications are on the formulary and steer them to the preferred ones.

Meanwhile, the vast trove of data being created through this patient's case—and millions of others like it—would be chronicled and analyzed ("mined"), searching for new patterns of disease, evidence of preferred strategies, and more. All of this would be iterative—as new information emerged from this and other research about disease risk factors or best practices, it would seamlessly flow into the system, spurring the next patient's care to be even better.

Contrast this vision of information nirvana with the prevailing state of most doctors' offices and hospitals.[1,2] Information is stored on paper charts, and thus unavailable to anyone who lacks physical possession of the relevant piece of paper (in some cases, the notes are sufficiently illegible that even physical custody of the paper does not insure information access). Notes are entered as free text, not in a format that facilitates analysis or productive interaction with other pieces of system data. When the patient moves across silos—from outpatient to inpatient, from state to state, from hospital to hospice—crucial information rarely moves with her. Communication of facts (e.g., medication lists, allergies, past medical history), which should be streamed through the system, instead lives at the mercy of person-to-person interactions or a haphazard pinball game of photocopies bouncing from place to place.

Even at the level of the individual practitioner, the impact of this chaos is profoundly demoralizing, wasteful, and dangerous. Just watch a nurse take a patient's vital signs on a typical hospital ward. The nurse looks at the numbers on the screen of a digital automated blood pressure cuff: **165/92**. She records them on an index card (or, sometimes, on her forearm or the cuff of her scrub suit), hopefully next to the correct patient's name. Later, she returns to the nurses' station and transcribes these numbers (again, hopefully belonging to the correct patient) onto the appropriate place in the chart (hopefully the right chart). Then, in a teaching hospital, an intern transcribes these vital signs onto another index card (or maybe, these days, an iPad) during morning rounds. He presents these data to his resident and later to his attending, who each do the same thing. Eventually, each of these practitioners writes, or dictates, notes for the medical record. Any wonder that this information (which, you'll recall, began life in digital form!) is frequently wrong? Or that busy healthcare professionals find that huge chunks of their valuable time are squandered? Or that the patient has the sense (particularly after she has been asked the same question by 10 different people) that the right hand has no idea what the left hand is doing?

Why has healthcare, the most information intensive of industries, entered the modern age of computers so sluggishly, reluctantly, and haphazardly? Part of the reason is that, until recently, the business or clinical case for healthcare information technology (HIT) was far from ironclad. Such justification was needed because HIT is extraordinarily expensive (about $50,000 per doctor in an ambulatory office, and up to $150 million to completely wire a large teaching hospital), unreimbursed, and extremely challenging to implement. Moreover, until the past few years, most healthcare computer systems were relatively clunky and user unfriendly, in part because the market for them was too weak to fund the research and development and generate the user feedback and refinement cycles needed for complex systems to mature.

We are now at a turning point for HIT. The patient safety movement has catalyzed the widespread recognition that a robust computer scaffolding is absolutely essential to efforts to improve quality, safety, efficiency, and coordination of care. There are striking examples of successes, such as that enjoyed by the huge Veterans Affairs (VA) system, whose early adoption of electronic health records (EHRs) and computerized provider order entry (CPOE) sparked a substantially improved quality of care.[3] A large and convincing literature demonstrates that well-designed and implemented electronic systems can lead to significant benefits for systems and patients.[4-8]

At the same time, there is a more troubling, though not entirely surprising, side of the story. A decade ago, my colleagues and I openly worried that the early glowing evidence about HIT's benefits had come from a handful of institutions that had lovingly built their own systems, had highly committed leaders, and had invested heavily in computerization.[9] As Shojania and I wrote in our 2004 book *Internal Bleeding*:

> But the average hospital will not share these conditions, any more than your local Gilbert and Sullivan troupe resembles the Metropolitan Opera...More than one CIO has tried to airlift a commercial system into her hospital, then stood scratching her head at how slick the system seemed to be during the vendor's demo, and how poorly it performed in real life.[10]

As you've already seen, our suspicions—that the implementation of commercial IT systems at thousands of hospitals and hundreds of thousands of ambulatory offices might not go quite so smoothly—have, sadly, been proven

Table 13-1	MECHANISMS BY WHICH INFORMATION TECHNOLOGY CAN IMPROVE PATIENT SAFETY

- Improving communication
- Making knowledge more readily accessible
- Prompting for key pieces of information
- Assisting with calculations
- Monitoring and checking in real time
- Providing decision support

Reproduced with permission from Bates DW, Gawande AA. Improving safety with information technology. *N Engl J Med* 2003;348:2526–2534.

correct. A growing literature tells stories of HIT implementation failures, unanticipated consequences, and even harm.[11–16] It is a sobering but useful tale, one that highlights the immense challenges of fundamental change in complex adaptive systems (Chapter 2), the critical need to use human factors design principles (Chapter 7), and the overwhelming complexity of the task itself.

This chapter will describe the main types of HIT systems, some of their safety advantages (Table 13-1), and some of the problems—including new kinds of errors—they can create. Because HIT addresses so many safety targets and is a component of so many solutions, considerable information about HIT's role in specific areas can also be found throughout the book.

ELECTRONIC HEALTH RECORDS

Because most medical errors represent failures in communication and data transmission (Figure 9-3), computerization of the medical record would seem like a safety lynchpin. (While the old term was "electronic medical record" [EMR], the term "EHR" is generally preferred, since it emphasizes the role of the patient in viewing and even contributing to the record and the fact that the EHR may chronicle and even influence health status, not just a patient's medications and diagnoses.) But to realize this benefit, attention must be paid to a variety of system and user factors. The system factors include the ease of use, the speed with which data can be entered and retrieved, the quality of the user interface, and the presence of value-added features such as order entry, decision support, sign-out and scheduling systems, links to all the necessary data (e.g., x-rays and electrocardiograms), and automatic reports. The user factors primarily relate to the training and readiness of the provider and nonprovider workforce (Chapters 7 and 16).

User efficiency is particularly important. Despite the hope that computerization would save time for providers, emerging evidence indicates that the opposite is often true, particularly for physicians.[17] Some of this cost in time may be repaid in more efficient information retrieval, but increasing attention will need to be focused on facilitating workflow. (Remember that digital blood pressure reading?—in the "wired" hospital, it will magically leap from blood pressure machine into the EHR, where it can be seamlessly imported into each provider's note.) Effective systems will, of course, provide huge efficiency benefits to administrators, researchers, and insurers by capturing data in standardized formats and allowing electronic transmission.

Unfortunately, this facilitated movement of bits and bytes has a dark side, in the form of the *"copy-and-paste" phenomenon*. One tongue-in-cheek essayist captured the problem beautifully:

> The copy-and-paste command allows one day's note to be copied and used as a template for the next day's note. Ideally, old information and diagnostic impressions are deleted and new ones added. In reality, however, there is no deletion, only addition. Daily progress notes become progressively longer and contain senescent information. The admitting diagnostic impression, long since discarded, is dutifully noted day after day. Last month's echocardiogram report takes up permanent residence in the daily results section. Complicated patients are on "post-op day 2" for weeks. One wonders how utilization review interprets such statements.[18]

A study of 167,000 computerized records in the U.S. Department of Veterans Affairs (VA) healthcare system found that physical examinations were completely copied (from one author to another) in 3% of the charts.[19] Some IT systems can disable the copy-and-paste function, although this may be unacceptable to providers (some information really *does* remain static from day to day, and having to retype or redictate it is wasteful and annoying), and resourceful providers can usually find a way to bypass such restrictions anyway.[20] In the end, copy-and-paste is like many elements of patient safety, in that introducing structural changes without ensuring that caregivers possess the requisite education and professionalism is likely to lead to new types of mischief, or even harm.

One important choice for EHR developers is the use of *structured versus unstructured data*. Physicians, in particular, have always preferred entering data as unstructured prose (captured through typing, transcription services, or increasingly, speech recognition software), which has the advantages of ease of use and familiarity, and is consistent with the long tradition of "telling the patient's story."[21,22] On the other hand, unstructured data are difficult to analyze for patterns, to use to support quality improvement and public reporting activities, and to link to computerized decision support. Structured, or coded, data (captured via templates or automatically fed into the EHR after being recorded by electronic devices) can support these functions, but they fail to comport with clinicians' mental model for data acquisition and analysis. Ongoing research is attempting to identify the best mix of structured and unstructured EHR inputs, and to develop new ways (through "natural language processing") to mine narrative prose for key data elements.[22] It is likely that high-quality EHRs of the future will combine the best of both types of data capture and analysis.

An important advance in EHRs is the ability to promote *patient engagement* (Chapter 21). At the very least, allowing patients access to their laboratory data and giving them the ability to schedule their own appointments represents real progress.[23] But patients, who are increasingly accustomed to managing their own affairs (financial, travel, dating) with the support of electronic systems, are interested in new kinds of tools to help with their medical care and overall health.[24] Many patients now keep *personal health records* (PHRs), although a minority do so electronically. Future developments in this area are likely to weave patient- and provider-facing electronic systems together, facilitate new kinds of information flow and communications (e-mails, text messaging, video consultations, and more), and raise a host of issues surrounding reimbursement, privacy, data integrity (what happens when the provider and patient disagree about what should be in a jointly created record?), and more.[25,26] Obviously, the implications of this on patient safety will be profound, with the capacity both for great leaps forward and some new hazards.

EHRs raise yet another challenge, one that is even more profound. As the physician-writer Abraham Verghese has observed, clinicians' focus is increasingly centered on the data in the computer, sometimes at the cost of the human connections so fundamental to the practice of medicine and the art of healing. After discussing the traditional approach to patients, in which "the [patient's] body is the text," Verghese writes of a new, more expedient approach that he sees in today's trainees:

> The patient is still at the center, but more as an icon for another entity clothed in binary garments: the "iPatient." Often, emergency room personnel have already scanned, tested, and diagnosed, so that interns meet a fully formed iPatient long before seeing the real patient. The iPatient's blood counts and emanations are tracked and trended like a Dow Jones Index, and pop-up flags remind caregivers to feed or bleed. iPatients are handily discussed (or "card-flipped") in the bunker [the conference room where the team does its work], while the

real patients keep the beds warm and ensure that the folders bearing their names stay alive on the computer.[27]

Taking full advantage of the remarkable potential for EHRs to improve safety and quality while heeding Verghese's cautionary tale may be one of the most subtle yet important challenges facing caregivers in the modern age.

COMPUTERIZED PROVIDER ORDER ENTRY

Because the prescribing process is one of the Achilles' heels of medication safety (Figure 4-3), efforts to computerize this process have long been a focus of safety efforts. In 1998, Bates et al. demonstrated that a CPOE system with decision support reduced serious medication errors by 55%, mediated by improved communication, better availability of information, constraints to prevent the use of inappropriate drugs, doses, and frequencies, and assistance with monitoring.[4,28] Another study of more sophisticated decision support found an 83% reduction in medication errors.[29] The advantages of CPOE over paper-based systems are many; in addition to those listed in Table 13-2, the

Table 13-2 **ADVANTAGES OF CPOE SYSTEMS OVER PAPER-BASED SYSTEMS**

- Free of handwriting identification problems
- Faster to reach the pharmacy
- Less subject to error associated with similar drug names
- More easily integrated into medical records and decision support systems
- Less subject to errors caused by use of apothecary measures
- Easily linked to drug–drug interaction warnings
- More likely to identify the prescribing physician
- Able to link to ADE reporting systems
- Able to avoid specification errors, such as trailing zeros
- Available and appropriate for training and education
- Available for immediate data analysis, including postmarketing reporting
- Claimed to generate significant economic savings
- With online prompts, CPOE systems can:
    Link to algorithms to emphasize cost-effective medications
    Reduce underprescribing and overprescribing
    Reduce incorrect drug choices

Abbreviation: ADE, adverse drug event.

Reproduced with permission from Koppel R, Metlay JP, Cohen A, et al. Role of computerized physician order entry systems in facilitating medication errors. *JAMA* 2005;293:1197–1203. Copyright © 2005 American Medical Association. All rights reserved.

Figure 13-1 ■ Example of a CPOE system's warning of a potentially fatal medication–allergy interaction. (Reproduced with permission from Bates DW, Gawande AA. Improving safety with information technology. *N Engl J Med* 2003;348:2526–2534.)

installation of CPOE systems inevitably leads organizations to standardize chaotic processes (the equivalent of cleaning out your closet before moving), which has its own safety benefits.[4]

Much of the value of CPOE systems comes from identifying out-of-range results or potentially unsafe interactions, and rapidly alerting providers so that they can decide whether their plan is correct.[30] For example, a CPOE system can alert a provider to a potentially fatal medication–allergy interaction (Figure 13-1) or a potentially dangerous laboratory result (Table 13-3). These systems can also be used at the healthcare system level to identify and track errors via trigger tools (Chapters 2 and 14).

In addition to helping clinicians avoid mistakes, CPOE systems can suggest actions that should always accompany certain orders. These "*corollary orders*" should be second nature, but our memories are fallible and we sometimes forget to check a creatinine and potassium after starting an angiotensin-converting enzyme (ACE) inhibitor, a digoxin level after beginning digoxin, or a glucose level after starting insulin. In one study, clinicians were twice as likely to accept a computerized prompt for a corollary

	Critical Values		
Lab Test	Low	High	Common Qualifications or Variations
Serum glucose	<40 or 45 mg/dL	>500 mg/dL	High value could have lower threshold in newborns (e.g., >200 mg/dL)
Serum sodium	<120 mEq/L	>160 mEq/L	High value could have lower threshold (e.g., >152 mEq/L)
Serum potassium	<2.5 mEq/L	>6.0 mEq/L	Either value could have slightly different threshold
Serum bicarbonate	≤10 mEq/L	≥40 mEq/L	Either value could have slightly different threshold
Serum calcium (total)	<7.0 mg/dL	>13.0 mg/dL	Either value could have slightly different threshold
White blood cell count	$<2 \times 10^{-9} \, L^{-1}$	$>50 \times 10^{-9} \, L^{-1}$	Low value could be specified in terms of absolute neutrophil count (e.g., ANC $<0.5 \times 10^{-9} \, L^{-1}$). High value could have threshold as high as $100 \times 10^{-9} \, L^{-1}$. Thresholds commonly vary across settings (inpatient vs. outpatient) and patient populations (oncology patients, pediatrics).
Hematocrit	<20%	>60%	Inpatient settings often omit critical threshold for high values
Platelet count	$<20 \times 10^{-9} \, L^{-1}$	$>1000 \times 10^{-9} \, L^{-1}$	Threshold for low value commonly varies across settings (inpatient vs. outpatient) and patient populations (oncology patients, pediatrics)
Prothrombin time	Not applicable	International normalized ratio (INR) >5	
Partial thromboplastin time	Not applicable	>100 seconds	High value may have higher threshold (e.g., >120 seconds) or may be specified relative to the normal range (e.g., >3 times upper limit of normal)
Blood culture	Not applicable	Positive result	
Cerebrospinal fluid culture or direct examination	Not applicable	Positive result	
Acid fast bacilli stain (any specimen)	Not applicable	Positive result	

Table 13-3 **SAMPLE CRITICAL LABORATORY VALUES***

*A typical policy for the appropriate response to a critical value is that someone from the laboratory must notify by telephone a physician, nurse, physician assistant, or medical assistant at the ordering location. In accordance with Joint Commission requirements, laboratory staff must ask the recipient of the results to read back the results to ensure that they were properly received. (Reproduced with permission from Astion M. The result stopped here. *AHRQ WebM&M* (serial online); June 2004. Available at: http://webmm.ahrq.gov/case.aspx?caseID=65.)

order than they were to place the order without the prompting.[31] I'll say more about these functions—which go under the general name of clinical decision support systems (CDSS)—later in this chapter.

Despite the great appeal of CPOE, one study at an academic medical center found 22 new error types caused or exacerbated by a commercial CPOE system, including long gaps in medication delivery because of a fragmented CPOE display, failure to discontinue medications or renew antibiotics, and delayed ordering caused by CPOE system downtime.[11] Even more worrisome, one prominent children's hospital experienced a threefold *increase* in the mortality rate of critically ill patients after a new CPOE system was installed.[12] There, caregivers noted inefficient order entry, too much time spent at the computer screen and away from the bedside, and several other workflow-related problems. While this study has been criticized on methodological grounds and a subsequent study of the same CPOE system at another children's hospital found improved mortality,[8] the cautionary notes it raises about human factors (Chapter 7) and unanticipated consequences merit our attention.

We can expect that, as the market for CPOE grows and commercial products experience many crucial user-feedback-generated improvement cycles, the systems will become better, errors associated with them will become less common, and the full safety benefits of CPOE will begin to be realized. Table 13-4 highlights the many categories of IT-related errors that have been identified and suggests a number of mitigating strategies.[15]

OTHER IT–RELATED SAFETY SOLUTIONS

Bar coding and radio-frequency identification systems

Even when rigorous safety checks are embedded into the prescribing process, errors at the time of drug administration can still lead to great harm (Chapter 4). To prevent these errors, many institutions are implementing bar coding or radio-frequency identification (RFID) solutions. In bar code medication administration (BCMA), a nurse must swipe a bar code on the medication, the patient's wristband, and her own badge to confirm a three-way match before a medication can be administered.[32] In RFID systems, the medication package has an implanted chip that transmits a signal, allowing for passive identification (like driving through an automated toll booth) rather than requiring a scan. Despite its intuitive appeal, RFID remains more expensive, and—because patients are taking multiple medications and nurses often have the medications for multiple patients on their carts—somewhat trickier to implement. For now, most hospitals seeking to improve their medication administration process have favored BCMA.

Table 13-4 **EXAMPLES OF INFORMATION TECHNOLOGY–RELATED ERRORS AND CORRESPONDING SUGGESTED MITIGATING PROCEDURES**

Sociotechnical Model Dimension	Examples of Types of Possible Errors	Examples of Potential Ways to Reduce Likelihood of These Errors
Hardware and software: required to run the healthcare applications	Computer or network is not functioning Input data truncated (i.e., buffer overflow): some entered data lost	Provide redundant hardware for all essential patient care activities Warn users when data entered exceed amount that can be stored
Clinical content: data, information, and knowledge entered, displayed, or transmitted	Allowable item cannot be ordered (e.g., no amoxicillin in the antibiotic pick list) Incorrect default dose for given medication	Conduct extensive prerelease testing on all system–system data interfaces and human–computer interfaces to ensure that new features are working as planned and that existing features are working as before
Human–computer interface: aspects of the system that users can see, touch, or hear	Data entry or review screen does not show complete data (e.g., missing patient name, medical record number, birthdate) Two buttons with same label but different functionality Wrong decision about KCI administration based on poor data presentation on the computer screen	Encourage and provide methods for clinicians to report when patient-specific screens do not contain key patient demographics so that the software can be fixed Prerelease inspection of all screens for duplicate button names Improve data displays and train users to routinely review and cross-validate all data values for appropriateness before making critical decisions
People: the humans involved in the design, development, implementation, and use of HIT	Two patients with same name: data entered for wrong patient Incorrect merge of two patients' data Nurses scan duplicate patient bar code taped to their clipboard rather than bar code on patient to save time	Alert providers to potential duplicate patient names and require reconfirmation of patient identity before saving data (e.g., display patient photo before signing) Develop tools to compare key demographic data and calculate a probability estimate of similarity Improve user training, user interfaces, work processes, and organizational policies to reduce need for workarounds

(continued)

Table 13-4   EXAMPLES OF INFORMATION TECHNOLOGY–RELATED ERRORS AND CORRESPONDING SUGGESTED MITIGATING PROCEDURES (*continued*)

Sociotechnical Model Dimension	Examples of Types of Possible Errors	Examples of Potential Ways to Reduce Likelihood of These Errors
Workflow and communication: the steps needed to ensure that each patient receives the care he or she needs at the time he or she needs it	Computer discontinues a medication order without notifying a human	Implement fail-safe communication (e.g., resend message to another hospital designee if no response from physician or nurse) for all computer-generated actions
	Critical abnormal test result alerts not followed up	Implement robust quality assurance systems to monitor critical alert follow-up rates; use dual notification for alerts judiciously
Organizational policies and procedures: internal culture, structures, policies, and procedures that affect all aspects of HIT management and healthcare	Policy contradicts physical reality (e.g., required bar code medicine administration readers not available in all patient locations)	Before and after implementation, conduct inspections and interviews and monitor feedback from users in all physical locations
	Policy contradicts personnel capability (e.g., one pharmacist to verify all orders entered via CPOE in large hospital)	Before and after implementation, conduct interviews with all affected users to better gauge workload
	Incorrect policy allows "hard stops" on clinical alerts, causing delays in needed therapy	Disallow "hard stops" on almost all alerts; users should be able to override the computer in all but the most egregious cases (e.g., ordering promethazine as intravenous push by peripheral vein)
External rules, regulations, and pressures: external forces that facilitate or place constraints on the design, development, implementation, use, and evaluation of HIT in the clinical setting	Billing requirements lead to inaccurate documentation in EHR (e.g., inappropriate copy and paste)	Highlight all "pasted" material and include reference to source of material
	Joint Commission—required medication reconciliation processes causing rushed development of new medication reconciliation applications that were difficult to use and caused errors: safety goal rescinded only to be reinstated July 1, 2011	Carefully consider potential adverse unintended consequences before making new rules or regulations: conduct interviews and observations of users to gauge effects of rules and regulations on patient safety, quality of care, and clinician work life

(continued)

Table 13-4 **EXAMPLES OF INFORMATION TECHNOLOGY–RELATED ERRORS AND CORRESPONDING SUGGESTED MITIGATING PROCEDURES** *(continued)*		
Sociotechnical Model Dimension	Examples of Types of Possible Errors	Examples of Potential Ways to Reduce Likelihood of These Errors
System measurement and monitoring: evaluation of system availability, use, effectiveness, and unintended consequences of system use	Incomplete or inappropriate (e.g., combining disparate data) data aggregation leads to erroneous reporting Incorrect interpretation of quality measurement data	Increase measurement and monitoring transparency by providing involved stakeholders with access to raw data, analytical methods, and reports

Abbreviations: CPOE, computerized provider order entry; EHR, electronic health record; HIT, health information technology; KCl, potassium chloride.

Reprinted with permission from Sittig DF, Singh H. Defining health information technology–related errors: new developments since 'to err is human'. *Arch Intern Med* 2011;171:1281–1284. Copyright © 2011 American Medical Association. All rights reserved.

Like all HIT systems, BCMA has its challenges. Nurses worry that it will take too much time (although one study demonstrated that it did not[33])—and some observers have already documented workarounds (such as when a nurse takes a handful of patient wristbands and scans them outside the patient's room to save time) that bypass the systems' safety features.[34] Another concern is whether BCMA systems can be sufficiently flexible to deal with acutely ill patients.[35]

Finally, BCMA must be rooted in an environment of robust safety processes. We documented one case in which two patients (one a poorly controlled diabetic) were mistakenly given each other's bar-coded wristbands, nearly leading to a fatal insulin overdose in the nondiabetic whose computerized record erroneously indicated that he had a stratospheric blood sugar.[14] Like all IT systems, BCMA can become a very efficient error propagator if the inputted data are incorrect.

These concerns notwithstanding, effective use of BCMA technology can substantially reduce medication dispensing errors. After a long period during which bar coding was supported more by face validity than hard evidence, two studies by Poon et al. have demonstrated that bar coding really does work. The first focused on a process invisible to most doctors and nurses: the drug dispensing system in the pharmacy. There, a bar code scanning system reduced both errors and potential adverse drug events.[36] The other study, of a bedside bar coding system, is probably the more important one for the field of patient safety.[7] In it, a "closed-loop" system that combined CPOE, BCMA, and an electronic medication administration record (eMAR) led to an approximately 50% decrease in drug administration errors and potential adverse drug events.

I have come to believe that bar coding may be even more important than CPOE for hospital medication safety, at least in the short term. In the last several years, there have been a number of high-profile medication errors in the United States, virtually all involving medication administration (including the heparin dosing error that nearly killed actor Dennis Quaid's newborn twins[37]). In these cases, the problem was that there was nothing standing between a nurse and a potentially fatal mistake: no layers of metaphorical "Swiss cheese" (Chapter 2). During this same period, I cannot recall a single prescribing error that garnered similar attention.

Does this mean that prescribing errors are a thing of the past? Sadly, of course not. But even in the many hospitals and offices that lack CPOE, many prescribing errors are now avoided because physicians have access to handheld or computerized prescribing aids, allowing them to quickly look up drug indications, interactions, and dose ranges. Moreover, some of the riskiest practices—such as writing "U" for "units"—are now banned by the Joint Commission (Chapter 4).

Whether my admittedly unscientific observation is true or not, it is comforting that BCMA, which seemed like a good idea for such a long time, is now supported by robust evidence. In the end, of course, hospitals will need both BCMA *and* CPOE. The studies of Poon et al.[7,36] demonstrate the synergistic value of blending these technologies together in a "closed loop."

Smart intravenous pumps

Progress in medication safety through BCMA still leaves a large gap: the safety of medications infused intravenously. Approximately 90% of hospitalized patients receive at least one intravenous medication. Because many of these medications are far more dangerous than pills, and their doses are more variable (often calculated by the hour, or through complex weight- and size-based formulae), the opportunity for harm is real. Here again, as with BCMA, the problem is that there is no downstream opportunity to catch errors at the administration phase. Because of this, there has been considerable interest in so-called "smart intravenous pumps."

Smart pumps are engineered to have built-in danger alerts, clinical calculators, and drug libraries that include information on the standard concentrations of frequently used drugs. They also can record every infusion, creating a database that can identify risky situations and medications for future interventions. Studies have shown that these pumps can prevent many infusion errors,[38–40] but that attention must be paid to seamlessly interfacing these systems with other computerized medication systems such as CPOE and BCMA.[41]

One group of researchers compared three types of pumps—traditional pumps, smart pumps, and smart pumps with bar coding technology—and found that the smart pumps were most effective either when they had bar coding (to ensure that the pharmacy-prepared bag was the correct one for a given patient) or when "hard" (i.e., unchangeable by the bedside nurse) dosing limits were used.[42] When one considers the increasing number and complexity of intravenous infusions in hospitalized (Figure 7-1), and now even homebound, patients, perfecting this technology and working through the complex machine–person interaction issues should be high priorities.

Other IT solutions

When people think of information technology and patient safety, they generally think of EHRs, CPOE, and perhaps BCMA. It is worth adding several others to the list of IT tools that can help improve medication safety, such as "smart pumps," eMARs, and automated drug dispensing systems.[43] Once the bugs are worked out of these systems, hospitals' challenges will be to find the money to purchase, maintain, and train people on all of them, and then to weave them together into a seamless whole (Chapter 7).

It is worth pointing out that a wide range of other IT-based solutions can help improve patient safety outside the sphere of medication safety. For example, in many hospitals, staff members now wear voice-activated wireless microphones, or use modern text paging or cell phone systems— even systems modeled on Facebook and Twitter—to facilitate instant communication among caregivers. The value of IT-based sign-out systems and computer-based simulation is discussed in Chapters 8 and 17, respectively. And we shouldn't forget the importance of more clinically oriented HIT, such as the picture archiving and communication systems (PACS) that allow digital radiographs to be reviewed from a few miles, or a few thousand miles, away from the hospital or clinic.[44] In addition to their convenience, PACS can decrease x-ray interpretation errors by facilitating double reads, computerized enhancements of images, and access to prior radiographs.[45] Moving even closer to the patient, the use of handheld ultrasound can lower the risks of central line placement or thoracentesis (Chapter 5).[46,47]

COMPUTERIZED CLINICAL DECISION SUPPORT SYSTEMS

Although much of HIT's emphasis has been on replacing the paper chart and moving information around, its ultimate value may lie more in computerized clinical decision support systems (CDSS) that can provide guidance to clinicians at the point of care. For example, some systems offer simple alerts such as drug–drug, drug–allergy, or drug–lab interactions (Figure 13-1),[48] or links to evidence-based guidelines (the clinician types in a diagnosis of "pneumonia" and a link to a recent pneumonia management guideline materializes).

But that is just the start. More prescriptive decision support systems can "hard wire" certain kinds of care. For example, order sets for common diagnoses can be loaded into a CPOE system, making it easy to do the right thing by simply clicking a few boxes.[6,49] Or an intensive care unit (ICU) system can alert the physician or nurse when a patient's vital signs veer outside preset parameters (Figure 13-2). Note that these prescriptive systems usually permit clinicians to deviate from recommended protocols, but this takes more time, because the doctor needs to type out the orders

Figure 13-2 ▪ "Smart" monitoring system in an ICU. This screen highlights physiologic changes that are occurring (in this case, a rapid pulse and a trend toward increasing pulse and decreasing blood pressure [BP]); such monitoring can help clinicians detect and respond to such changes before an adverse event occurs. The heart-rate (HR) limit alert is triggered when the heart rate crosses a high (H) or low (L) limit, which are determined according to the patient's active medical conditions. Patient 5 (thick arrow) has had surgery and is at risk for perioperative coronary events. The limit value is given in brackets, followed by the patient's current value. The heart-rate or blood-pressure trend alert is triggered if the heart rate or blood pressure changes substantially over a period of several hours. Patient 4 (thin arrows) has an increasing heart rate and a decreasing blood pressure; on evaluation, this patient was found to have hypovolemia. The baseline value is given in brackets, followed by the current value. (Reproduced with permission from Bates DW, Gawande AA. Improving safety with information technology. *N Engl J Med* 2003;348:2526–2534.)

instead of accepting an order set, and may even be asked to document the reason for deviation. Even more prescriptively, the computer could all but force a given practice, making the clinician jump through several hoops (such as "call a specialist for approval") before being allowed to bypass a recommendation.

Of course, this is tricky stuff, as humans worry both about machines taking over their lives and that guidelines embedded in computer systems may not completely apply to the situation and patient at hand. Many health-care experts and providers are also troubled by the possibility that prescriptive guidelines may stand in the way of innovation or "out of the box thinking." These issues are real and will need to be worked through over time, but for healthcare systems, which are increasingly being judged on their adherence to evidence-based processes of care (Chapters 3 and 19), the level of tolerance for individual practice differences that vary from established best practices is likely to fall.

More pragmatically, one of the great challenges of CDSS systems has been *alert fatigue,* as clinicians rapidly tire of being bombarded by warnings and sometimes fail to notice even the important ones.[50] One study of approximately 5000 computerized alerts showed that clinicians overrode "critical drug interaction" and "allergy–drug interaction" alerts approximately 75% of the time.[51] And these alerts may anger clinicians, particularly if they are time-consuming to address. In one famous case, an expensive CPOE system failed partly because physicians rebelled against all the alerts.[13] As systems become more prescriptive, clinicians may also bristle at hardwired care protocols that appear to lack flexibility ("*cookbook medicine*").

All of this creates a daunting calibration challenge for designers of CDSS: making sure clinicians are alerted when appropriate but not so much that they simply learn to ignore or click out of every alert (especially the important ones). A recent *JAMA* commentary even raised the specter of physicians or health systems forestalling their purchase of CDSS systems because they fear being held liable for ignoring alerts (Chapter 18).[52] Because the experience of virtually every HIT implementation has been that the vast majority of alerts are ignored, most modern installations begin with a "less is more" philosophy: retaining the truly life-threatening, mission-critical alerts while jettisoning the "nice to know" ones. This philosophy, which has been taken to high art by Google (think about how uncluttered your Google search page is) and Apple (ditto your iPad), is deeply rooted in human factors thinking and also has implications for alarm systems in ICUs and hospital wards (Chapter 7).

Along with our growing awareness of the human factors implications of alerts, we are also starting to see the blending together of computerized systems and multidisciplinary patient safety and quality improvement programs. In

Chapter 11, I discussed a fall prevention protocol that was embedded in a computerized environment: the IT system calculated the patient's risk of falling and created a customized educational program for the patient and family, while also targeting actions for the various providers (Figure 11-2).[53] We can expect to see more of this type of integration—an exciting development.

Just as exciting, a new philosophy of "*measure-vention*" is emerging, in which real-time computerized measurement of performance is not fed back to providers one or two weeks (or one or two years) later, but immediately, allowing for "just in time" improvements. For example, one program aims to improve adherence with venous thromboembolism prophylaxis (Chapter 11) by using an electronic dashboard that captures and reports each patient's VTE prophylaxis status in real time (Figure 13-3).[54] In another application of the same principle, a real-time electronic surveillance dashboard

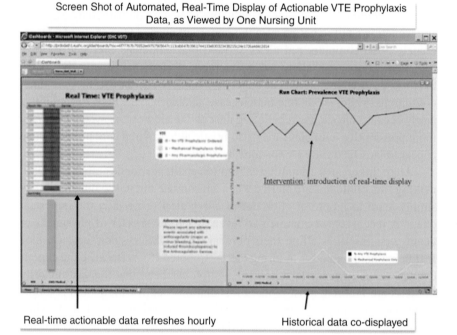

Screen Shot of Automated, Real-Time Display of Actionable VTE Prophylaxis Data, as Viewed by One Nursing Unit

Real-time actionable data refreshes hourly   Historical data co-displayed

Figure 13-3 ▪ The measure-vention strategy depicted in this figure is a real-time dashboard formatted to classify patient's VTE prophylaxis status. Each patient's status is categorized as red (no VTE prophylaxis ordered), yellow (mechanical prophylaxis only, with no pharmacologic prophylaxis), and green (pharmacologic or therapeutic anticoagulation). (Reproduced with permission from Maynard G, Stein J. Designing and implementing effective venous thromboembolism prevention protocols: lessons from collaborative efforts. *J Thromb Thrombolysis* 2009;4:81–89.)

allows pharmacists to intercept and prevent medication errors and optimize therapy.[55] These innovative strategies hold real promise for improving safety.

IT SOLUTIONS FOR IMPROVING DIAGNOSTIC ACCURACY

Finally, another type of decision support focuses on improving diagnostic accuracy (Chapter 6). Early clinical artificial intelligence programs—in which clinicians entered key elements from the history, physical examination, and laboratory studies and the computer fashioned a list of diagnosis—were disappointing, because the computer-generated diagnostic lists mixed plausible possibilities with nonsensical ones, and the data entry time (which came over and above clinical charting time) was prohibitive.[56]

Recent advances have generated new interest in diagnostic decision support. Some programs now pull data directly from the EHR, bypassing the need for redundant data entry. Others mine textbooks and journal articles to find diagnoses most frequently associated with citations of certain symptoms and signs.[57] Most modern programs not only suggest possible diagnoses but also link to helpful resources and references. The accuracy of today's top programs, such as Isabel (Figure 13-4) and DxPlain, far surpasses that of earlier models.[58,59]

Diagnostic decision support systems are likely to be judged on the seamlessness of the inputting process and the helpfulness of the diagnostic possibilities they offer. As of yet, no studies convincingly prove that these systems improve patient outcomes, but this is probably more reflective of the challenges of measuring the frequency and impact of diagnostic errors (Chapter 6) than it is of the quality or usefulness of the tools.

One can envision future computerized decision aids that draw their information directly from the EHR (though this will be challenging if patient histories remain mostly unstructured, as I discussed earlier in the chapter), produce possible diagnoses that are automatically updated with new information, and actually "learn" by integrating prior experiences from the system itself, making them ever more accurate over time. In a world in which Amazon.com helpfully suggests, "People who bought book X also liked book Y," how about a decision support system that says, "Patients at our hospital with this constellation of findings often turned out to have diagnoses X or Y"? While this might have seemed like fantasy a decade ago, anyone who observed the IBM computer "Watson" defeat the world's top *Jeopardy!* contestants became convinced that it may be just a matter of time before this kind of computerized firepower transforms the diagnostic process. Oh, and by the way, IBM is working on a medical version of its *Jeopardy!*-playing computer: "Dr. Watson."[60]

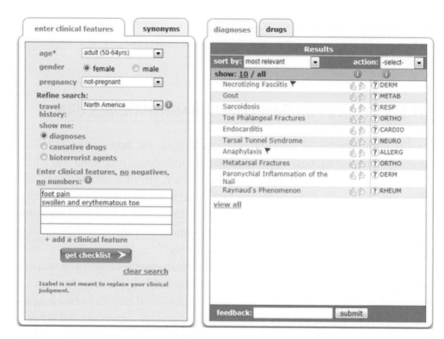

Figure 13-4 ▪ Screenshot from the Isabel diagnostic system. Signs, symptoms, and laboratory abnormalities are entered on the list on the left, and a differential diagnosis is generated. Clicking on any of the diagnoses takes the user to textbook chapters and online literature with additional information. (From http://isabelhealthcare.files.wordpress.com/2011/07/isabelblog-pic.png.)

THE POLICY ENVIRONMENT FOR HIT

The story of HIT neatly follows along the lines of what has been called the "Technology Hype Cycle" (Figure 13-5).[61] The Cycle, originally described by the consulting firm Gartner, is made up of a predictable series of phases that technologies tend to traverse after their introduction:

- "Technology Trigger": after its initial launch, the technology reaches the attention of the public and industry.
- "Peak of Inflated Expectations": A few successful applications of the technology (often by highly selected individuals or organizations—sound familiar?) catalyze unrealistic expectations, often pushed along by word of mouth, the blogosphere, or the marketing prowess of the vendor.
- "Trough of Disillusionment": Virtually no technology can live up to its initial hype. As negative experience grows, the balloon is pricked and

Figure 13-5 ▪ The Technology Hype Cycle. (Reproduced with permission from Gartner. Gartner Hype Cycle. Available at: http://www.gartner.com/technology/research/methodologies/hype-cycle.jsp.)

air rushes out. The media move on to cover another "hotter" technology, and the cycle repeats.

- ▪ "Slope of Enlightenment": A few hardy individuals and organizations, seeing the technology's true potential, begin experimenting with it, no longer burdened by inflated expectations. Assuming that the technology is worthwhile, they begin to see and demonstrate its value.
- ▪ "Plateau of Productivity": As more organizations ascend the "Slope of Enlightenment," the benefits of the technology (which has improved from its initial clunky phase based on user feedback and the self-preserving instincts of the developers) become widely demonstrated and accepted. The height of the plateau, of course, depends on the quality of the technology and the size of its market.

This cycle perfectly describes the history of CPOE (over the last 15 years) and diagnostic artificial intelligence tools (over the past 30–40 years). The hope is that these technologies—all HIT, really—are now somewhere on either the Slope of Enlightenment or the Plateau of Productivity.

In any case, while I believe that we are now more realistic about HIT's warts (and that's a good thing), there is no doubt that we *do* need to wire our healthcare system, that some speed bumps are inevitable, and that the

HIT story represents a market failure. No federal intervention was needed to get United Airlines or Wal-Mart to computerize—the business case to do so was compelling. But in healthcare, the fact that HIT systems are so complex and expensive, that many of the benefits accrue to parties other than those shelling out the money (such as insurers), and that HIT systems need to "talk to each other" (interoperability) creates a compelling case for some degree of government involvement.[62]

In the United States, the federal government is in the process (in 2012) of distributing approximately $30 billion to hospitals and community physicians who implement HIT systems that meet a variety of functionality and interoperability standards known as *"Meaningful Use"* (Table 13-5).[63,64] The presence of such support in nearly all developed countries (more directly in countries with government-run healthcare systems) signals the start of a very rapid implementation phase for HIT worldwide. Implementation is also being catalyzed by studies illustrating a positive business case[65,66] and by pressure from patient safety advocacy groups, such as the Leapfrog Group, a coalition of major business purchasers that has deemed HIT to be one of the "evidence-based safety practices" that it uses to judge hospitals.[67]

As self-help guru Tony Robbins once observed, most people overestimate what they can do in a year, and underestimate what they can do in a decade.

Table 13-5 THE CORE OBJECTIVES OF THE "MEANINGFUL USE" STANDARDS*

- Use computerized physician order entry (CPOE) for medication orders
- Implement drug–drug and drug–allergy checks
- Generate and transmit permissible prescriptions electronically
- Maintain an up-to-date problem list, active medication list, and allergy list
- Record demographics, vital signs, and smoking status
- Implement at least one clinical decision rule
- Report ambulatory clinical quality measures to CMS or to states
- Provide patients with an electronic copy of their health information, including:
  - diagnostic test results, problem list, medication lists, and medication allergies
- Provide clinical summaries of each office visit (or, for hospitals, a summary of the hospitalization)
- Have the capability to exchange key clinical information among providers of care and patient-authorized entities electronically
- Protect electronic protected health information (ePHI) created or maintained by the EHR through implementation of appropriate technical capabilities

Abbreviations: CMS, Centers for Medicare & Medicaid Services.

*Specific features of an EHR that providers will be required to use to qualify for incentive payments under the HITECH Act.[63,64]

In the case of HIT, this is likely to be an accurate assessment. While adoption will continue to occur in fits and starts for the next few years, a decade from now HIT systems will have transformed much of the safety enterprise, if not all of healthcare. If the systems mature and developers and implementers learn from past mistakes, this will be decidedly for the better.

KEY POINTS

- The implementation of HIT has been remarkably slow until recently, but the pace is beginning to accelerate, driven by a growing business case and government incentives.
- Many healthcare activities require multiple providers (and others) to view patient-level information simultaneously, a powerful argument for EHRs.
- CPOE can ensure that physicians' orders are legible and respect preset parameters.
- Bar coding or other similar systems can help decrease the frequency of medication administration (and other patient identification–related) errors.
- Ultimately, much of the benefit of HIT will come through the thoughtful implementation of computerized decision support, which ranges from simply providing information to clinicians at the point of care to more prescriptive systems that "hardwire" certain care processes.
- While HIT has tremendous appeal, its history to date has been characterized by a surprising number of failures and unanticipated consequences, illustrating the importance of human factors and the challenges of implementing major changes in complex organizations.

REFERENCES

1. Jha AK, Desroches CM, Campbell EG, et al. Use of electronic health records in US hospitals. *N Engl J Med* 2009;360:1628–1638.
2. DesRoches CM, Campbell EG, Rao SR, et al. Electronic health records in ambulatory care—a national survey of physicians. *N Engl J Med* 2008;359:50–60.
3. Jha AK, Perlin JB, Kizer KW, Dudley RA. Effect of the transformation of the Veterans Affairs Health Care System on the quality of care. *N Engl J Med* 2003;348:2218–2227.
4. Bates DW, Gawande AA. Improving safety with information technology. *N Engl J Med* 2003;348:2526–2534.

5. Rothschild JM, Keohane CA, Cook EF, et al. A controlled trial of smart infusion pumps to improve medication safety in critically ill patients. *Crit Care Med* 2005;33: 533–540.

6. Kucher N, Koo S, Quiroz R, et al. Electronic alerts to prevent venous thromboembolism among hospitalized patients. *N Engl J Med* 2005;352:969–977.

7. Poon EG, Keohane CA, Yoon CS, et al. Effect of bar-code technology on the safety of medication administration. *N Engl J Med* 2010;362:1698–1707.

8. Longhurst CA, Parast L, Sandborg CI, et al. Decrease in hospital-wide mortality rate after implementation of a commercially sold computerized physician order entry system. *Pediatrics* 2010;126:14–21.

9. Shojania KG, Duncan BW, McDonald KM, et al. Safe but sound: patient safety meets evidence-based medicine. *JAMA* 2002;288:508–513.

10. Wachter RM, Shojania KG. *Internal Bleeding: The Truth Behind America's Terrifying Epidemic of Medical Mistakes.* New York, NY: Rugged Land; 2004.

11. Koppel R, Metlay JP, Cohen A, et al. Role of computerized physician order entry systems in facilitating medication errors. *JAMA* 2005;293:1197–1203.

12. Han YY, Carcillo JA, Venkataraman ST, et al. Unexpected increased mortality after implementation of a commercially sold computerized physician order entry system. *Pediatrics* 2005;116:1506–1512.

13. Wachter RM. Expected and unanticipated consequences of the quality and information technology revolutions. *JAMA* 2006;295:2780–2783.

14. McDonald CJ. Computerization can create safety hazards: a bar-coding near miss. *Ann Intern Med* 2006;144:510–516.

15. Sittig DF, Singh H. Defining health information technology–related errors: new developments since 'to err is human'. *Arch Intern Med* 2011;171:1281–1284.

16. Nanji KC, Rothschild JM, Salzberg C, et al. Errors associated with outpatient computerized prescribing systems. *J Am Med Inform Assoc* 2011;18:767–773.

17. Poissant L, Pereira J, Tamblyn R, et al. The impact of electronic health records on time efficiency of physicians and nurses: a systematic review. *J Am Med Inform Assoc* 2005;12:505–516.

18. Hirschtick RE. A piece of my mind. Copy-and-paste. *JAMA* 2006;295:2335–2336.

19. Thielke S, Hammond K, Helbig S. Copying and pasting of examinations within the electronic medical record. *Int J Med Inform* 2007;76(suppl 1):122–128.

20. Siegler EL, Adelman R. Copy and paste: a remediable hazard of electronic health records. *Am J Med* 2009;122:495–496.

21. Rosenbloom ST, Denny JC, Xu H, et al. Data from clinical notes: a perspective on the tension between structure and flexible documentation. *J Am Med Inform Assoc* 2011;18:181–186.

22. Johnson SB, Bakken S, Dine D, et al. An electronic health record based on structured narrative. *J Am Med Inform Assoc* 2008;15:54–64.

23. Tang PC, Lansky D. The missing link: bridging the patient–provider health information gap. *Health Aff (Millwood)* 2005;24:1290–1295.

24. Tang PC, Lee TH. Your doctor's office or the Internet? Two paths to personal health records. *N Engl J Med* 2009;360:1276–1278.

25. Archer N, Fevrier-Thomas U, Lokker C, et al. Personal health records: a scoping review. *J Am Med Inform Assoc* 2011;18:515–522.

26. Halamka JD, Mandl KD, Tang PC. Early experiences with personal health records. *J Am Med Inform Assoc* 2008;15:1–7.
27. Verghese A. Culture shock—patient as icon, icon as patient. *N Engl J Med* 2008; 359:2748–2751.
28. Bates DW, Leape LL, Cullen DJ, et al. Effect of computerized physician order entry and a team intervention on prevention of serious medication errors. *JAMA* 1998;280:1311–1316.
29. Bates DW, Teich JM, Lee J, et al. The impact of computerized physician order entry on medication error prevention. *J Am Med Inform Assoc* 1999;6:313–321.
30. Boling B, McKibben M, Hingl J, et al.; Clinical Informatics Outcomes Research Group. Effectiveness of computerized provider order entry with dose range checking on prescribing errors. *J Patient Saf* 2005;1:190–194.
31. Overhage JM, Tierney WM, Zhou XH, et al. A randomized trial of "corollary orders" to prevent errors of omission. *J Am Med Inform Assoc* 1997;4:364–375.
32. Wright AA, Katz IT. Bar coding for patient safety. *N Engl J Med* 2005;454:329–331.
33. Poon EG, Keohane CA, Bane A, et al. Impact of barcode medication administration technology on how nurses spend their time providing patient care. *J Nurs Adm* 2008;38:541–549.
34. Koppel R, Wetterneck T, Telles JL, et al. Workarounds to barcode medication administration systems: their occurrences, causes, and threats to patient safety. *J Am Med Inform Assoc* 2008;15:408–423.
35. Patterson ES, Cook RI, Render ML. Improving patient safety by identifying side effects from introducing bar coding in medication administration. *J Am Med Inform Assoc* 2002;9:540–553.
36. Poon EG, Cina JL, Churchill W, et al. Medication dispensing errors and potential adverse drug events before and after implementing bar code technology in the pharmacy. *Ann Intern Med* 2006;145:426–434.
37. Grant M. Dennis Quaid's quest. *AARP The Magazine.* September/October 2010;53: 48–51, 90–91.
38. Keohane CA, Hayes J, Saniuk C, et al. Intravenous medication safety and smart infusion systems: lessons learned and future opportunities. *J Infus Nurs* 2005;28: 321–328.
39. Larsen GY, Parker HB, Cash J, et al. Standard drug concentrations and smart-pump technology reduce continuous-medication-infusion errors in pediatric patients. *Pediatrics* 2005;116:e21–e25.
40. Williams CK, Maddox RR, Heape E, et al. Application of the IV Medication Harm Index to assess the nature of harm averted by "smart" infusion safety systems. *J Patient Saf* 2006;2:132–139.
41. Husch M, Sullivan C, Rooney D, et al. Insights from the sharp end of intravenous medication errors: implications for infusion pump technology. *Qual Saf Health Care* 2005;14:80–86.
42. Trbovich PL, Pinkney S, Cafazzo JA, et al. The impact of traditional and smart pump infusion technology on nurse medication administration performance in a simulated inpatient unit. *Qual Saf Health Care* 2010;19:430–434.
43. Chapuis C, Roustit M, Bal G, et al. Automated drug dispensing system reduces medication errors in an intensive care setting. *Crit Care Med* 2010;38:2275–2281.

44. Wachter RM. International teleradiology. *N Engl J Med* 2006;354:662–663.

45. Bryan S, Weatherburn G, Buxton M, et al. Evaluation of a hospital picture archiving and communication system. *J Health Serv Res Policy* 1999;4:204–209.

46. Rothschild JM. Ultrasound guidance of central vein catheterization. In: Shojania KG, Duncan BW, McDonald KM, et al., eds. *Making Health Care Safer: A Critical Analysis of Patient Safety Practices.* Evidence Report/Technology Assessment No. 43, AHRQ Publication No. 01-E058. Rockville, MD: Agency for Healthcare Research and Quality; July 2001.

47. Duncan DR, Morgenthaler TI, Ryu JH, et al. Reducing iatrogenic risk in thoracentesis: establishing best practice via experiential training in a zero-risk environment. *Chest* 2009;135:1315–1320.

48. Classen DC, Phansalkar S, Bates DW. Critical drug–drug interactions for use in electronic health records systems with computerized physician order entry: review of leading approaches. *J Patient Saf* 2011;7:61–65.

49. Garg AX, Adhikari NK, McDonald H, et al. Effects of computerized clinical decision support systems on practitioner performance and patient outcomes: a systematic review. *JAMA* 2005;293:1223–1238.

50. Kuperman GJ, Bobb A, Payne TH, et al. Medication-related clinical decision support in computerized provider order entry systems: a review. *J Am Med Inform Assoc* 2007;14:29–40.

51. Payne TH, Nichol WP, Hoey P, et al. Characteristics and override rates of order checks in a practitioner order entry system. *Proc AMIA Symp* 2002;2002:602–606.

52. Greenberg M, Ridgely MS. Clinical decision support and malpractice risk. *JAMA* 2011;306:90–91.

53. Dykes PC, Carroll DL, Hurley A, et al. Fall prevention in acute care hospitals. A randomized trial. *JAMA* 2010;304:1912–1918.

54. Maynard G, Stein J. Designing and implementing effective venous thromboembolism prevention protocols: lessons from collaborative efforts. *J Thromb Thrombolysis* 2009;4:81–89.

55. Waitman LR, Phillips IE, McCoy AB, et al. Adopting real-time surveillance dashboards as a component of an enterprise-wide medication safety strategy. *Jt Comm J Qual Patient Saf* 2011;37:326–332.

56. Berner ES, Webster GD, Shuerman AA, et al. Performance of four computer-based diagnostic systems. *N Engl J Med* 1994;330:1792–1796.

57. Ramnarayan P, Winrow A, Coren M, et al. Diagnostic omission errors in acute paediatric practice: impact of a reminder system on decision-making. *BMC Med Inform Decis Mak* 2006;6:37.

58. Bond WF, Schwartz LM, Weaver KR, et al. Differential diagnosis generators: an evaluation of currently available computer programs. *J Gen Intern Med* July 26, 2011 [Epub ahead of print].

59. Graber ML, Mathew A. Performance of a web-based clinical diagnosis support system for internists. *J Gen Intern Med* 2008;23(suppl 1):37–40.

60. Dolan PL. Fresh from "Jeopardy!" victory, Watson to take on health care. *American Medical News.* March 14, 2011. Available at: http://www.ama-assn.org/amednews/2011/03/14/bisa0314.htm.

61. Gartner Hype Cycle. Available at: http://www.gartner.com/technology/research/ methodologies/hype-cycle.jsp.

62. Poon EG, Blumenthal D, Jaggi T, et al. Overcoming barriers to adopting and implementing computerized physician order entry systems in U.S. hospitals. *Health Aff (Millwood)* 2004;23:184–190.

63. Blumenthal D. Launching HITECH. *N Engl J Med* 2010;362:382–385.

64. Blumenthal D, Tavenner M. The "meaningful use" regulations for electronic health records. *N Engl J Med* 2010;363:501–504.

65. Kaushal R, Jha AK, Franz C, et al. Return on investment for a computerized physician order entry system. *J Am Med Inform Assoc* 2006;13:261–266.

66. Byrne CM, Mercincavage LM, Pan EC, et al. The value from investments in health information technology at the U.S. Department of Veterans Affairs. *Health Aff (Millwood)* 2010;29:629–638.

67. Galvin RS, Delbanco S, Milstein A, et al. Has the Leapfrog Group had an impact on the health care market? *Health Aff (Millwood)* 2005;24:228–233.

ADDITIONAL READINGS

Agency for Healthcare Research and Quality. *Advances in Patient Safety: New Directions and Alternative Approaches.* Rockville, MD: Agency for Healthcare Research and Quality; July 2008. AHRQ Publication No. 080034 (1–4).

Ash JS, Berg M, Coiera E. Some unintended consequences of information technology in health care: the nature of patient care information system-related errors. *J Am Med Inform Assoc* 2004;11:104–112.

Aspden P, Wolcott J, Bootman JL, et al., eds. *Preventing Medication Errors: Quality Chasm Series.* Committee on Identifying and Preventing Medication Errors. Washington, DC: National Academy Press; 2007.

Black AD, Car J, Pagliari C, et al. The impact of eHealth on the quality and safety of health care: a systematic overview. *PLoS Med* 2011;8:e1000387.

Classen DC, Bates DW. Finding the meaning in meaningful use. *N Engl J Med* 2011; 365:855–858.

Committee on Patient Safety and Health Information Technology, Board on Health Care Services, Institute of Medicine. *Health IT and Patient Safety: Building Safer Systems for Better Care.* Washington, DC: National Academies Press; 2011.

Cutler DM, Feldman NE, Horwitz JR. U.S. adoption of computerized physician order entry systems. *Health Aff (Millwood)* 2005;24:1654–1663.

Hunt DL, Haynes RB, Hanna SE, et al. Effects of computer-based clinical decision support systems on physician performance and patient outcomes: a systematic review. *JAMA* 1998;280:1339–1346.

Jha AK. The promise of electronic records. Around the corner or down the road? *JAMA* 2011;306:880–881.

Kuperman GJ, Gibson RF. Computerized physician order entry: benefits, costs, and issues. *Ann Intern Med* 2003;39:31–39.

Shekelle PG, Morton SC, Keeler EB. *Costs and Benefits of Health Information Technology.* Evidence Report/Technology Assessment No. 132. Prepared by the Southern California Evidence-based Practice Center under contract no. 290-02-0003. Rockville, MD: Agency for Healthcare Research and Quality; April 2006. AHRQ Publication No. 06-E006.

Singh H, Thomas EJ, Mani S, et al. Timely follow-up of abnormal diagnostic imaging test results in an outpatient setting: are electronic medical records achieving their potential? *Arch Intern Med* 2009;169:1578–1586.

Stires D. Technology has transformed the VA. *Fortune Magazine.* May 15, 2006:130–132, 134, 136.

REPORTING SYSTEMS, ROOT CAUSE ANALYSIS, AND OTHER METHODS OF UNDERSTANDING SAFETY ISSUES

14

OVERVIEW

In the late 1990s, as patients, reporters, and legislators began to appreciate the scope of the medical errors problem, the response was nearly Pavlovian: we need more reporting! This commonsensical appeal had roots in several places, including the knowledge that transparency often drives change, the positive experiences with reporting in the commercial aviation industry,[1] the desire by many interested parties (patients, legislators, the media, healthcare leaders) to understand the dimensions of the safety problem, and the need of individual healthcare organizations to know which problems to work on.

I'll begin this chapter by focusing on reporting within the walls of a healthcare delivery organization such as a hospital or clinic. I'll then widen the lens to consider extra-institutional reporting systems. Further discussion on these issues, from somewhat different perspectives, can be found in Chapters 3, 20, and 22.

The systems to capture local reports are generally known as *incident reporting* (IR) *systems*. Incident reports come from frontline personnel (e.g., the nurse, pharmacist, or physician caring for a patient when a medication error occurred) rather than, say, from supervisors. From the perspective of those receiving the data, IR systems are *passive* forms of surveillance, relying on involved parties to choose to report. More *active* methods of surveillance, such as retrospective chart review, direct observation, and trigger tools, have already been addressed in Chapter 1, though I'll have more to say about them later in this chapter.

Although IR systems capture only a fraction of incidents, they have the advantages of relatively low cost and the involvement of caregivers in the process of identifying important problems for the organization. Yet the experience with them has been disappointing—while well-organized IR systems can yield important insights, they can also waste substantial resources, drain provider goodwill, and divert attention from more important problems.[2]

I believe that the following realities should frame discussions of the role of reporting in patient safety:

- Errors occur one at a time, to individual patients—often already quite ill—scattered around hospitals, nursing homes, and doctors' offices. This generates tremendous opportunity to cover up errors, and requires that providers be engaged in efforts to promote transparency.
- Because reporting errors takes time and can lead to shame and (particularly in the United States) legal liability, providers who choose to report need to be protected from unfair blame, public embarrassment, and legal risk.
- Reporting systems need to be easy to access and use, and reporting must yield palpable improvements. Busy caregivers are not likely to report if systems are burdensome to use or reports seem to disappear into the dark corners of a bureaucracy.
- Many different stakeholders need to hear about and learn from errors. However, doctors, nurses, hospital administrators, educators, researchers, regulators, legislators, the media, and patients all have different levels of understanding and may need to see very different types of reports. This diversity makes error reporting particularly challenging.
- Although most errors do reflect systems problems, some *can* be attributed to bad providers. The public—and those charged with defending the public's interest, such as licensing and credentialing boards—have a legitimate need to learn of these cases and take appropriate (including disciplinary) action (Chapter 19).
- Similarly, even when the problem is systemic and not one of "bad apples," the public has a right to know about systems that are sufficiently unsafe that a reasonable person would hesitate before receiving care from them.
- Medical errors are so breathtakingly common that the admonition to "report everything" is silly. In the care of the average intensive care unit patient, 1.7 errors are made each day, and the average hospitalized patient experiences one medication error per day.[3] A system that captured every error and near miss would quickly accumulate unmanageable mountains of data, require boatloads of analysts, and result in caregivers spending much of their time reporting and digesting the results instead of caring for patients.

Taken together, these "facts on the ground" mean that error reporting, while conceptually attractive, must be approached thoughtfully. IR systems need to be easy to use, nonpunitive, and manned by people skilled at analyzing the data and putting them to use. The energy and resources invested in designing action plans that respond to IRs should match the level of energy and resources invested in the IR system itself. After all, the goal of an IR system is not data collection but meaningful improvements in safety and quality.

There is yet another cautionary note to be sounded regarding IR systems: voluntary reporting systems cannot be used to derive rates—of errors, or harm, or anything, really.[4] I know this because I periodically visit hospitals and look at their IR reporting trends. If the reports have gone up by, let's say, 20% in the past year, they invariably tell me, "Look at these numbers. You see, we've established a culture of reporting, and people are confident that reports lead to action. We're getting safer!"

That sounds great until I visit a comparable institution, but one whose IR volume has fallen recently. "This is great," they always say. "We've had fewer errors!" The problem is obvious: I have absolutely no way of knowing which explanation is correct, and neither do you.

Given the limitations of IR systems, healthcare organizations need to employ other techniques to capture errors and identify risky situations.[5,6] This chapter will cover a few of them, including *failure mode and effects analysis* and *trigger tools*. Errors and adverse events that *are* reported must be put to good use, such as by turning them into stories that are shared within organizations, in forums such as *Morbidity and Mortality (M&M) conferences*. Finally, errors that are of particular concern—often called *sentinel events*—must be analyzed in a way that rapidly generates the maximum amount of institutional learning and catalyzes the appropriate changes. The method of doing this is known as *root cause analysis* (RCA). The following sections discuss each of these issues and techniques.

GENERAL CHARACTERISTICS OF REPORTING SYSTEMS

Error reports, whether filed on paper or through the Web, and whether routed to the hospital's safety officer or to a federal regulator, can be divided into three main categories: anonymous, confidential, and open. *Anonymous reports* are ones in which there is no identifying information asked of the reporter. Although they have the advantage of encouraging reporting, anonymous systems have the disadvantage of preventing necessary follow-up questions from being answered. In a *confidential reporting system,* the identity of the reporter is known but shielded from authorities such as regulators and representatives of the legal system (except in cases of clear professional misconduct or criminal acts). Such systems tend to capture more useful data than anonymous systems, because follow-up questions can be asked. The key to these systems, of course, is that reporters must trust that they are truly confidential. Finally, in *open reporting systems* all people and places are publicly identified. These systems have a relatively poor track record in healthcare, because the potential for unwanted publicity and blame is very strong, and it is often easy for individuals to cover up errors (even with "mandatory" reporting).

Another distinguishing feature of reporting systems is the organizational entity that receives the reports. With that in mind, let's first consider the local hospital system—the IR system—before expanding the discussion to systems that move reports to other entities beyond the clinical organization's walls.

HOSPITAL INCIDENT REPORTING SYSTEMS

Hospitals have long had IR systems, but prior to the patient safety movement these systems received little attention. Traditional IR systems relied on providers—nearly always nurses (most studies show that nurse reports outnumber physician reports by at least five to one[7])—to fill out paper reports. The reports generally went to the hospital's risk manager, whose main concern was often to limit his or her institution's potential legal liability (Chapter 18). There was little emphasis on systems improvement, and dissemination of incidents to others in the system (other managers, caregivers, educators) was unusual. Most clinicians felt that reporting was a waste of time, and so few did it.

IR systems have become far more important in the past decade, but until recently have been studied insufficiently. Based on a 2008 survey of 1600 U.S. hospitals' error reporting systems, Farley et al. described four key components of effective systems (Table 14-1). Unfortunately, they found that only a minority of hospitals met these criteria.[8] Specifically, only a small fraction of hospitals showed evidence of a safety culture that encouraged

Table 14-1   **CHARACTERISTICS OF AN EFFECTIVE REPORTING SYSTEM**
▪ Institution must have a supportive environment for event reporting that protects the privacy of staff who report occurrences.
▪ Reports should be received from a broad range of personnel.
▪ Summaries of reported events must be disseminated in a timely fashion.
▪ A structured mechanism must be in place for reviewing reports and developing action plans.

Reproduced with permission from Farley DO, Haviland A, Champagne S, et al. Adverse-event-reporting practices by US hospitals: results of a national survey. *Qual Saf Health Care* 2008;17:416–423.

reporting, properly analyzed error reports, and effectively disseminated the results of these analyses.

These failures are not for lack of effort or, in many hospitals, lack of investment. In fact, many hospitals have invested heavily in their IR systems, mostly in the form of new computerized infrastructure. However, the resources and focus needed to change the culture around incident reporting and management, to properly analyze reports, and to create useful and durable action plans have been less forthcoming.[2]

That said, the computerized systems do have their advantages. For example, most systems now allow any provider to submit an incident and categorize it by error type (e.g., medication error, patient fall; Table 14-2) and level of harm (e.g., no harm, minimal harm, serious harm, death). In confidential systems, the reporter can be contacted electronically to provide additional detail

---

Table 14-2   TYPICAL MAJOR CATEGORIES IN A HOSPITAL IR SYSTEM

- Anesthesia issues
- Behavior management (including restraint use/seclusion)
- Cardiac and respiratory arrest
- Confidentiality and consent issues
- Controlled substance issues
- Diagnosis/treatment issues
- Dietary services
- Environmental safety
- Falls/injuries (involving patients)
- Home care issues
- Infection control (including blood-borne pathogens, isolation issues)
- IVs, tubes, catheter, and drain issues (including broken, infiltrated catheters)
- Laboratory results (including result errors, tests not performed, wrong specimens)
- Medical devices (including device malfunction, improper use)
- Medication-related events (including errors, delays, and adverse drug reactions)
- Patient flow issues
- Patient property loss
- Radiology issues
- Security issues
- Skin issues (including pressure ulcers)
- Surgical issues (including death in operating room, retained objects, unplanned return to OR)
- Sterile processing issues
- Skin issues
- Transfusion issues
- Unprofessional staff behavior

if needed. Computerized systems also make it easy to create aggregate statistics about reports, although it is important to reemphasize that voluntary systems are incapable of providing accurate error rates.[3]

Probably most importantly, incident reports can be routed to the managers positioned to take action or spot trends (unfortunately, not all computerized IR systems have this functionality). For example, when an error pertaining to the medical service is reported through the hospital's computerized IR system at UCSF—my hospital—the system automatically sends an e-mail to me as chief of the service, as well as the service's head nurse, the hospital's risk manager, the "category manager" (an appropriate individual is assigned to each item in Table 14-2), and the hospital's director of patient safety. Each of us can review the error, have a discussion about it (orally or within the IR system's computerized environment), and document the action we took in response.

Although this represents great progress, it is important to appreciate the amount of time, skill, and energy all of these functions require. Many hospitals have built or purchased fancy IR systems, exhorted their staff to "report everything—errors, near misses, everything," and then found themselves overwhelmed by thousands of reports. I'd much rather see a system that received fewer reports but acted on those reports promptly and effectively than one with far more reports that end up in the black hole of a hospital's hard drive. As you see, developing thoughtful ways to manage data overload—whether the goal is to prevent alert fatigue in a CPOE system (Chapter 13) or to handle thousands of error reports—is an overarching theme in the field of patient safety.

In an increasingly computerized environment and with the advent of trigger tools and other new methods of identifying cases of error and harm, some patient safety experts are starting to question the role of voluntary error reporting by frontline personnel. For example, some wonder whether every medication error and every fall really need to be reported through an IR system. My answer is no. Perhaps we should be sampling common error categories in depth for short periods of time (i.e., monthly). I can envision a system in which January is Falls Month, February is Pressure Ulcer Month, and so on. I am confident that a hospital employing this strategy would learn everything it needed to know about its latent errors (Chapter 1) in these areas after such a sampling.[9]

On the other hand, organizations *do* need ways to disseminate the lessons they have learned from serious errors and to understand their error patterns in order to plan strategically (Chapter 22), to meet regulatory reporting requirements (Chapter 20), and to pursue their risk management and error disclosure responsibilities (Chapter 18). Given these realities, IR systems must be improved, not abolished. This is clearly an area sorely in need of fresh thinking.

THE AVIATION SAFETY REPORTING SYSTEM

Turning to reports that "leave the building," the pressure to build statewide or federal reporting systems grew in part (like so much of the patient safety field) from the experience of commercial aviation.[1,10] As we consider extra-institutional reporting systems, it is worth reflecting on whether this particular aviation analogy is apt.

On December 1, 1974, a Trans World Airlines (TWA) flight crashed into the side of a small mountain in Virginia, killing all 92 passengers and crew. As tragic as the crash was, the subsequent investigation added insult to injury, because the problems leading to the crash (poorly defined minimum altitudes on the Dulles Airport approach) were well known to many pilots but not widely disseminated. A year later, the Federal Aviation Administration (FAA) launched the *Aviation Safety Reporting System* (ASRS). Importantly, recognizing that airline personnel might be hesitant to report errors and near misses to their primary regulator, FAA contracted with a third party (NASA) to run the system and broadcast its lessons to the industry.

There is general agreement that the ASRS is one of the main reasons for aviation's remarkable safety record (a 10-fold decrease in fatalities over the past generation; Figure 9-1). Five attributes of the ASRS have helped create these successes: ease of reporting, confidentiality, third-party administration, timely analysis and feedback, and the possibility of regulatory action. The ASRS rules are straightforward: if anyone witnesses a near miss (note an important difference from healthcare: non-near misses in aviation—that is, crashes—don't need a reporting system, because they appear on the news within minutes), that person *must* report it to ASRS within 10 days. The reporter is initially identified so that he or she can be contacted, if needed, by ASRS personnel; the identifying information is subsequently destroyed. In over 30 years of operation, there have been no reported confidentiality breaches of the system. Trained ASRS personnel analyze the reports for patterns, and they have several pathways to disseminate key information or trigger actions (including grounding airplanes or shutting down airports, if necessary).

Even as healthcare tries to emulate these successes, it is worth highlighting some key differences between its problems and those of commercial aviation. The biggest is the scale of the two enterprises and their errors.[10] Notwithstanding its extraordinary effort to encourage reporting, the ASRS receives about 35,000 reports per year, across the entire U.S. commercial aviation system.[11,12] If all errors and near misses were being reported in American healthcare, this would almost certainly result in more than 35,000 reports *per day*—over 10 million reports per year! My own 600-bed hospital generates 15,000 yearly reports, and (a) we don't report everything, (b) we are one of

6000 hospitals in the country, and (c) you would need to add in the errors and adverse events from nonhospital facilities and ambulatory practices to come up with an overall estimate. There are simply many more things that go wrong in the healthcare system than in the aviation system. This makes prioritizing and managing error reports a much knottier problem for us than it is in aviation.

REPORTS TO ENTITIES OUTSIDE THE HEALTHCARE ORGANIZATION

As the patient safety field gained momentum, the pressure to report errors or harm beyond the walls of provider institutions grew rapidly, driven in part by the inspiring example of the ASRS. By 2008, 26 U.S. states had implemented mandatory reporting programs, to which some hospital errors must be reported.[13,14] Of these, 23 states used the data to hold individual hospitals accountable (such as by inspecting hospitals after reports or levying fines) and 18 states had established learning systems, drawn largely from error reports.

The best approach to reporting outside the walls of the provider institution—to states, federal authorities, or other regulators and accreditors—remains unsettled and controversial. In most cases, states have mandated reporting of only serious errors or adverse events, such as those on the National Quality Forum's list of serious reportable events (sometimes called the "Never Events" list; Appendix VI and Chapter 20).

Other regulators have taken a broader approach to reporting. For example, Pennsylvania requires hospitals to report all "serious events," "incidents," and hospital-acquired infections. In 2009, it received its one millionth submission. Similarly, the UK's National Patient Safety Agency (NPSA) has had a national reporting system for "patient safety incidents" in England and Wales since 2004. The NPSA (which was slated for decommissioning by the Cameron government in 2012) received one million reports *in the year 2007 alone!* Of course, these reporting systems (which were created by legislative action) employ good people trying to do their best to manage these overwhelming data and turn them into something useful. Pennsylvania, for example, publishes a quarterly newsletter that describes important errors and patterns gleaned from the reports.[15]

But I remain skeptical that broad-scale, "report everything"–type state or federal systems will be worth the substantial resources they require. I am much more enthusiastic about the limited approach to reporting pioneered by Minnesota, which in 2005 began to require hospitals (and later ambulatory surgical centers) to report only those cases of error or harm that rose to the level of the "Never Events" list (Appendix VI). In 2010, Minnesota received 305 such reports, a much more manageable number than Pennsylvania's hundreds of thousands. In my view, Minnesota's analyses of its database, and the programs it has developed in response to these reports,[16] are as useful as Pennsylvania's, with a savings of many thousands of person-hours of both reporting and analysis time.

Before leaving the subject of outside reporting systems, it is worth highlighting several specialized reporting systems that have made important contributions to patient safety. For example, the MEDMARX voluntary error reporting system and the system maintained by the Institute for Safe Medication Practices (ISMP) have led to valuable insights about medication errors (Chapter 4).[17,18] Useful research and analysis has also come out of specialty reporting systems such as the ICU Safety Reporting System developed by Johns Hopkins and an online surgical reporting system at Northwestern University.[19,20] Finally, my colleagues and I produce a Web site, *AHRQ WebM&M*,[21] which is, at its core, a reporting and learning system.[22] We receive confidential anonymous reports of cases of medical errors or adverse events, and choose three interesting ones to post each month, accompanied by an expert commentary (Figure 14-1). The site receives approximately 1.5 million unique visits yearly. Further illustrating the point that the question is not how many reports you receive but what you do with them, over the eight year history of *WebM&M* we have received only about 600 case report submissions, not a huge number but easily enough to cull three useful cases each month.

To this observer, the lessons are clear: as with hospital IR systems, reporting is not a numbers game where the person or system with the most reports "wins." Rather, the goal is the most efficient system that produces the greatest amount of learning and productive change. I believe that external reporting works best when the reports are confidential and cover only a limited universe of serious events (i.e., events on the NQF list). This too is an area that is begging for innovative approaches and rigorous research.

PATIENT SAFETY ORGANIZATIONS

In 2005, the U.S. Congress passed the Patient Safety and Quality Improvement Act, which authorized the creation of *patient safety organizations* (PSOs) to encourage "voluntary, provider-driven initiatives to improve the safety and quality of patient care." The U.S. Agency for Healthcare Research and Quality (AHRQ) was charged with overseeing the development of PSOs, private or public entities that agree to adhere to common reporting standards and are granted federal protection for shared data.[23]

AHRQ has published its criteria for becoming a PSO: they include a signed commitment to collect and analyze patient safety data for the purposes of improving healthcare and the presence of robust confidentiality and privacy

Figure 14-1 ■ Screenshot of the home page of the July 2011 edition of *AHRQ WebM&M*. (Available at: http://webmm.ahrq.gov/. Reproduced with permission.)

Table 14-3 **EXAMPLES OF PATIENT SAFETY ORGANIZATIONS (PSOs) CERTIFIED BY AHRQ***	
Type of Organization	**Representative Examples**
State hospital associations or state safety organizations	Maryland Patient Safety Center, Texas PSO
Large healthcare delivery systems	Baptist Health Patient Safety Partnership, Ascension Health PSO
Malpractice carriers	MCIC Vermont, Academic Medical Center PSO (an entity of the Risk Management Foundation of Harvard Medical Institutions)
Medical specialty societies	Society of Hospital Medicine PSO, Society for Vascular Surgery PSO
Private provider networks	Cogent PSO, Emergency Consultants PSO
Private vendors	GE PSO (information technology vendor), Quantros Patient Safety Center (computerized incident reporting system vendor)

*As of December 2011, 76 organizations had been officially listed as PSOs by the Agency for Healthcare Research and Quality. The full list is available at: http://www.pso.ahrq.gov/listing/psolist.htm.

protections.[24] As of December 2011, 76 organizations, including state hospital associations, large healthcare provider networks, and information technology and data management companies, had been certified (Table 14-3).[25] In addition, AHRQ has developed a set of common definitions and reporting formats (the "Common Format") to facilitate the collection and analysis of safety events.

In exchange for voluntarily becoming a PSO, organizations receive robust legal protections for their patient safety and quality data. This is particularly important in some states, which—in a misguided effort to promote public accountability—have stripped away all prior protections for peer review and quality improvement data. In one (Florida), the passage of such legislation promptly led most hospitals, fearful of liability, to discontinue error analysis and learning sessions such as M&M conferences.[26]

While PSOs are a welcome option (particularly in light of these legal issues), their impact on safety remains unclear. Given how difficult it is for even a single hospital to effectively manage its own incident reports and disseminate the lessons from them without being overwhelmed by an avalanche of data, a healthy skepticism about the ability of 5 hospitals—or 50—to do this successfully is warranted.

ROOT CAUSE ANALYSIS AND OTHER INCIDENT INVESTIGATION METHODS

After we learn of a significant error, what should we do? The technique of *root cause analysis* (RCA) involves a deliberate, comprehensive dissection of an error, laying bare all of the relevant facts and searching assiduously for underlying ("root") causes rather than being satisfied by facile explanations (such as "the doctor pulled the wrong chart" or "the pharmacist stocked the wrong medicine"). Some U.S. states now require RCAs after serious events (and require that reports from them be submitted along with error notifications),[13,14] and the Joint Commission mandates an RCA after every "sentinel event."

To ensure that RCAs are maximally productive, certain elements appear to be important:

1. *Strong leadership and facilitation*: it is easy for an RCA to drift away from the search for root causes and toward the assignment of blame. The leader must be skilled at steering the conversation toward key systems defects, including complex and potentially charged issues involving culture and communication. The use of a structured tool to prompt participants to consider the full range of potential contributing factors can be helpful (Table 2-1).[27–29]

2. *An interdisciplinary approach*: the RCA committee should include representatives of all of the relevant disciplines (at a minimum, physicians, nurses, pharmacists, and administrators). In addition, a risk manager is often present and generally helpful, although the discussion should focus on what can be learned from the error rather than on how to reduce the institution's liability. In larger organizations, content experts (such as in information technology and human factors) can add their insights.

3. *Individuals who participated in the case should be invited to "tell their stories."* These discussions can be highly emotional, and the RCA leader needs to skillfully manage the presentation of facts to ensure maximum benefit, paying particular attention to avoiding finger-pointing and the defensiveness it invariably engenders. It is often useful for someone (usually the patient safety officer or risk manager) to have gathered many of the key facts and timelines and present them to the RCA committee to streamline the discussion. However, even when this has been done, it is important to confirm the facts with the participants early in the meeting and offer them the opportunity to share their perspectives. In most cases, all the involved caregivers should be present at the same meeting to share their views; in rare instances, this will be too emotionally charged and sequential presentations may be preferable.

4. *Some institutions routinely invite other frontline workers (such as an uninvolved nurse or physician) to RCAs to help educate them in the process and demystify the ritual.* The hope is that they can serve as ambassadors for the process with their colleagues. Other organizations have found that the participation of lay individuals adds an important perspective.

5. *Focus more on the process than the report.* A recent ethnographic analysis of RCAs in England concluded that the process often failed to meet its goals because much of the focus was on the production of a final report.[29] In their important cautionary note, Nicolini et al. found that RCAs were being used:

> as a governance tool and a way to re-establish organizational legitimacy in the aftermath of incidents.... This risks transforming RCA from a process of learning and service improvement into a bureaucratized and routine management chore. What was conceived as a 'means to an end' (producing organizational learning and change) becomes an 'end in itself' regulated by a number of well-known bureaucratic principles. This stands in conflict with the espoused learning agenda.

The goal of the RCA is to identify systems factors that led to the error, and to suggest solutions that can prevent similar errors from causing harm in the future.[30–33] Some have suggested that the term "root cause analysis" is misleading since—as we learned from the discussion of the Swiss cheese model (Chapter 1)—most adverse events and errors have multiple "holes in the cheese." In fact, it is nearly unheard of for an effective RCA to identify a single root cause of an error, particularly if the committee has deeply considered all the potential systems issues.

In its zeal to emphasize contributory systems factors, an RCA committee should not shy away from identifying human error, nor from taking appropriate steps to ensure accountability (such as when there is evidence of repetitive errors by a single individual or failure to adhere to sensible safety rules) (Chapter 19). Often, these findings signal a need to move this part of the discussion to a more appropriate venue, such as a medical staff credentialing or a peer review committee. As with many aspects of trying to improve patient safety, finding the appropriate balance between a systems approach and individual accountability is the most challenging aspect of the RCA process.

At UCSF Medical Center, we transformed our RCA process several years ago, and I believe that this was one of the most important things we have done to improve safety.[34] These changes are described in Table 14-4. Unfortunately, we do not have data that prove the effectiveness of this process, and there

Table 14-4	THE UCSF MEDICAL CENTER ROOT CAUSE ANALYSIS PROCESS	
Prior Structure	**New Model**	**Comment or Rationale**
RCAs were scheduled in a haphazard way following a safety-related event	A weekly, scheduled 2-hour meeting, with the first hour devoted to performing an RCA of a recent event	New structure insures same committee members (including senior administrators) present, and permits rapid RCA (within days of event)
Frontline caregivers invited to participate in RCA	Clear directive from hospital leadership to attend any RCA that discusses a case provider was involved in	E-mail to involved caregivers (after initial fact-finding by staff member) directing them to attend next meeting; substantial pressure to do so
Lots of time spent fact-finding before RCA meeting	Less time on fact-finding; first segment of RCA meeting relatively free-form discussion by involved personnel about "what happened"	Prior requirement for detailed fact-finding often delayed RCA by weeks. We have found it better to get the right people to the table and let them tell their story
Action plan often fuzzy as to next steps and who was responsible for carrying them out	No meeting ends without clear action plan and assigned responsibilities	Often requires additional meetings of assigned personnel, but clarity regarding what is to be done (or needs to be learned) and who is responsible for doing it is crucial
No discussion of disclosure to patient/family	No meeting ends without discussion about how/whether disclosure was accomplished, whether more needs to be done, and whether payment was (or should be) waived	Important to make this issue visible and demonstrate support for full disclosure and payment waiver policies
Follow-up reports not expected, haphazard process	Second hour of RCA meeting reserved for 15-minute follow-up reports from previously charged groups	Standing committee members become better at learning what did and didn't work; follow-up requirement forces accountability for those charged with carrying out action plan and allows senior administrators to intervene if implementation stalled by need for resources or political pressure

are few studies in the literature comparing different ways of conducting, and following up on, RCAs.

In the face of this informational vacuum, a few commentators have voiced skepticism about the value of RCAs. Some have argued that the process is wasteful, in part because, as each examines similar errors, individual hospitals frequently find themselves discovering the same root causes.[35] The formation of PSOs may help us test whether, in fact, aggregating RCAs across many institutions improves efficiency, or, by removing so much of the local context and including fewer directly involved participants, it strips away some of its effectiveness. As with so many of the elements of error reporting and analysis, we have much more to learn.

MORBIDITY AND MORTALITY CONFERENCES

While the RCA process is confidential, many institutions have recognized the value of presenting cases of medical errors to diverse groups of providers, usually in an *M&M conference*. Cases of medical errors are often quite interesting and dramatic, and a well-constructed "M&M" can quickly become one of the premier educational sessions in an institution. As with RCAs, it is vital that the leader be a skilled facilitator—striving to protect the presenter (if he or she participated in the care of the patient) from public humiliation, and working to elucidate system factors that bear improvement or general lessons for the audience.

Traditionally, most M&M conferences have involved physicians only, focused on a single discipline (i.e., surgery or medicine), and not comported with modern patient safety thinking. One UCSF study demonstrated that internal medicine M&M conferences rarely classify errors as errors (tending instead to divert into academic discussions of pathophysiology or more traditional aspects of diagnosis and therapy), while surgical conferences often focus on individual fault at the cost of insufficient discussion of system issues.[36] In another study, the leaders of 12 clinical departments at Johns Hopkins Hospital were interviewed about their M&Ms. Patient safety and quality improvement were an explicit goal in only 42%. Only one department (8%) used a structured tool to elicit systems issues, and only seven (58%) had a plan for assigning individuals to follow-up on recommendations.[37]

Some innovative approaches have recently been brought to this time-honored exercise, including interdisciplinary M&M conferences (e.g., with both physicians and nurses), cross-specialty M&M conferences (e.g., surgeons and internists), and conferences that involve institutional administrators and catalyze action and follow-up.[38–40] In the latter model, after systems issues are uncovered in the M&M, a group is charged with returning later to present what was learned about them and how they were fixed. One teaching hospital applied a systems audit framework (Table 14-5) to its M&M conferences, and found that this change led to an improved safety culture and enhanced resident awareness of systems issues.[41]

Unfortunately, many hospitals (particularly nonacademic ones) and departments lack M&M conferences, and they are rare in outpatient settings. Reasons cited include fear of medicolegal risk (although the content of M&M

Table 14-5 **SIX STEPS OF THE SYSTEMS AUDIT USED IN AN INNOVATIVE M&M CONFERENCE FORMAT**
1. Review all documentation related to the case and identify all involved providers.
2. Interview stakeholders, including those who directly provided care and those involved in the system.
3. Use a quality improvement tool (such as a fishbone diagram or mind map*) to conduct a root cause analysis.
4. Determine overall cost of care and the cost of the adverse outcome.
5. Identify a systems issue that contributed to the outcome.
6. Propose systems-level interventions and prioritize based on effort–yield projections.

*Fishbone diagram: a cause-and-effect diagram where the "head" of the fish represents the adverse outcome or systems problem and the "bones" represent contributing factors. **Mind map**: A diagram representing the relationships between a systems problem and its root causes. The adverse outcome or problem is typically depicted in the center with contributing factors branching outward to multiple levels. (Reproduced with permission from Baker S, Darin M, Lateef O. Multidisciplinary morbidity and mortality conferences: improving patient safety by modifying a medical tradition. *Jt Comm Perspect Patient Saf* 2010;10:8–10.)

conferences is protected from legal exposure in most U.S. states [the exception of Florida was cited earlier[26]] if they are performed under the hospital's quality assurance umbrella[42]) and the absence of time or expertise. Luckily, there are now several academic series—both print and on-line—that provide M&M-type analyses of errors.[21,32,43–45]

OTHER METHODS OF CAPTURING SAFETY PROBLEMS

It is important to recognize that IR systems are only one of several methods to capture safety problems. Increasingly, methods to identify "system safety" through certain measurable structures, processes, and outcomes (Donabedian's Triad, Chapter 3) have been developed that do not depend on voluntary reporting. Over time, more and more (though certainly not all) of these measures will be captured via an institution's information technology system (Chapter 13). A detailed discussion of these methods, including the increasingly popular *Global Trigger Tool* (GTT) to identify adverse events, can be found in Chapters 1 and 3. Table 1-3 shows the test characteristics (sensitivity and specificity) of voluntary incident reports, the AHRQ Patient Safety Indicators, and the GTT, illustrating that the GTT is by far the most sensitive.[46] Table 1-4 highlights some of the advantages and disadvantages of the most common methods of measuring errors and harm. The take-away message is that there are various ways of measuring the safety of an organization, and a well-constructed safety program will use several of them to get a robust picture of its challenges and opportunities.[5,6,47]

Just as IRs are not the only way to identify safety problems, RCAs are not the sole means of analyzing such problems and developing fixes. For example, the technique of failure mode and effects analysis (FMEA), borrowed from engineering, is being used by many healthcare institutions to identify active and latent threats to safety.[48] In an FMEA, the likelihood that a particular process will fail is combined with an estimate of the relative impact of that failure to produce a "criticality index." This index allows one to assign priorities to specific processes as improvement targets.

As one illustration, an FMEA of the medication dispensing process on a hospital ward might break down all the steps, from receipt of orders in the central pharmacy to filling automated dispensing machines by pharmacy technicians (Chapter 4). Each step would be assigned a probability of failure and an impact score, allowing it to be ranked according to the product of these two numbers. Steps ranked at the top would be prioritized for error-proofing. The strength of the FMEA technique is that it taps into the insights of both experts and frontline workers to prioritize hazards and create an agenda for improvement. Anecdotally, some institutions have reported that FMEAs led to useful insights not obtainable from other methods, but this has not been subject to rigorous analysis.[49–51]

KEY POINTS

- Although it is natural to favor reporting as an important component of improving patient safety, several factors (including the ubiquity of errors, the difficulty capturing errors without voluntary reporting, and the multiple perspectives and stakeholders) make error reporting quite challenging.
- The most common reporting systems are institutionally-based voluntary IR systems. Increasingly, hospitals and other healthcare organizations are required to submit certain reports to extra-institutional entities such as states, the federal government, and regulators, with mixed results.
- Significant errors should be deeply investigated through an RCA, seeking system problems that merit improvement.
- Sharing stories of errors is an important part of improving safety. This is usually done through an institutional M&M conference, though there are now outside resources that carry out similar functions. Recent innovations in the M&M format are bringing the conference in line with modern patient safety thinking.
- Other methods of capturing safety problems include identifying the lack of evidence-based safety structures, processes, and outcomes, and using trigger tools and FMEA. A robust institutional safety program will integrate multiple methods to get a broad view of its safety challenges and opportunities.

REFERENCES

1. Helmreich RL. On error management: lessons from aviation. *BMJ* 2000;320:781–785.
2. Shojania KG. The frustrating case of incident-reporting systems. *Qual Saf Health Care* 2008;17:400–402.
3. Donchin Y, Gopher D, Olin M, et al. A look into the nature and causes of human errors in the intensive care unit. *Crit Care Med* 1995;23:294–300.
4. Pronovost PJ, Miller MR, Wachter RM. Tracking progress in patient safety: an elusive target. *JAMA* 2006;296:696–699.
5. Levtzion-Korach O, Frankel A, Alcalai H, et al. Integrating incident data from five reporting systems to assess patient safety: making sense of the elephant. *Jt Comm J Qual Patient Saf* 2010;36:402–410.
6. Shojania KG. The elephant of patient safety: what you see depends on how you look. *Jt Comm J Qual Patient Saf* 2010;36:399–401, AP1–AP3.
7. Rowin EJ, Lucier D, Pauker SG. Does error and adverse event reporting by physicians and nurses differ. *Jt Comm J Qual Patient Saf* 2008;34:537–545.
8. Farley DO, Haviland A, Champagne S, et al. Adverse-event-reporting practices by US hospitals: results of a national survey. *Qual Saf Health Care* 2008;17: 416–423.
9. Wachter RM. Hospital incident reporting systems: time to slay the beast. *Wachter's World* (blog). Available at: http://community.the-hospitalist.org/2009/09/20/hospital-incident-reporting-systems-time-to-slay-the-monster/.
10. Wilf-Miron R, Lewenhoff I, Benvamini Z, et al. From aviation to medicine: applying concepts of aviation safety to risk management in ambulatory care. *Qual Saf Health Care* 2003;12:35–39.
11. Barach P, Small SD. Reporting and preventing medical mishaps: lessons from non-medical near miss reporting systems. *BMJ* 2000;320:759–763.
12. Aviation Safety Reporting System. *About ASRS Data.* Available at: http://asrs.arc.nasa.gov/search/dbol/aboutdata.html.
13. Rosenthal J, Booth M. *Maximizing the Use of State Adverse Event Data to Improve Patient Safety.* Portland, ME: National Academy for State Health Policy; 2005.
14. Levinson DR. *Adverse Events in Hospitals: State Reporting Systems.* Washington, DC: US Department of Health and Human Services, Office of the Inspector General; December 2008. Report No. OEI-06-07-00471.
15. Patient Safety Authority. *2010 Annual Report.* Harrisburg, PA: Patient Safety Authority; April 2011. Available at: http://patientsafetyauthority.org/PatientSafetyAuthority/Pages/AnnualReports.aspx.
16. Minnesota Department of Health. *Adverse Health Events in Minnesota, Seventh Annual Public Report.* St. Paul, MN: Minnesota Department of Health; January 2011. Available at: http://www.health.state.mn.us/patientsafety/ae/2011ahereport.pdf.
17. Zhan C, Smith SR, Keyes MA, et al. How useful are voluntary medication error reports? The case of warfarin-related medication errors. *Jt Comm J Qual Patient Saf* 2008;34:36–45.
18. Institute for Safe Medication Practices. *ISMP Medication Errors Reporting Program.* Available at: https://www.ismp.org.

19. Wu AW, Holzmueller CG, Lubomski LH, et al. Development of the ICU safety reporting system. *J Patient Saf* 2005;1:23–32.

20. Bilimoria KY, Kmiecik TE, DaRosa DA, et al. Development of an online morbidity, mortality, and near-miss reporting system to identify patterns of adverse events in surgical patients. *Arch Surg* 2009;144:305–311.

21. *AHRQ WebM&M: Morbidity and Mortality Rounds on the Web.* Available at: http://webmm.ahrq.gov/.

22. Wachter RM, Shojania KG, Minichiello T, et al. AHRQ WebM&M, online medical error reporting and analysis. In: Henriksen K, Battles JB, Marks ES, Lewin DI, eds. *Advances in Patient Safety: From Research to Implementation (Volume 4: Programs, Tools, and Products).* Rockville, MD: Agency for Healthcare Research and Quality; February 2005.

23. In conversation with William B. Munier, MD, MBA. *AHRQ WebM&M* (serial online); July 2011. Available at: http://www.webmm.ahrq.gov/perspective.aspx?perspectiveId=105.

24. Jaffe R. Becoming a patient safety organization. *AHRQ WebM&M* (serial online); July 2011. Available at: http://www.webmm.ahrq.gov/perspective.aspx?perspectiveId=106.

25. Agency for Healthcare Research and Quality. *Listed Patient Safety Organizations.* Available at: http://www.pso.ahrq.gov/listing/psolist.htm.

26. Barach P. The unintended consequences of Florida medical liability legislation. *AHRQ WebM&M* (serial online); December 2005. Available at: http://www.webmm.ahrq.gov/perspective.aspx?perspectiveID=14.

27. Vincent C. Understanding and responding to adverse events. *N Engl J Med* 2003;348:1051–1056.

28. Vincent C, Taylor-Adams S, Stanhope N. Framework for analyzing risk and safety in clinical medicine. *BMJ* 1998;316:1154–1157.

29. Nicolini D, Waring J, Mengis J. Policy and practice in the use of root cause analysis to investigate clinical adverse events: mind the gap. *Soc Sci Med* 2011;73:217–225.

30. Bagian JP, Gosbee J, Lee CZ, et al. The Veterans Affairs root cause analysis system in action. *Jt Comm J Qual Improv* 2002;28:531–545.

31. Rex JH, Turnbull JE, Allen SJ, et al. Systematic root cause analysis of adverse drug events in a tertiary referral hospital. *Jt Comm J Qual Improv* 2000;26:563–575.

32. Chassin MR, Becher EC. The wrong patient. *Ann Intern Med* 2002;136:826–833.

33. Flanders SA, Saint S. Getting to the root of the matter. *AHRQ WebM&M* (serial online); July 2005. Available at: http://webmm.ahrq.gov/case.aspx?caseid=98.

34. Wachter RM. How UCSF's root cause analysis process became our most useful safety activity. *Wachter's World* (blog). Available at: http://community.the-hospitalist.org/2009/12/17/how-ucsf-s-root-cause-analysis-process-became-our-most-useful-patient-safety-activity/.

35. Wu AW, Lipshutz AKM, Pronovost PJ. Effectiveness and efficiency of root cause analysis in medicine. *JAMA* 2008;299:685–687.

36. Pierluissi E, Fischer MA, Campbell AR, et al. Discussion of medical errors in morbidity and mortality conferences. *JAMA* 2003;290:2838–2842.

37. Aboumatar HJ, Blackledge CG Jr, Dickson C, et al. A descriptive study of morbidity and mortality conferences and their conformity to medical incident analysis models: results of the morbidity and mortality conference improvement study, phase 1. *Am J Med Qual* 2007;22:232–238.

38. Berenholtz SM, Hartsell TL, Pronovost PJ. Learning from defects to enhance morbidity and mortality conferences. *Am J Med Qual* 2009;24:192–195.

39. Ksouri H, Balanant PY, Tadié JM, et al. Impact of morbidity and mortality conferences on analysis of mortality and critical events in intensive care practice. *Am J Crit Care* 2010;19:135–145.

40. Baker S, Darin M, Lateef O. Multidisciplinary morbidity and mortality conferences: improving patient safety by modifying a medical tradition. *Jt Comm Perspect Patient Saf* 2010;10:8–10.

41. Szostek JH, Wieland ML, Loertscher LL, et al. A systems approach to morbidity and mortality conference. *Am J Med* 2010;123:663–668.

42. Stewart RM, Corneille MG, Johnston J, et al. Transparent and open discussion of errors does not increase malpractice risk in trauma patients. *Ann Surg* 2006;243: 645–651.

43. Wachter RM, Shojania KG, Markowitz AJ, et al. Quality grand rounds: the case for patient safety. *Ann Intern Med* 2006;145:629–630.

44. Wachter RM, Shojania KG. *Internal Bleeding: The Truth Behind America's Terrifying Epidemic of Medical Mistakes.* New York, NY: Rugged Land; 2004.

45. Wachter RM, Shojania KG. The faces of errors: a case-based approach to educating providers, policy makers, and the public about patient safety. *Jt Comm J Qual Saf* 2004;31:665–670.

46. Classen DC, Resar R, Griffin F, et al. 'Global Trigger Tool' shows that adverse events in hospitals may be ten times greater than previously measured. *Health Aff (Millwood)* 2011;30:581–589.

47. Lipczak H, Knudsen JL, Nissen A. Safety hazards in cancer care: findings using three different methods. *BMJ Qual Saf* 2011;20:1052–1056.

48. McDermott RE, Mikulak RJ, Beauregard MR. *The Basics of FMEA.* Portland, OR: Resources Engineering, Inc; 1996.

49. DeRosier J, Stalhandske E, Bagian JP, et al. Using health care failure mode and effect analysis: the VA National Center for Patient Safety's prospective risk analysis system. *Jt Comm J Qual Improv* 2002;28:248–267.

50. Linkin DR, Sausman C, Santos L, et al. Applicability of healthcare failure mode and effects analysis to healthcare epidemiology: evaluation of the sterilization and use of surgical instruments. *Clin Infect Dis* 2005;41:1014–1019.

51. Bonnabry P, Cingria L, Ackermann M, et al. Use of a prospective risk analysis method to improve the safety of the cancer chemotherapy process. *Int J Qual Health Care* 2006;18:9–16.

| ADDITIONAL READINGS

Classen DC, Lloyd RC, Provost L, et al. Development and evaluation of the Institute for Healthcare Improvement global trigger tool. *J Patient Saf* 2008;4:169–177.

Evans SM, Berry JG, Smith BJ, et al. Attitudes and barriers to incident reporting: a collaborative hospital study. *Qual Saf Health Care* 2006;15:39–43.

Longo DR, Hewett JE, Ge B, et al. The long road to patient safety: a status report on patient safety systems. *JAMA* 2005;294:2858–2865.

Lyons M, Adams S, Woloshynowych M, et al. Human reliability analysis in healthcare: a review of techniques. *Int J Risk Safe Med* 2004;16:223–237.

Milch CE, Salem DN, Pauker SG, et al. Voluntary electronic reporting of medical errors and adverse events. *J Gen Intern Med* 2006;21:165–170.

Pronovost PJ, Holzmueller CG, Young J, et al. Using incident reporting to improve patient safety: a conceptual model. *J Patient Saf* 2007;3:27–33.

Vincent C. *Patient Safety.* 2nd ed. London: Elsevier; 2010.

Weissman JS, Annas CL, Epstein AM, et al. Error reporting and disclosure systems: views from hospital leaders. *JAMA* 2005;293:1359–1366.

CREATING A CULTURE OF SAFETY | 15

OVERVIEW

In Chapter 9, I discussed the tragic collision of two 747s on a foggy morning in Tenerife, the crash that vividly illustrated to everyone in the field of commercial aviation the risks associated with steep and unyielding *authority gradients*. In response to Tenerife and similar accidents, aviation began a series of training programs, generally called "crew resource management" or "cockpit resource management" (CRM) programs, designed to train diverse crews in communication and teamwork. Some of these programs also incorporate communication skills, such as training in Situation, Background, Assessment, and Recommendations (SBAR) and briefing/debriefing techniques (Chapter 9). There is widespread agreement that these programs helped transform the culture of aviation, a transformation that was largely responsible for the remarkable safety record of commercial airlines over the past generation (Figure 9-1).

As the healthcare field began to tackle patient safety, it naturally looked to other organizations that seemed to have addressed their error problems effectively.[1] The concept of *high reliability organizations* (HROs) became shorthand for the relatively mistake-free state enjoyed by airlines, computer chip manufacturers, nuclear power plants, and naval aircraft carriers—but certainly not healthcare organizations.[2,3] According to Weick and Sutcliffe, HROs share the following characteristics:[2]

- *Preoccupation with failure*: the acknowledgment of the high-risk, error-prone nature of an organization's activities and the determination to achieve consistently safe operations.
- *Commitment to resilience*: the development of capacities to detect unexpected threats and contain them before they cause harm, or to recover from them when they do occur.

255

- *Sensitivity to operations*: an attentiveness to the issues facing workers at the frontline, both when analyzing mistakes and in making decisions about how to do the work. Management units at the frontline are given some autonomy in identifying and responding to threats, rather than being forced to work under a rigid top-down approach.
- *A culture of safety*: in which individuals feel comfortable drawing attention to potential hazards or actual failures without fear of censure from management.

Over the past few years, the patient safety world has embraced the concept of HROs. Personally, I find the concept intriguing, but wonder whether it is something of a healthcare "MacGuffin." Legendary film director Alfred Hitchcock used to love to insert a MacGuffin—a plot device, such as a piece of jewelry, a stack of important-looking papers, or a suitcase, that "motivates the characters or advances the story, but the details of which are of little or no importance otherwise"—into his films. Similarly, when I hear a healthcare organization pledge to become an HRO, I wonder whether they are trying to advance their own "patient safety story" without committing themselves to an actionable or measurable target. In this, I find myself agreeing with British safety expert Charles Vincent, who wrote, "Put simply, reading the HRO literature offers a great deal of inspiration, but little idea of what to do in practice to enhance safety."[4,5]

This hints at an overarching challenge we face as we enter the crucial but hazy world of safety culture, which can sometimes feel like the weather—*everybody talks about it but nobody does anything about it*. When it comes to safety culture, everyone seems to have an opinion. As with many complex matters in life, the truth lies somewhere between the commonly polarized viewpoints. Is a safe culture top down or bottom up? Both. Is it "no blame" or dependent on a strong framework for accountability? Both. Is it a local phenomenon ("microculture") or an attribute of an entire organization? Both. Is it enhanced by following a set of rules and standards or by creating a nimble frontline staff, able to innovate, think on its feet, and even break a rule or two when that's required for safe care? Well, both.

The gossamer nature of safety culture—sometimes defined as "the way we do things around here"—can be frustrating to those entering the field, whether their goal is to improve the safety of their own practice or that of an entire hospital. It seems to be nowhere and everywhere. Yet the past few years have seen real progress in the area of safety culture: our understanding of what it means is growing richer and more nuanced, and we are discovering robust ways of measuring it and, to a degree, improving it. This, thankfully, provides something for even the pragmatist to grab on to.

AN ILLUSTRATIVE CASE

In a large teaching hospital, an elderly woman ("Joan Morris"*) is waiting to be discharged after a successful neurosurgical procedure. A floor away, another woman with a similar last name ("Jane Morrison") is scheduled to receive the day's first cardiac electrophysiology study (EPS), a procedure in which a catheter is threaded into the heart to start and stop the heart repetitively to find the cause of a potentially fatal rhythm disturbance. The EPS laboratory calls the floor to send "Morrison" down, but the clerk hears "Morris" and tells that patient's nurse that the EP lab is ready for her patient. That's funny, she thinks, my patient was here for a neurosurgical procedure. Well, she assumes, one of the docs must have ordered the test and not told me. So she sends the patient down.

Later that morning, the neurosurgery resident enters Joan Morris's room to discharge his patient, and is shocked to learn that his patient is in the EPS laboratory. He sprints there, only to be told by the cardiologists that they are in the middle of a difficult part of the procedure and can't listen to his concerns. Assuming that his attending physician ordered the test without telling him, he returns to his work.

Luckily, the procedure, which was finally aborted when the neurosurgery attending came to discharge his patient and learned she was in the EPS laboratory, caused no lasting harm (in fact, the patient later remarked, "I'm glad my heart checked out OK").[6]

The case illustrates several process problems, and it would be easy, even natural, to focus on them. Many hospitals would respond to such a case by mandating that procedural units use complete patient names, hospital numbers, and birthdays when calling for a patient; by requiring a written order from the physician before allowing his or her patient to leave a floor for a procedure; by directing that important information be read back to ensure accuracy; or by implementing a bar coding system that matches a patient's identity with the name in the computerized scheduling system. And these would all be good things to do.

But these changes would leave an important layer of Swiss cheese (Chapter 1)—perhaps the most crucial one of all—unaddressed, the one related to the cultural issues that influence, perhaps even determine, the actions of

---

*Joan Morris and Jane Morrison are fictitious names, but are designed to illustrate the fact that the two patients' real last names were similar to each other, but not identical.

many of the participants. A closer look at the case, now through a safety culture lens, reveals issues surrounding hierarchies, the "culture of low expectations," production pressures, and rules.[6] After a brief discussion about measuring safety culture, I'll address each of these topics in turn, and then consider solutions such as teamwork training and checklists. Rapid Response Teams and dealing with disruptive behavior are covered in Chapters 16 and 19, respectively.

MEASURING SAFETY CULTURE

While one could try to assess safety culture by directly observing provider behavior (and some studies do just that[7,8]), the usual method is through self-reports of caregivers and managers, collected via a survey instrument. The two most popular instruments are the *AHRQ Patient Safety Culture Survey* and the *Safety Attitudes Questionnaire* (SAQ).[9–11] A core benefit of using one of these validated instruments is that they have been administered to tens of thousands of healthcare workers and leaders, which means that benchmarks (for various types of clinical units and healthcare organizations) have been established. There has also been considerable research performed using these instruments, with results that have been surprising, sometimes even eye-popping. They include:

- Safety culture is mostly *a local phenomenon*. Pronovost and Sexton administered the SAQ to clinicians at 100 hospitals.[12] While they found considerable variation in safety culture *across* hospitals (with positive scores ranging from 40% to 80%, Figure 15-1), there was even more variation when they looked at 49 individual units *within* a single hospital (positive scores ranging from 0% to 100%, Figure 15-2). It is not too much of an oversimplification to say that your *hospital* doesn't have a safety culture—rather, your fourth floor ICU has one, your step-down unit 50 ft away has a different one, and your emergency department has still another one. This is liberating in a way, since one need not look far afield for the secrets of a strong safety culture—it's likely that some unit in your organization has already figured them out.
- Safety culture *varies markedly among different providers*, and it is important to query all of them to paint a complete picture of a unit's culture. In a seminal 2000 study, Sexton et al. administered the SAQ to members of operating room teams (Figure 15-3).[13] Whereas nearly 80% of the surgeons felt that teamwork was strong in their OR, only one in four nurses and 10% of the residents felt the same way. More recent studies have found that these differences persist.[14,15]
- Safety culture is *perceived differently by caregivers and administrators*. Singer et al. found that problematic views of culture were much more

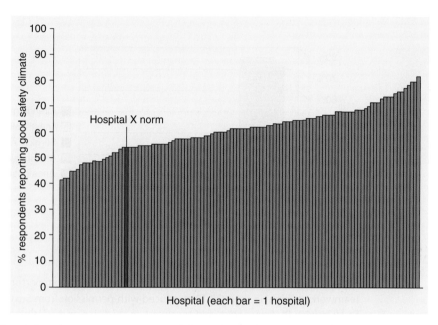

Figure 15-1 ▪ Safety climate scores across 100 different hospitals. (Reproduced with permission from Pronovost PJ, Sexton B. Assessing safety culture: guidelines and recommendations. *Qual Saf Health Care* 2005;14:231–233. © 2005 by BMJ Publishing Group Ltd.)

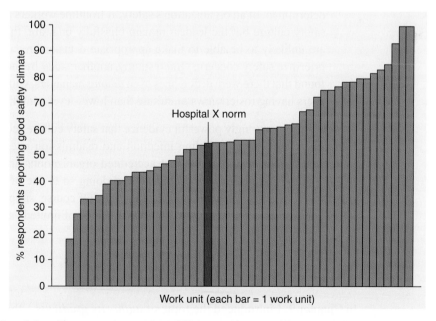

Figure 15-2 ▪ Safety climate scores across 49 different work units within a single hospital. (Reproduced with permission from Pronovost PJ, Sexton B. Assessing safety culture: guidelines and recommendations. *Qual Saf Health Care* 2005;14:231–233. © 2005 by BMJ Publishing Group Ltd.)

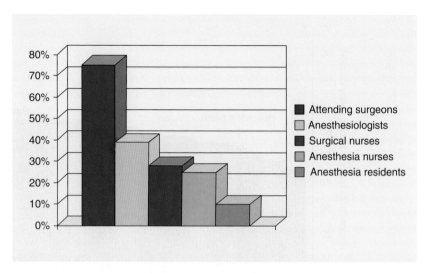

Figure 15-3 ■ Members of different groups of operating room personnel who rated teamwork as "high" in their OR. (Reproduced with permission from Sexton JB, Thomas EJ, Helmreich RL. Error, stress, and teamwork in medicine and aviation: cross-sectional surveys. *BMJ* 2000;320:745–749.)

common among frontline providers than hospital managers working in the same facilities.[16] They argue that this difference may be an important determinant of an organization's safety: if frontline workers perceive poor safety culture but the leaders remain blissfully unaware, the two groups are unlikely to be able to make appropriate decisions regarding how to prioritize safety concerns. Interestingly, another study by the same group found that there were differences even *among* managers, with senior managers having rosier views of culture than lower-level administrators.[17]

There is increasingly powerful evidence that safety culture scores correlate with clinical outcomes, including infection and readmission rates.[10,18–21] The Joint Commission now requires that accredited organizations administer and analyze safety culture surveys each year, and doing so is one of the National Quality Forum's "safe practices" (Appendix VII). Of course, simply measuring safety culture without a strategy to improve it will be of limited value.

HIERARCHIES, SPEAKING UP, AND THE CULTURE OF LOW EXPECTATIONS

In Chapter 9, I introduced the topic of *authority gradients*—the psychological distance between a worker and his or her supervisor. These gradients are often referred to in terms of hierarchies; an organization is said to have *steep hierarchies* if these gradients tend to be large. In the wrong patient case described at the start of this chapter, the nurse's reluctance to raise concerns when told that her patient was being called for a procedure she didn't know about, or the neurosurgery resident's decision to acquiesce after getting pushback from the cardiology staff, can be attributed at least partly to steep authority gradients. So too can the tragic events that doomed the KLM 747 in Tenerife (Chapter 9). You may also recall the case that begins Chapter 9, in which a Code Blue is aborted when a physician finds a "no code" order in the wrong patient's chart. There too, a young nurse was reluctant to question the resident's confident proclamation, even though she had received sign-out an hour earlier that portrayed the patient's status as "full code."

Authority gradients are natural and, to a degree, healthy. But when they prevent caregivers with important knowledge or concerns from sharing them with superiors for fear of being wrong or angering the boss, they become dangerous. This issue pertains not only to direct clinical care but also to whether the ward clerk, pharmacist, or intern will point out hazardous conditions to his or her floor manager, pharmacy director, or department chair. Safe organizations find ways to tamp down hierarchies at all levels, encouraging individuals (including patients, Chapter 21) to speak up when they see unsafe conditions or suspect that something might be awry.

In their masterful discussion of the wrong patient case in our *Quality Grand Rounds* series in the *Annals of Internal Medicine* (Appendix I), Chassin and Becher introduced the concept of "the culture of low expectations."[6] In reflecting on the actions—or inactions—of the nurse and the resident, they wrote:

> We suspect that these physicians and nurses had become accustomed to poor communication and teamwork. A 'culture of low expectations' developed in which participants came to expect a norm of faulty and incomplete exchange of information [which led them to conclude] that these red flags signified not unusual, worrisome harbingers but rather mundane repetitions of the poor communication to which they had become inured.[6]

Fighting the culture of low expectations is a crucial step in creating a safety culture. Doing this requires a change in default setting of all the providers, from:

A. If you're not sure it is wrong, assume it is right (*it's probably just another glitch, we have them all the time around here*) **to**

B. If you're not sure it is right, assume that it is wrong—and do whatever it takes to become sure, even at the cost of delaying the first case in the operating room or making someone important a little irritated.

There is no shortcut to fighting the culture of low expectations. Yes, it is important to clean up communications with tools such as SBAR (Chapter 9) and information technology (Chapter 13)—making the instinct to think, "another glitch, but it must be right," less automatic. (I often tell healthcare leaders that they can improve their organization's safety immediately by simply purging the four words—*it must be right*—from their staff's vocabulary.)

But healthcare organizations will always have examples of faulty, ambiguous communication or rapid changes that cannot be communicated to everyone. Therefore, changing the dominant mindset from "A" to "B" requires a powerful and consistent message from senior leadership (Chapter 22). As importantly, when a worker *does* take the time to perform a double check after noticing something that seems amiss—and it turns out that everything was okay—it is vital for senior leaders to vocally and publicly support that person. If praise is reserved for the "great save" but withheld for the clerk who voiced a concern when nothing later proved to be wrong, staff are unlikely to adopt mindset "B," because they will still fret about the repercussions of being mistaken.[22]

PRODUCTION PRESSURES

Another, perhaps more subtle, culprit in the EPS case—and in safety culture more generally—is *production pressure*.[23,24] In a nutshell, every industry, whether it produces hip replacements or SUVs, has to deal with the tension between safety and throughput. The issue is not whether they experience this tension—that would be like asking if they experience the Laws of Gravity. Rather, it is how they balance these twin demands.

When my children were small, we often went to a well-known pancake restaurant on weekend mornings for breakfast. I was in awe of the establishment's speed: customers were seated promptly, their orders were taken rapidly, putting a fork down on a cleaned plate immediately cued the server to politely ask "is there anything else I can get you today?," and the cleanup was brisk. The reason for this pace is obvious: in the fast food business, with large boluses of customers arriving en masse and relatively low profit margins per customer, corporate survival depends on throughput. The food is fine but not great, and there are periodic errors (of the two-forks, no-knife type). But that's what happens when production trumps safety and reliability.

Only a couple of miles from this particular restaurant is San Francisco International Airport (SFO). The tension between production and safety is particularly acute at SFO, since its two main runways are merely 738 ft apart—I often feel like I can read the newspaper headlines of a passenger in an adjacent plane when both runways are operating.

The Federal Aviation Administration (FAA) enforces inviolable rules about throughput at SFO and every other airport. For example, when the cloud cover falls below 3000 ft (which, in foggy San Francisco, happens often), one of the two runways is closed, gumming up the entire U.S. air traffic control system. And whatever the weather, planes cannot land more often than one each minute. The explanation for these rules is as simple as the explanation for the restaurant's speed: when the aviation industry has to choose between production and safety, safety wins. The result: despite 400,000 takeoffs and landings each year, there has not been a fatal crash at SFO in over 50 years.

I've used this metaphor many times in speeches to hospital staff and leaders, usually capping it by asking audiences: "As it balances production and safety, does your hospital look more like the pancake restaurant or SFO?" Although things have improved a bit in the last few years, the answers still run about 10:1 in favor of the restaurant.

Addressing production pressures sometimes involves creating more efficient processes that free up time to do the work safely (just recall the description in Chapter 13 of the maddening waste of time and effort that often occurs when a nurse has to chart a blood pressure measurement). But it also involves choices, such as slowing down the operating rooms when they reach a state of chaos. This is expensive and disruptive, but so is closing a runway. In aviation, our society willingly pays this price to ensure safety, but we have not done so in healthcare.

As always, it is vital to appreciate the limits of analogies between healthcare and other industries. When SFO closes Runway 10R, planes sit on the ground (or circle overhead) and passengers are inconvenienced. But if we close our emergency department to new ambulances ("go on divert") because of safety concerns, patients, some quite ill, need to be taken to other facilities. This carries its own safety cost, one that needs to be weighed as we address this challenging balance.

Charles Vincent quotes an oil industry executive who captured the tension beautifully; I think of this statement every time I hear a hospital CEO or board member earnestly declare, "safety is our top priority." The executive said:

> Safety is not our top priority. Our top priority is getting oil out of the ground. However, when safety and productivity conflict, then safety takes priority.[4]

I saw the sign in Figure 15-4 on the gate outside a construction site in London. Can you imagine a similar sign in the entrance to your hospital's operating room or emergency department? Until you can, we need to reflect more on the nexus between production pressures and patient safety.

Figure 15-4 ■ A sign outside a roadway construction site in London. Can you imagine a similar sign outside a clinical unit in a hospital?

TEAMWORK TRAINING

It should be clear from the above discussion that safety culture involves far more than what happens in the operating room, in the labor and delivery suite, or on the wards. It is influenced, and sometimes determined, by the organizational culture, leadership, context, incentives, and more. For this reason, there has been increasing emphasis on the engagement of healthcare boards and other leaders.[25,26] I will return to their crucial role at the end of this section and again in Chapter 22.

But much of the discussion around safety culture *does* center on the world of caregivers. You have already heard a fair amount about this in our discussions of handoffs and teamwork (Chapters 8 and 9). But let's now turn to efforts to improve culture, most specifically through team training, checklists, and the thoughtful use of rules.

As I've noted, one of the key ways that the commercial aviation industry transformed its culture in the 1980s was through team training (CRM) programs.[1] Healthcare was relatively slow to embrace this kind of training for several reasons: it was not required by regulators or accreditors (Chapter 20), it was often challenging to get clinicians (particularly physicians) to participate, many people found the concept unattractive (I've had colleagues ask me whether teamwork training will require them to hug their colleagues and sing "Kumbaya"), and the evidence for its effectiveness was relatively weak.

The last objection has been largely answered by the experience of the U.S. Veterans Affairs (VA) healthcare system. Neily et al. compared surgical outcomes of 74 VA hospitals in which surgical teams had undergone team training with those of 34 facilities that had not yet implemented such training.[27] They found that the risk-adjusted mortality rate had fallen 50% more in team training hospitals than in controls. Moreover, there was evidence of a dose–response curve, with additional training yielding even further cuts in mortality. The particular training program used by the VA emphasized four core areas of competency: team leadership, situation monitoring, mutual support, and communication.[28] Several other studies have also demonstrated the benefits of team training,[29–33] but there have been negative trials.[34] Still, after a period of high hopes but substantial uncertainty, the weight of the evidence now supports the premise that teamwork training improves both safety culture and clinical outcomes.

Healthcare CRM programs come in a variety of shapes and sizes, though all focus on improving communication skills, forging a more cohesive environment, encouraging caregivers to speak up when they have concerns, addressing errors in a nonjudgmental fashion, and implementing tools such as time outs and briefs/debriefs (Chapter 5). The general experience is that, even when using an "off the shelf" program, it is best to allow for some local customization. In Table 15-1, Mayer et al. outline a number of implementation factors that help determine success[29] and, in Table 15-2, Weaver et al. enumerate 12 best practices for evaluating team training programs.[35]

From the literature and my own experience in implementing team training at UCSF[36] (the outline of our program is shown in Table 15-3), I'd emphasize the following practices and strategies:

1. *Employ strong leadership and "champions"*: Changing a culture is hard, and one person's "empowerment" might be another's loss of power and status. The case for culture change has to be clearly articulated, and buy-in—particularly from the physicians, nurses, and hospital executives at the top of the authority ladder—is vital. Luckily, thoughtful leaders now appreciate the safety risks associated with poor teamwork and steep authority gradients, and many are welcoming CRM-type programs.

2. *Use aviation and other relevant nonhealthcare analogies, but don't overdo them*: At UCSF, we used actual airline pilots in some of our training, and this was helpful. Pilots can confess to medical audiences that their culture was previously similar to that of physicians, and that they participated in team training programs reluctantly at first, but that they now have come to believe that such training is essential to improving culture and decreasing errors. The Tenerife story and others like it are powerful ways to energize a healthcare audience, and—particularly for physicians—the pilots' experiences are quite relevant.

   However, healthcare providers will be quick to highlight differences between an operating room and a cockpit. The biggest difference: a cockpit "team" is made up of two or three individuals with similar training, expertise, income, and social status—operating in quiet behind a sealed door. Dampening this hierarchy is easy compared

Table 15-1	IMPLEMENTATION FACTORS FOR SUCCESSFUL TEAM TRAINING
Success Factor	**Implementation Strategy**
1. Align team training objectives and safety aims with organizational goals	Communication to organizational leaders and unit staff linked potential impact of teamwork on meeting organizational goals for employee satisfaction, patient satisfaction, and quality of care.
2. Provide organizational support for the team training initiative	The patient safety officer and a program manager each dedicated 40% effort to this project. Physician, nurse, and respiratory therapy senior leaders approved change team members' time on the project. Continuing education units for nurses, physicians, and respiratory therapists was approved and provided.
3. Get frontline care leaders on board	Both formal and informal unit leaders were recruited for active involvement in the project, either through inclusion in change team or by determining best approach and timing for training. Individuals were recognized for involvement by wearing TeamSTEPPS badges that identified them as TeamSTEPPS Master Trainers (Coach badge) or participants (Ready badge).
4. Prepare the environment and trainees for team training	Before training and during regular staff meetings, we provided trainees with information about why the unit was selected, what training would be provided, and expected outcomes. In addition, TeamSTEPPS was framed as a way to standardize and increase consistency of already good team performance as opposed to implementation for remediation purposes.
5. Determine required resources and time commitment and ensure their availability	Training sessions were scheduled at times that would minimize schedule disruptions for staff and were offered on all shifts and days of the week. If needed, overtime training hours were budgeted and approved.
6. Facilitate application of trained teamwork skills on the job	Staff were trained together in interdisciplinary groups to remove hierarchy barriers. The training included an opportunity to practice, and, following training, unit-based change team leaders modeled and encouraged use of TeamSTEPPS skills. Multiple reinforcement aids were developed and used (e.g., chocolates with TeamSTEPPS labels were handed out after good teamwork events and TeamSTEPPS note cards were printed to provide a handwritten note of recognition for good teamwork).
7. Measure the effectiveness of the team training program	Metrics of success were identified early and periodically reported back to staff. Training effectiveness was measured on multiple levels.

Reproduced with permission from Mayer CM, Cluff L, Lin WT, et al. Evaluating efforts to optimize TeamSTEPPS implementation in surgical and pediatric intensive care units. *Jt Comm J Qual Patient Saf* 2011;37:365–374.

Table 15-2 **BEST PRACTICES FOR EVALUATING TEAM TRAINING PROGRAMS**

Planning
- **Best Practice 1.** Before designing training, start backwards: think about traditional frameworks for evaluation in reverse.
- **Best Practice 2.** Strive for robust, experimental design in your evaluation: it is worth the headache.
- **Best Practice 3.** When designing evaluation plans and metrics, ask the experts—your frontline staff.
- **Best Practice 4.** Do not reinvent the wheel; leverage existing data relevant to training objectives.
- **Best Practice 5.** When developing measures, consider multiple aspects of performance.
- **Best Practice 6.** When developing measures, design for variance.
- **Best Practice 7.** Evaluation is affected by more than just training itself. Consider organizational, team, or other factors that may help (or hinder) the effects of training (and thus evaluation outcomes).

Implementation
- **Best Practice 8.** Engage socially powerful players early. Physician, nursing, and executive engagement is crucial to evaluation success.
- **Best Practice 9.** Ensure evaluation continuity: have a plan for employee turnover at both the participant and evaluation administration team levels.
- **Best Practice 10.** Environmental signals before, during, and after training must indicate that the trained knowledge, skills, and attitudes and the evaluation itself are valued by the organization.

Follow-up
- **Best Practice 11.** Get in the game, coach! Feed evaluation results back to frontline providers and facilitate continual improvement through constructive coaching.
- **Best Practice 12.** Report evaluation results in a meaningful way, both internally and externally.

Reproduced with permission from Weaver SJ, Salas E, King HB. Twelve best practices for team training evaluation in health care. *Jt Comm J Qual Patient Saf* 2011;37:341–349.

with doing so in a busy operating or delivery room, where the authority ladder might span from the chief of neurosurgery or obstetrics to a ward clerk who is a recent immigrant with a high school degree (Chapter 9). Moreover, the process of flying is now so automated that pilots are mostly in the cockpit (like control room workers at nuclear power plants) to react to emergencies. Medicine is a long way from being that routinized. These differences mean that aviation examples should rapidly give way to medical ones.

Table 15-3   ELEMENTS OF THE UCSF CREW RESOURCE MANAGEMENT ("TRIAD FOR OPTIMAL PATIENT SAFETY," TOPS) CURRICULUM

Topic	Description	Time (minutes)
Welcome	From a system leader (i.e., chief medical officer)	10
"Laying the foundation"	Brief overview, goals of the day	15
*First, Do No Harm**	Video shown, followed by facilitated discussion to serve as icebreaker	40
Lecture on healthcare team behaviors and communication skills	Delivered by a commercial airline pilot. Introduces key principles of safety culture, communication, inc. SBAR, CUS words (Chapter 9)	60
Small-group facilitated "scenarios"	Two case scenarios, groups of ~8 people (must be interdisciplinary) to teach and practice standardized communication, team behaviors	80

The TOPS project was funded by the Gordon and Betty Moore Foundation. Reproduced with permission from Sehgal NL, Fox M, Vidyarthi AR, et al.; TOPS Project. A multidisciplinary teamwork training program: the Triad for Optimal Patient Safety (TOPS) experience. *J Gen Intern Med* 2008;23: 2053–2057.

*Powerful video based on actual events from malpractice claim files of a perinatal mistake that results in a mother's death. Can be obtained from the Partnership for Patient Safety. Available at: http://www.p4ps.org/interactive_videos.asp.

3. *Consider whether to use simulation*: Experts debate the utility of adding simulation to culture and communication training programs (there is less debate on the utility of simulation for improving technical skills; Chapters 5 and 17).[37,38] Proponents of simulation in CRM training argue that it "raises the stakes," allows participants to suspend disbelief more readily, and makes lessons more memorable.[39] Others feel that simulation (particularly high-fidelity, realistic simulation, as opposed to role-playing case scenarios) is not worth the added cost and complexity, and might even distract providers from the lessons regarding communication and collaboration.[40] Whether simulation is or is not used, it is critical to "get everybody in the room" to work through case-based scenarios, and to provide an opportunity for skillful debriefing and interdisciplinary cross-talk. Didactics can go only so far in transforming deep-seated attitudes and beliefs.

4. *Programs must live on beyond the initial training*: Although a brief (e.g., 4–6 hours) CRM program can sensitize workers to some of the key cultural and communication issues, effective programs outlive their initial training phase. Whether the programs live on in the form of "unit-based safety teams" or other vehicles, the new emphasis on teamwork and collaboration must be supported by structures that endure (see also Chapter 22).[41,42]

Before leaving the topic of teamwork training, I'd like to loop back to where we began this section. Team training may seem like a convenient solution to poor safety culture, and the evidence now confirms that it does help. But, as Salas et al. point out, such training likely accounts for a small fraction of a team's effectiveness; the rest is determined by the culture and actions of the organization.[43] They continue:

The organizational system matters. What the top leadership does, matters. What policies and procedures are in place to support teamwork, matters. The formal and informal signs and symbols of what is important in the organization—as conveyed through the norms, conditions, policies, procedures, metrics in place, and the messages that top leadership sends—make or break transformational culture change. One cannot forget that organizations tend to obtain the behaviors, cognitions, and attitudes that they measure and reinforce. We need to shift from thinking about a "team training intervention" to creating and sustaining an organizational system that supports teamwork. The best team training in the world will not yield the desired outcomes unless the organization is aligned to support it.

CHECKLISTS AND CULTURE

I've mentioned checklists several times throughout this book, mostly as a method to ensure adherence to key care processes. It may seem strange to now see a section on checklists in a chapter on safety culture. Yet in his book, *The Checklist Manifesto*, surgeon and author Atul Gawande reminds us that checklists can address a number of safety targets.[44] In leading the multicenter study that established the value of the World Health Organization's surgical checklist (Figure 5-2),[45] Gawande came to appreciate that the value of "the lowly checklist" was not simply in ensuring that the team gave the right preoperative antibiotics at the correct time, but in prompting team members in the operating room to introduce themselves to each other before a procedure begins. In other words, it was as much a culture-changing intervention as a cookbook.

Of course, concerns about "cookbook medicine" explain much of the resistance to the use of checklists, particularly among physicians. Gawande writes:

> ... we have the means to make some of the most complex and dangerous work we do ... more effective than we ever thought possible. But the prospect pushes against the traditional culture of medicine, with its central belief that in situations of high risk and complexity what you want is a kind of expert audacity.... Checklists and standard operating procedures feel like exactly the opposite, and that's what rankles many people.[44]

Reflecting further on the intersection between checklists and physician culture, Gawande writes; "All learned occupations have a definition of professionalism, a code of conduct ... [with] at least three common elements": selflessness, an expectation of skill, and an expectation of trustworthiness. He continues:

> Aviators, however, add a fourth expectation, discipline; discipline in following prudent procedure and in functioning with others. This is a concept almost entirely outside the lexicon of most professions, including my own. In medicine, we hold up 'autonomy' as a professional lodestar, a principle that stands in direct opposition to discipline.... The closest our professional codes come to articulating the goal [of discipline] is an occasional plea for 'collegiality. ' What is needed, however, isn't just that people working together be nice to each other. It is discipline.[44]

Gawande would doubtless agree that checklists can't solve all our problems, but they—and other safety-oriented activities such as standardization, simplification, forcing functions, and double checks—*can* help us deliver healthcare that is safer and more reliable. In applying these solutions, though, we need to grapple with the fact that checklists challenge some of physicians' most deeply held beliefs about what it means to be an excellent doctor.

The relationship between checklists and culture is a two-way street: checklists can influence culture, but their success can also be determined by an organization's ambient culture. While today's enthusiasm for checklists is well grounded, it is worth reading descriptions by Bosk et al.[46] and Dixon-Woods et al.[47] of the co-interventions crucial to the remarkable success of the Michigan central line–associated bloodstream infection study (which is often characterized—too simplistically—as a "checklist intervention"; Chapter 10).[48] We are already beginning to see failures of interventions that were organized around the naive assumption that simply embedding a checklist into a complex clinical process, without addressing matters of culture, will enhance safety.

One other point about checklists has emerged from recent research. After participating in the WHO surgical safety intervention, 21% of clinicians disagreed with or gave neutral responses to the statement, "The checklist prevents errors in the operating room." Yet 93% of the same respondents stated that they would want the checklist to be used *if they themselves were having an operation.*[49] This is Lake Wobegon Meets Patient Safety: humans naturally believe they are above average in their carefulness.[50] Accordingly, tools such as checklists might seem useful for "the other guy"—you know, the one who isn't quite as careful as I am. But life doesn't work that way. Inserting checklists—to be used by everyone—into error-prone processes as part of a comprehensive strategy to improve culture represents one of the major recent advances in patient safety.

Developing a great checklist is not a trivial undertaking. Like many good checklists, the WHO surgical checklist went through scores of iterations before the final version was produced.[44] Through experiences like this and collaboration with other industries that have been using checklists for decades, we are beginning to understand some of the design principles for effective healthcare checklists. Figure 15-5, from McLaughlin, depicts a poor and an improved surgical checklist, illustrating some of these tenets.[51]

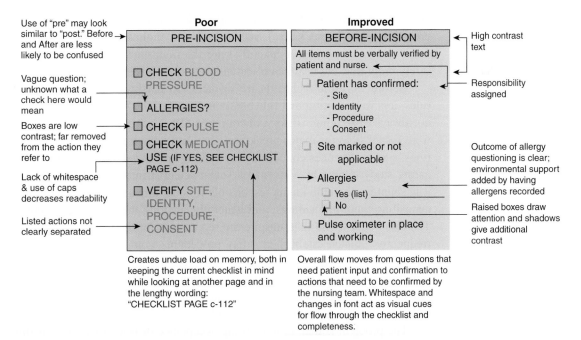

Figure 15-5 ■ Examples of a poor and improved surgical checklist. (Reproduced with permission from McLaughlin AC. What makes a good checklist? *AHRQ WebM&M* (serial online); October 2010. Original image at: http://webmm. ahrq.gov/media/perspectives/images/persp92_f01.gif.)

RULES, RULE VIOLATIONS, AND WORKAROUNDS

Gawande's comments on discipline naturally lead us into a discussion of rules and standard procedures. Healthcare providers are, of course, familiar with clinical rules: treat hypovolemia with fluids, don't give gadolinium to patients in renal failure, abscesses need to be drained. Although such rules were developed informally in the past and handed down by experts to trainees, our modern paradigm is to base clinical guidelines on firm scientific evidence (Chapter 3).

The field of patient safety is not agnostic about such clinical guidance. Providing high-quality, safe care requires that we pay attention to evidence-based rules and guidelines while allowing clinicians the flexibility to deviate when their patients do not fit the template (such as in patients with multiple and overlapping diseases).[52] In Chapter 13, we discussed the role of computerized clinical decision support systems, which should make it easier for clinicians to follow such rules by providing up-to-date guidance at the point of care.

But these clinical rules fall largely in the domain of quality of care (Chapter 3). In the safety field, we are more concerned with rules and policies enacted to prevent patient harm. Examples might include: perform a "time out" prior to the first incision (Chapter 5), read back a critical lab value (Table 13-3), use a checklist before inserting a central line (Chapter 10), and check the patient's identity before sending her off to a potentially dangerous procedure (this chapter's case). Such rules (e.g., "flight attendants, please arm doors and cross check for takeoff") are the mainstays of many industries' safety programs, but healthcare's attention to them has been sporadic, at best.

Before we criticize healthcare workers too harshly for breaking safety rules, it is worth noting that rule breaking is part of the human condition, and not always a bad thing. History, of course, is filled with stories of gadflies who were responsible for major breakthroughs. And who among us never breaks rules, such as the ones concerning jaywalking and speed limits?[53] In a fascinating study quoted by Vincent,[4] a social scientist interviewed British railway shunters, the individuals responsible for coupling and uncoupling trains, depositing them into sidings, and generally ensuring their safe movement.[54] The researcher found that, despite the risky nature of the work, the shunters frequently violated established safety procedures, sometimes for reasons of inexperience, sometimes because they felt a rule was unnecessary or silly, and sometimes because they believed their action did not pose any serious risk (Table 15-4). James Reason calls the last category a *routine rule violation*, and most times they are harmless enough.[55]

The problem is that an unblinking acceptance of rule violations has diffused throughout medicine, particularly among physicians, whose status atop the hierarchy and, at least in the United States, as independent entrepreneurs (rather than employees of the hospital or healthcare system) has traditionally

Table 15-4 **RAILWAY SHUNTERS' REASONS FOR VIOLATING RULES**	
Reason for Violation	Percent
This is a quicker way of working	39
Inexperienced shunter	38
Time pressure	37
High workload	30
The shunter is lazy	19
A skilled shunter can work safely this way	17
The rule can be impossible to work to	16
Design of the sidings makes the violation necessary	16
Management turns a blind eye	12
Physical exhaustion	7
No one understands the rule	6
It is a more exciting way of working	6
It is a macho way to work	5
The rule is outdated	5

Reproduced with permission from Lawton R. Not working to rule: understanding procedural violations at work. *Saf Sci* 2004;28:199–211.

given them license to ignore rules. But, just as with the broken windows theory of policing (which holds that letting people get away with minor violations, such as breaking windows in abandoned houses, tacitly encourages them to try their hand at larger crimes),[56] it can be argued that our permissiveness toward healthcare rule violators is responsible for the high rate of violations of some very important rules, such as hand hygiene. As Henry Kissinger famously said, "History teaches that weakness is provocative…."[57]

Yet before we embrace a more punitive approach to rule-breakers (which I discuss more fully in Chapter 19), it is worth recognizing the extraordinary complexity swirling around this area. Vincent[4] highlights the contributions of Diana Vaughan (whose study of the Challenger shuttle disaster introduced the concept of *normalization of deviance*) and Rene Amalberti (whose studies have illuminated the frequent migration of workers from the "legal" to the "illegal-normal," sometimes driven by differences in risk perception by individuals).[58,59] Vincent and coworkers also describe a fascinating study by French anesthesiologists documenting the brief lifespan of many safety rules.[60] "They are born," Vincent writes, "they have a vigorous youth where most people take note of them, they begin to get old and less notice is taken of them, and finally they die."[4]

As our quest to improve safety drives us to pay more attention to rules and procedures, we need to be sure that the rules we promulgate are important enough to be worth paying attention to, that we distinguish "must follow" from "nice to follow" rules (some organizations call the inviolable ones "*Red Rules*"),[61] and that we enlist teams and peers to help enforce crucial rules. One aspect of high functioning teams is that they reach consensus that deviations from certain rules will not be tolerated, and then enforce such decisions with everything from gentle reminders to outright sanctions. You'll know you've achieved a safe culture when you see someone low in the hierarchy—say, a new nurse—reminding a senior physician to wash his or her hands, and the physician responds by simply saying, "thank you," then turns to the sink or gel dispenser.

SOME FINAL THOUGHTS ON SAFETY CULTURE

I end the chapter with a few general reflections on the remarkably rich and challenging issue of safety culture. Rather than emphasizing the issues above (promoting teamwork and collaboration, dampening down authority gradients, fighting the culture of low expectations, staying attuned to production pressures, mandating adherence to key rules and policies), some institutions define a safety culture in terms of the following questions:

- Do workers report errors?
- Is there a "no blame" culture?
- Is "improving patient safety" listed in the strategic plan?

Let's consider these points one by one.

As I discussed in Chapter 14, I don't believe that pushing workers to report, report, and report some more (particularly to an institutional or governmental reporting system) is likely to generate a safety culture. That said, local reporting (especially when there is a supportive unit leader who listens to problems and helps fix them, and when reports fuel engaging M&M conferences and unit-based problem solving) is important, and reporting can be a useful part of a broader effort to discover problems and engage frontline workers.

The issue of "no blame" is one of the most complex in the safety field. Throughout the book, I have discussed the importance of a systems approach, fighting the instinct to blame and replacing it with a focus on identifying system flaws that allow our inevitable human errors to cause harm. I believe that this new mental model has been responsible for much of the progress that we have made in the first decade of the patient safety movement.

That said, the "no blame" mantra has been taken by some to absurd levels. Blame *is* appropriate for individuals who make frequent, careless errors, who fail to keep up with their specialty, who come to work intoxicated, or who choose to ignore reasonable safety rules. David Marx and others have promoted the concept of a "*Just Culture*" (rather than a "no blame" culture) as a way to reconcile an appropriate focus on "no blame" when caring, competent workers make errors with the need to hold individuals (and institutions) accountable for blameworthy errors or conditions.[62] This concept is explored more fully in Chapter 19.

Finally, placing patient safety in, or even atop, an institution's strategic plan is no guarantee of a safe culture (Chapter 22). Senior leadership and hospital boards make an important statement when they prioritize patient safety among their values and missions, but too many organizations and leaders offer lip service without promoting the effort and allocating the resources to make this commitment real.[25,26] Creating a safe culture is hard work. But once it is created, it is easy to identify its presence, as well as its absence.

KEY POINTS

- Safe cultures are ones in which people willingly speak up when they see risky situations and behaviors, there are relatively flat hierarchies, workers follow critical safety rules, and the need for throughput is balanced against the need for safety.
- Many institutions are employing teamwork training programs, usually modeled on aviation's CRM programs, and emerging research on the results of well-implemented programs is promising.
- Validated survey instruments are available to measure safety culture and to benchmark against like clinical units or organizations.
- One aspect of a safe culture is fighting "the culture of low expectations," in which workers assume faulty communication and therefore fail to perform double checks despite clear warning signs.
- Checklists can not only encourage compliance with safe processes of care but also facilitate culture change by improving teamwork and communication. Their success, in turn, can also be influenced by the ambient culture.
- The concept of a "Just Culture" has been advanced to emphasize the importance of blending a systems focus with appropriate individual and institutional accountability.

REFERENCES

1. Helmreich RL. On error management: lessons from aviation. *BMJ* 2000;320:781–785.
2. Weick KE, Sutcliffe KM. *Managing the Unexpected: Assuring High Performance in an Age of Complexity*. 2nd ed. San Francisco, CA: John Wiley & Sons; 2007.
3. Pronovost PJ, Berenholtz SM, Goeschel CA, et al. Creating high reliability in health care organizations. *Health Serv Res* 2006;41:1599–1617.
4. Vincent C. *Patient Safety*. 2nd ed. West Sussex, UK: Wiley-Blackwell; 2010:282.
5. Vincent C, Benn J, Hanna GB. High reliability in healthcare. *BMJ* 2010;340:c84.
6. Chassin MR, Becher EC. The wrong patient. *Ann Intern Med* 2002;136:826–833.
7. Berridge EJ, Mackintosh NJ, Freeth DS. Supporting patient safety: examining communication within delivery suite teams through contrasting approaches to research observation. *Midwifery* 2010;26:512–519.
8. Catchpole K, Mishra A, Handa A, et al. Teamwork and error in the operating room: analysis of skills and roles. *Ann Surg* 2008;247:699–706.
9. Agency for Healthcare Research and Quality. *Patient Safety Culture Surveys*. Rockville, MD: Agency for Healthcare Research and Quality; November 2010. Available at: http://www.ahrq.gov/qual/patientsafetyculture/.
10. Sexton JB, Helmreich RL, Neilands TB, et al. The Safety Attitudes Questionnaire: psychometric properties, benchmarking data, and emerging research. *BMC Health Serv Res* 2006;6:44.
11. Colla JB, Bracken AC, Kinney LM, et al. Measuring patient safety climate: a review of surveys. *Qual Saf Health Care* 2005;14:364–366.
12. Pronovost PJ, Sexton B. Assessing safety culture: guidelines and recommendations. *Qual Saf Health Care* 2005;14:231–233.
13. Sexton JB, Thomas EJ, Helmreich RL. Error, stress, and teamwork in medicine and aviation: cross sectional surveys. *BMJ* 2000;320:745–749.
14. Huang DT, Clermont G, Sexton JB, et al. Perceptions of safety culture vary across the intensive care units of a single institution. *Crit Care Med* 2007;35:165–176.
15. Makary MA, Sexton JB, Freischlag JA, et al. Operating room teamwork among physicians and nurses: teamwork in the eye of the beholder. *J Am Coll Surg* 2006;202:746–752.
16. Singer SJ, Gaba DM, Geppert JJ, et al. The culture of safety: results of an organization-wide survey in 15 California hospitals. *Qual Saf Health Care* 2003;12:112–118.
17. Singer SJ, Falwell A, Gaba DM, et al. Patient safety climate in US hospitals: variation by management level. *Med Care* 2008;46:1149–1156.
18. Huang DT, Clermont G, Kong L, et al. Intensive care unit safety culture and outcomes: a US multicenter study. *Int J Qual Health Care* 2010;22:151–161.
19. Singer S, Lin S, Falwell A, et al. Relationship of safety climate and safety performance in hospitals. *Health Serv Rev* 2009;44:399–421.
20. Mardon RE, Khanna K, Sorra J, et al. Exploring relationships between hospital patient safety culture and adverse events. *J Patient Saf* 2010;6:226–232.
21. Hansen LO, Williams MV, Singer SJ. Perceptions of hospital safety climate and incidence of readmission. *Health Serv Res* 2011;46:596–616.
22. Wachter RM. Low on the totem pole. *AHRQ WebM&M* (serial online); December 2005. Available at: http://webmm.ahrq.gov/case.aspx?caseID=110.

23. Carayon P. Production pressures. *AHRQ WebM&M* (serial online); May 2007. Available at: http://webmm.ahrq.gov/case.aspx?caseID=150.

24. Gaba DM, Howard SK, Jump B. Production pressure in the work environment. California anesthesiologists' attitudes and experiences. *Anesthesiology* 1994;81:488–500.

25. Joshi MS, Hines SC. Getting the board on board: engaging hospital boards in quality and patient safety. *Jt Comm J Qual Patient Saf* 2006;32:179–187.

26. Goeschel CA, Wachter RM, Pronovost PJ. Responsibility for quality improvement and patient safety: hospital board and medical staff leadership challenges. *Chest* 2010;138:171–178.

27. Neily J, Mills PD, Young-Xu Y, et al. Association between implementation of a medical team training program and surgical mortality. *JAMA* 2010;304:1693–1700.

28. Dunn EJ, Mills PD, Neily J, et al. Medical team training: applying crew resource management in the Veterans Health Administration. *Jt Comm J Qual Patient Saf* 2007;33:317–325.

29. Mayer CM, Cluff L, Lin WT, et al. Evaluating efforts to optimize TeamSTEPPS implementation in surgical and pediatric intensive care units. *Jt Comm J Qual Patient Saf* 2011;37:365–374.

30. Weaver SJ, Rosen MA, DiazGranados D, et al. Does teamwork improve performance in the operating room? A multilevel evaluation. *Jt Comm J Qual Patient Saf* 2010; 36:133–142.

31. Wolf FA, Way LW, Stewart L. The efficacy of medical team training: improved team performance and decreased operating room delays: a detailed analysis of 4863 cases. *Ann Surg* 2010;252:477–485.

32. Morey JC, Simon R, Jay GD, et al. Error reduction and performance improvement in the emergency department through formal teamwork training: evaluation results of the MedTeams project. *Health Serv Res* 2002;37:1553–1581.

33. Riley W, Davis S, Miller K, et al. Didactic and simulation nontechnical skills team training to improve perinatal patient outcomes in a community hospital. *Jt Comm J Qual Patient Saf* 2011;37:357–364.

34. Nielsen PE, Goldman MB, Mann S, et al. Effects of teamwork training on adverse outcomes and process of care in labor and delivery: a randomized controlled trial. *Obstet Gynecol* 2007;109:48–55.

35. Weaver SJ, Salas E, King HB. Twelve best practices for team training evaluation in health care. *Jt Comm J Qual Patient Saf* 2011;37:341–349.

36. Sehgal NL, Fox M, Vidyarthi AR, et al.; TOPS Project. A multidisciplinary teamwork training program: the Triad for Optimal Patient Safety (TOPS) experience. *J Gen Intern Med* 2008;23:2053–2057.

37. Shapiro MJ, Morey JC, Small SD, et al. Simulation based teamwork training for emergency department staff: does it improve clinical team performance when added to an existing didactic teamwork curriculum? *Qual Saf Health Care* 2004;13:417–421.

38. Cook DA, Hatala R, Brydges R, et al. Technology-enhanced simulation for health professions education. *JAMA* 2011;306:978–988.

39. Gaba DM. What does simulation add to teamwork training? *AHRQ WebM&M* (serial online); March 2006. Available at: http://www.webmm.ahrq.gov/perspective.aspx?perspectiveID=20.

40. Pratt SD, Sachs BP. Team training: classroom training vs. high-fidelity simulation. *AHRQ WebM&M* (serial online); March 2006. Available at: http://www.webmm.ahrq.gov/perspective.aspx?perspectiveID=21.

41. Pronovost P, Weast B, Rosenstein B. Implementing and validating a comprehensive unit-based safety program. *J Patient Saf* 2005;1:33–40.

42. Pronovost P, King J, Holzmueller CG, et al. A web-based tool for the Comprehensive Unit-based Safety Program (CUSP). *J Comm J Qual Patient Saf* 2006;32:119–129.

43. Salas E, Gregory ME, King HB. Team training can enhance patient safety—the data, the challenge ahead. *J Comm J Qual Patient Saf* 2011;37:339–340.

44. Gawande A. *The Checklist Manifesto: How to Get Things Right*. New York, NY: Metropolitan Books; 2009.

45. Haynes AB, Weiser TG, Berry WR, et al.; for the Safe Surgery Saves Lives Study Group. A surgical safety checklist to reduce morbidity and mortality in a global population. *N Engl J Med* 2009;360:491–499.

46. Bosk CL, Dixon-Woods M, Goeschel CA, et al. Reality check for checklists. *Lancet* 2009;374:444–445.

47. Dixon-Woods M, Bosk CL, Aveling EL, et al. Explaining Michigan: developing an ex post theory of a quality improvement program. *Milbank Q* 2011;89:167–205.

48. Pronovost P, Needham D, Berenholtz S, et al. An intervention to decrease catheter-related bloodstream infections in the ICU. *N Engl J Med* 2006;355:2725–2732.

49. Haynes AB, Weiser TG, Berry WR, et al.; Safe Surgery Saves Lives Study Group. Changes in safety attitude and relationship to decreased postoperative morbidity and mortality following implementation of a checklist-based surgical safety intervention. *BMJ Qual Saf* 2011;20:102–107.

50. Kruger J. Lake Wobegon be gone! The "below-average effect" and the egocentric nature of comparative ability judgments. *J Pers Soc Psychol* 1999;77:221–232.

51. McLaughlin AC. What makes a good checklist? *AHRQ WebM&M* (serial online); October 2010. Available at: http://webmm.ahrq.gov/perspective.aspx?perspectiveID=92.

52. Boyd CM, Darer J, Boult C, et al. Clinical practice guidelines and quality of care for older patients with multiple comorbid diseases. Implications for pay for performance. *JAMA* 2005;294:716–724.

53. McKenna FP, Horswill MS. Risk taking from the participant's perspective: the case of driving and accident risk. *Health Psychol* 2006;25:163–170.

54. Lawton R. Not working to rule: understanding procedural violations at work. *Saf Sci* 1998;28:77–95.

55. Reason JT. *Human Error*. New York, NY: Cambridge University Press; 1990.

56. Wilson JQ, Kelling GL. Broken windows: the police and neighborhood safety. *The Atlantic Monthly*. March 1982.

57. Nuclear Age Peace Foundation. *Statement of the Honorable Henry A. Kissinger Before the Senate Foreign Relations Committee*. May 26, 1999. Available at: http://nuclearfiles.org/menu/key-issues/missile-defense/history/kissinger_statement-senate-foreign-relations.htm.

58. Vaughan D. *The Challenger Launch Decision: Risky Technology, Culture, and Deviance at NASA*. Chicago, IL: University of Chicago Press; 1997.

59. Amalberti R, Vincent C, Auroy Y. Violations and migrations in health care: a framework for understanding and management. *Qual Saf Health Care* 2006;15:166–171.

60. de Saint Maurice G, Auroy Y, Vincent C, et al. The natural lifespan of a safety policy: violations and system migration in anaesthesia. *Qual Saf Health Care* 2010;19:327–331.

61. Scharf WR. Red rules: an error-reduction strategy in the culture of safety. *Focus Patient Saf* 2007;10:1–2.

62. Marx D. *Patient Safety and the "Just Culture": A Primer for Health Care Executives.* April 17, 2001. Available at: http://www.mers-tm.org/support/Marx_Primer.pdf.

ADDITIONAL READINGS

Adler-Milstein JR, Singer SJ, Toffel MW. *Speaking Up Constructively: Managerial Practices that Elicit Solutions from Front-Line Employees.* Cambridge, MA: Harvard Business School; August 25, 2010. HBS Working Paper No. 11-005.

Donaldson L. *An Organisation with a Memory: Report of an Expert Group on Learning from Adverse Events in the NHS Chaired by the Chief Medical Officer.* London: The Stationery Office; 2000.

Kotter JP. Leading change: why transformation efforts fail. *Harv Bus Rev* 1995;73:59–67.

Lyndon A, Sexton JB, Simpson KR, et al. Predictors of likelihood of speaking up about safety concerns in labour and delivery. *BMJ Qual Saf* July 1, 2011 [Epub ahead of print].

Sexton JB, Berenholtz SM, Goeschel CA, et al. Assessing and improving safety climate in a large cohort of intensive care units. *Crit Care Med* 2011;39:934–939.

Shortell SM, Singer SJ. Improving patient safety by taking systems seriously. *JAMA* 2008;299:445–447.

Sorokin R, Riggio JM, Moleski S, et al. Physicians-in-training attitudes on patient safety: 2003 to 2008. *J Patient Saf* 2011;7:132–137.

Spath PL, ed. *Error Reduction in Health Care: A Systems Approach to Improving Patient Safety.* 2nd ed. San Francisco, CA: Jossey-Bass; 2011.

Lucian Leape Institute at the National Patient Safety Foundation. *Unmet Needs: Teaching Physicians to Provide Safe Patient Care.* Boston, MA: Lucian Leape Institute at the National Patient Safety Foundation; March 2010.

WORKFORCE ISSUES | 16

OVERVIEW

In many discussions of patient safety, it is assumed that the workforce is up to the task—in training, competency, and numbers. In these formulations, a combination of the right processes, information technology, and culture is enough to ensure safe care.

However, as any frontline worker can tell you, neglecting issues of workforce sufficiency and competency omits an important part of the equation. For example, a nursing or physician staff that is overworked and demoralized will breed unsafe conditions, even if good communication, sound policies, and efficient computers are in place.

In this chapter, I will discuss some key issues in workforce composition and organizational structure, including the nursing workforce, Rapid Response Teams, and trainee-related matters such as duty-hour restrictions and the so-called "July effect." I'll close with a discussion of the "second victim" phenomenon: the toll that errors take on caregivers themselves. In the next chapter, I'll discuss issues of training and competency.

NURSING WORKFORCE ISSUES

Much of our understanding of the interaction between workforce and patient outcomes and safety comes from studies of nursing. The combination of pioneering research exploring these associations,[1-5] a U.S. nursing shortage that emerged in the late 1990s, and effective advocacy by nursing organizations (because most hospital nurses in the United States are salaried and employed by the hospitals, they have a strong incentive to advocate for sensible workloads; contrast this to physicians, most of whom are self-employed and therefore calibrate their own workload) has created this focus.

Substantial data suggest that medical errors increase with higher ratios of patients to nurses. One study found that surgical patients had a 31% greater chance of dying in hospitals when, on average, a nurse cared for more than seven patients. For every additional patient added to a nurse's average

Table 16-1 **REASONS FOR FAILURE TO RESCUE**
Monitoring technology is used only in the intensive care unit or step-down units
Hospital-ward monitoring is only intermittent (vital sign measurements)
Intervals between measurements can easily be eight hours or longer
Regular visits by a hospital-ward nurse vary in frequency and duration
Visits by a unit doctor may occur only once a day
When vital signs are measured, they are sometimes incomplete
When vital signs are abnormal, there may be no specific criteria for activating a higher-level intervention
Individual judgment is applied to a crucial decision
Individual judgment varies in accuracy according to training, experience, professional attitude, working environment, hierarchical position, and previous responses to alerts
If an alert is issued, the activation process goes through a long chain of command (e.g., nurse to charge nurse, charge nurse to intern, intern to resident, resident to fellow, fellow to attending physician)
Each step in the chain is associated with individual judgment and delays
In surgical wards, doctors are sometimes physically unavailable because they are performing operations
Modern hospitals provide care for patients with complex disorders and coexisting conditions, and unexpected clinical deterioration may occur while nurses and doctors are busy with other tasks

Reproduced with permission from Jones DA, DeVita MA, Bellomo R. Rapid-response teams. *N Engl J Med* 2011;365:139–146.

At the present time, the optimal criteria to trigger an RRT response are unknown.[19] Some institutions use strict objective criteria, while others emphasize that anyone with concerns should feel free to activate the RRT. Some hospitals even allow patients and families to call the team. One Australian hospital's poster illustrating its vital sign criteria for activating its Medical Emergency Team (another name for RRT) is shown in Figure 16-1.[19]

Similarly, the optimal composition of the responding team remains uncertain. Some hospitals have used physician-led teams, while other RRTs are led by nurses, often with respiratory therapists as partners.[19] RRTs have a positive impact on nursing satisfaction and perhaps retention, although the magnitude of this benefit has not been fully quanified.[28]

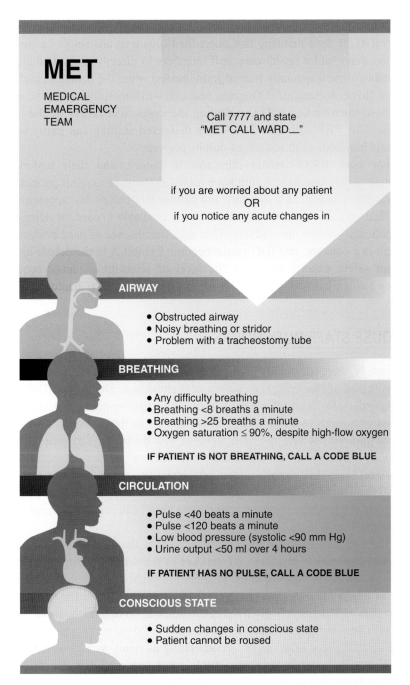

Figure 16-1 ■ An Australian hospital poster listing criteria for activation of a Rapid Response Team. (Reproduced with permission from Jones DA, DeVita MA, Bellomo R. Rapid-response teams. *N Engl J Med* 2011;365:139–146.)

While the Joint Commission does not specifically require the presence of an RRT, it does mandate that accredited organizations select "a suitable method that enables health care staff members to directly request additional assistance from a specially trained individual(s) when the patient's condition appears to be worsening."[29] Ongoing research will hopefully answer the many questions surrounding RRTs, including the cost-effectiveness of the intervention. An RRT with round-the-clock dedicated staffing can easily cost a hospital hundreds of thousands of dollars per year.

For now, RRTs remain attractive in theory, and their underlying rationale—that hospitals should have robust systems to monitor patients for deterioration as well as a structure and culture that ensure that appropriately qualified staff and necessary technology are available to care for deteriorating patients—seems unassailable. That said, the absence of hard evidence of benefit is a concern, and RRTs have become Exhibit A in the debate among patient safety experts regarding the level of scientific evidence required before a so-called "safe practice" is promoted or required (Chapter 22).[30–32]

HOUSE STAFF DUTY HOURS

Amazingly, there is virtually no research linking safety or patient outcomes to the workload of practicing (i.e., nontrainee) physicians. Dr. Michael DeBakey, the legendary Texas heart surgeon, was once said to have performed 18 cardiac bypass operations in a single day! The outcomes of the patients (particularly patient number 18) have not been reported. But the implicit message of such celebrated feats of endurance is that "real doctors" do not complain about their workload; they simply soldier on. With little research to question this attitude and with the dominant payment system in the United States continuing to reward productivity over safety, there have been few counterarguments to this machismo logic.

The one area in which this has changed is in the workload of physician trainees, particularly residents. At the core of residency training is the ritual of being "on call"—staying in the hospital overnight to care for sick patients. Bad as things are now, they have markedly improved since the mid-1900s, when many residents actually *lived* at the hospital (giving us the term "house officer") for months at a time. Even as recently as 20 years ago, some residents were on call every other night, accumulating as many as 120 weekly work hours—which is particularly remarkable when one considers that there are only 168 hours in a week.

Although resident call schedules became more reasonable over the past generation, until recently many residents continued to be on call every third night, with workweeks of more than 100 hours. But change has not come easily. As efforts to limit house staff shifts gained momentum, some physician leaders argued that traditional schedules were necessary to mint competent, committed physicians. For example, in 2002 the editor of the *New England Journal of Medicine* wrote that long hours:

> ... have come with a cost, but they have allowed trainees to learn how the disease process modifies patients' lives and how they cope with illness. Long hours have also taught a central professional lesson about personal responsibility to one's patients, above and beyond work schedules and personal plans. Whether this method arose by design or was the fortuitous byproduct of an arduous training program designed primarily for economic reasons is not the point. Limits on hours on call will disrupt one of the ways we've taught young physicians these critical values ... We risk exchanging our sleep-deprived healers for a cadre of wide-awake technicians.[33]

Therein lies the tension: legitimate concerns that medical professionalism might be degraded by "shift work" and that excellence requires lots of practice and the ability to follow many patients from clinical presentation through work-up to denouement, balanced against worries regarding the effects of fatigue on performance and morale.[34–37] The latter concerns are well grounded. One study showed that 24 hours of sustained wakefulness results in performance equivalent to that of a person with a blood alcohol level of 0.1%—above the legal limit for driving in every state in the United States.[38]

Although early researchers felt that this kind of impairment occurred only after very long shifts, we now know that chronic sleep deprivation is just as harmful. Healthy volunteers performing math calculations were just as impaired after sleeping 5 hours per night for a week as they were after a single 24-hour wakefulness marathon.[39] The investigators in this study didn't check to see what happened when both these disruptions occurred in the *same* week, the norm for many residents operating under traditional training models.

Although it defies common sense to believe that sleep-deprived brains and bad medical decisions are not related, hard proof of this intuitive link has been surprisingly hard to come by. Most studies using surgical simulators or videotapes of surgeons during procedures show that sleep-deprived residents have problems with both precision and efficiency, yet studies of nonsurgical trainees are less conclusive. One showed that interns who averaged less than 2 hours of sleep in the previous 32 hours made nearly twice as many errors reading ECGs and had to give each tracing more attention, especially when reading several in a row.[40] Another found that medical interns performed better on a simulated clinical scenario after a 16-hour shift than after a traditional extended duration shift.[41] Yet other studies showed that tired radiology residents made no more mistakes reading x-rays than well-rested ones, and sleepy ER residents performed physical examinations and recorded patient histories with equal reliability in both tired and rested conditions.[42]

In 2003, the Accreditation Council for Graduate Medical Education (ACGME, the group that blesses the 7800 residency programs in the United States, involving over 100,000 trainees) stepped into the breach, limiting residents to a maximum of 80 hours per week, with no shift lasting longer than 30 consecutive hours and at least one day off per week (Table 16-2).[43] Studies that followed these changes yielded surprisingly mixed results, with the weight of the evidence showing no significant change in patient safety or overall outcomes, but improved quality of life for residents.[43–47]

Notwithstanding the ambiguous evidence, pressure on the ACGME to do more continued to mount, driven by public and professional advocacy and by the results of a prominent study that found that residents on ICU rotations who worked in shifts averaging 16 hours committed fewer errors than those working traditional overnight shifts.[43,48] In 2008, the Institute of Medicine released a study recommending that overnight shifts for all residents be eliminated and that round-the-clock supervision be required.[49] In 2010, the ACGME responded by codifying the IOM's recommended supervision requirements, but prohibiting overnight shifts only for interns (first-year residents), not all residents (Table 16-2).[43,50]

As with the 2003 regulations, time will tell whether these changes, which went into effect in July 2011, will have the desired effects. We already know that they are unpopular with training program directors, who fear that they will soon begin to graduate undertrained physicians.[37] Residents, interestingly, are conflicted—confident that the new rules will improve their own quality of life but skeptical that they will improve their training and patient safety.[47] This debate is likely to continue, particularly since most other developed countries have duty-hour limits far more stringent than even the new U.S. standards (Table 16-3).[49]

In discussions regarding duty hours and fatigue, analogies are often made to other industries that have far more severe limits on consecutive work hours. For example, U.S. commercial pilots cannot fly for more than eight hours straight without relief, and truck drivers must pull off the road after 10 hours for a mandatory break. But between these shifts, the machines either sit idle or are operated by another crew. Fumbles may occur in the handoffs of the machines but they are unusual, and no one hands over the reins in the middle of a critical function (such as an airport landing approach). In medicine, on the other hand, handoff errors are routine (Chapter 8). This means that the real patient safety question is not whether fatigued doctors make more mistakes (they probably do), but whether the errors caused by fumbled handoffs and more subtle information seepage will exceed those caused by fatigue.

Table 16-2 **COMPARISON OF THE 2010 ACGME RESIDENT DUTY-HOUR STANDARDS WITH THE 2008 IOM RECOMMENDATIONS AND THE 2003 ACGME REQUIREMENTS***

Standards	2003 ACGME Requirements	Institute of Medicine 2008 Recommendations	2010 ACGME Standards
Maximum hours of work per week	80-hour week, averaged over 4 weeks	No change	No change
Maximum shift length	30 hours (admitting patients up to 24 hours, and then 6 additional hours for transitional and educational activities)	▪ 30 hours (admitting patients for up to 16 hours, plus 5-hour protected sleep period between 10 PM and 8 AM with the remaining hours for transition and educational activities) ▪ 16 hours with no protected sleep period	▪ Duty periods of PGY-1 residents must not exceed 16 hours in duration ▪ Intermediate-level and senior residents may be scheduled to a maximum of 24 hours of continuous duty. Strategic napping, especially after 16 hours of continuous duty and between 10 PM and 8 AM, is strongly suggested
Maximum in-hospital on-call frequency	Every third night, on average	Every third night, no averaging	Intermediate-level and senior residents: every third night (no averaging)
Minimum time off between scheduled shifts	10 hours after shift	▪ 10 hours after day shift ▪ 12 hours after night shift ▪ 14 hours after any extended duty period of 30 hours and not return until 6 AM the next day	▪ PGY-1 residents should have 10 hours off and must have 8 hours free from duty between scheduled duty periods ▪ Intermediate-level residents should have 10 hours off and must have 8 hours between duty periods and 14 hours free from duty after 24 hours of in-hospital duty ▪ Residents in the final year of training should have 10 hours free from duty and must have 8 hours between scheduled duty periods
Maximum frequency of in-hospital night shifts	Not addressed	Four nights maximum; 48 hours off after three or four nights of consecutive duty	Residents must not be scheduled for more than six consecutive nights of night duty (night float)

(continued)

Table 16-2   COMPARISON OF THE 2010 ACGME RESIDENT DUTY-HOUR STANDARDS WITH THE 2008 IOM RECOMMENDATIONS AND THE 2003 ACGME REQUIREMENTS* *(continued)*

Standards	2003 ACGME Requirements	Institute of Medicine 2008 Recommendations	2010 ACGME Standards
Mandatory time off-duty	■ 4 days off per month ■ 1 day (24 hours) off per week, averaged over 4 weeks	■ 5 days off per month ■ 1 day (24 hours) off per week, no averaging ■ One 48-hour period off per month	24 hours off per 7-day period when averaged over 4 weeks; home call cannot be assigned on these free days
Moonlighting	Internal moonlighting is counted against 80-hour weekly limit	■ Internal and external moonlighting is counted against 80-hour weekly limit ■ All other duty-hour limits apply to moonlighting in combination with scheduled work	■ Internal and external moonlighting count against 80-hour weekly limit ■ PGY-1 residents must not be permitted to moonlight, internally or externally
Limit on hours for exceptions	Maximum of 88 hours for individual programs with a sound educational rationale	No change	No change. Before submitting the request to review committee, the program director must obtain permission from the designated institutional official and the graduate medical education committee
Home call	■ Frequency of home call is not subject to the every-third-night, or 24 + 6 limitation ■ Residents on home call must have 1 day in 7 free from all responsibilities, averaged over 4 weeks ■ Hours logged when residents are called into the hospital are counted toward the 80-hour limit	Not addressed	■ Time on home call spent by residents in hospital must count toward the 80-hour maximum weekly limit ■ Frequency of home call is not subject to the every-third-night limitation ■ Residents are permitted to return to the hospital while on home call to care for new or established patients; each episode of this type of care, although it must be included in the 80-hour weekly maximum, will not initiate a new off-duty period

(continued)

Table 16-2 COMPARISON OF THE 2010 ACGME RESIDENT DUTY-HOUR STANDARDS WITH THE 2008 IOM RECOMMENDATIONS AND THE 2003 ACGME REQUIREMENTS* (continued)

Standards	2003 ACGME Requirements	Institute of Medicine 2008 Recommendations	2010 ACGME Standards
Supervision	▪ Programs must ensure that qualified faculty provide appropriate supervision	▪ Residency review committee should establish measurable standards of supervision according to specialty and level of training ▪ Residents in the first year must have immediate access to in-house supervision	▪ Program-specific trainee supervising physician communication guidelines and policies will be required ▪ Faculty assignments to teaching services need to be of sufficient length

*The 2010 standards went into effect July 2011. ACGME, Accreditation Council for Graduation Medical Education; IOM, Institute of Medicine; PGY-1, first-year resident ("intern").

Reproduced with permission from Pastores SM, O'Connor MF, Kleinpell RM, et al. The Accreditation Council for Graduate Medical Education resident duty hour new standards: history, changes, and impact on staffing of intensive care units. *Crit Care Med* 2011;39:2540–2549.

Table 16-3 HOUSE STAFF WORK HOUR REGULATIONS IN SELECTED COUNTRIES OUTSIDE THE UNITED STATES, 2008

	Maximum Hours/Week	Maximum Hours/Shift
European Union	48, averaged	13
United Kingdom	56–64, averaged	14–24
Denmark	37	13–16
France	52.5	10
New Zealand	72 (not averaged)	16
Australia	Unrestricted	N/A
Canada	Unrestricted nationally	Varies by province
Manitoba	89	24 + 2
Ontario	60 (intensive care unit, emergency department)	24 + 1 (certain rotations only)

Adapted with permission from Ulmer C, Wolman DM, Johns MME, eds. Committee on Optimizing Graduate Medical Trainee (Resident) Hours and Work Schedule to Improve Patient Safety. *Resident Duty Hours: Enhancing Sleep, Supervision, and Safety.* Institute of Medicine. Washington, DC: National Academies Press; 2008.

Moreover, a full accounting of the safety impact of duty-hour limits must also weigh the quality of care that physicians deliver *after* they enter full-time practice, and the substantial costs (well into the billions of dollars) to pay for new nonteaching services staffed by hospitalists, nurse practitioners, and physician assistants.[51] Finally, there is another, more subtle risk of the new standards: as the *New England Journal* editor feared, the new rules will contribute to a change in culture among physicians, from a "do whatever it takes" mindset to a "shift work" mentality. Residents themselves remain torn by their understandable desire for more rest and their deeply felt ethical commitment to their patients.[52,53]

Even as we ponder the implications of the duty-hour changes, there can be little debate on one issue: 100-hour workweeks *must* be bad for young doctors (and older ones too, although no one is regulating their hours presently), their loved ones, and ultimately their patients. Because of this, some form of duty-hour limits are welcome, as long as they are accompanied by active efforts to make handoffs safer, to relieve residents of superfluous paperwork, to provide decent rest facilities in hospitals, to hire alternate providers to pick up the slack, and to promote professionalism among trainees. Moreover, these changes must be accompanied by rigorous research to assess both their benefits and harms.

THE "JULY EFFECT"

Though not as vocal as the debate over duty hours, another potential patient safety risk associated with trainees has received more attention of late: the safety of patients cared for by new residents. Dubbed the "July effect" in the United States and the more macabre "August killing season" in the United Kingdom,[54] the evidence supporting the association between new residents and harm has long been debated. However, a 2011 systematic review of 39 studies by Young et al. found that the more methodologically rigorous studies did, in fact, find increased mortality (averaging about 8%) and decreased efficiency (longer lengths of stay).[55] The July effect could likely be mitigated by a number of interventions, including improved supervision, a limitation on trainees' workload in the first few weeks, and staggered starting times for new residents.

Young and his colleagues (including me) also recently raised concerns about another trainee-related transition: the year-end handover of outpatients that occurs in teaching settings.[56] Residents typically accrue large ambulatory panels, and then abruptly hand these patients off to new interns at the completion of training. With this handoff, patients experience a vast drop in the experience level of their physicians—both clinical experience and practical knowledge regarding the inner workings of the healthcare organization. We estimate that nearly 13,000 trainees hand their clinic populations off every July, so this handoff affects about 2 million unsuspecting patients.

The solutions to this problem are likely to be similar to those described above, including improved supervision and limited initial schedules. But here, the safety issues surrounding handoffs also assume great importance (Chapter 8), which means that fixes will also involve Web-based ambulatory sign-out systems and mandatory discussions between outgoing residents and incoming interns, at least regarding the most active and challenging patients. This issue may well be addressed by healthcare system or training program accreditors in the not-so-distant future.[57]

NIGHTS AND WEEKENDS

It is self-evident that hospitals are 24-7-365 enterprises, yet few hospitals staff the nights and weekends the way they do daytimes and weekdays. This is not completely without rationale: while the patients don't change, staffing needs partly relate to patients' requirements for transport or the intensity of testing and consultations. If more is being done to and for patients during the day or on weekdays because of the greater availability of personnel and equipment, richer staffing on these shifts may be appropriate.

That said, there are likely to be other explanations for lighter staffing on nights and weekends, relating to caregiver preferences or constrained hospital budgets. Such understaffing could easily put patients at risk on these "off hours." One hospital CEO put it well, after making a series of late-night administrative rounds.[58] "I've come to appreciate the fact that I work in two distinct places," the CEO, Dr. David Shulkin, observed, a "day hospital" and a "night and weekend hospital." He continued:

> The weekday hospital has a full administrative team, department chairs and service chiefs, experienced nurse managers, and a full complement of professional staff. The off-hours hospital, on the other hand, rarely, if ever, has senior managers present. Nurse-to-patient ratios are significantly lower. Even the number of residents is considerably lower—certainly lower than during my days of training—because of mandated work-hour restrictions.

Empirical data generally support Shulkin's concerns. The majority of studies that have scrutinized the outcomes of care on weekends and nights have documented higher death rates, higher readmission rates, and more surgical complications.[59–63] Moreover, survival rates after in-hospital cardiac arrest are lower, and medical mistakes are more common.[64,65] The evidence regarding the hazards of nights is slightly less robust than that of the weekends, but still of concern.[66,67]

The challenge will be to find the resources to provide adequate staffing on nights and weekends. In areas such as radiology or critical care, telemedicine may provide a partial answer by making physician expertise available without requiring on-site presence. In others, physicians will need to provide in-house coverage. Many hospitals have augmented their weekend and night staffing with a combination of hospitalists and intensivists. Selected groups of patients might benefit from being managed in specialized centers that offer adequate staffing at all times. For example, a recent study found that while stroke patients fared worse when admitted on weekends to general hospitals, this difference was eliminated when patients were admitted to specialized stroke centers.[68]

Some experts have argued for a more regulatory approach, and several states do in fact regulate nurse-to-patient ratios (see earlier discussion); these standards typically do not vary by time of day or day of the week. Ultimately, an integrated approach—including adequate staffing, appropriate oversight of trainees, and thoughtful use of technology, guided by evidence and supported by appropriate transparency and, when needed, regulatory or accreditation standards—will be needed to address the "two hospitals" problem.

"SECOND VICTIMS": SUPPORTING CAREGIVERS AFTER MAJOR ERRORS

While the healthcare system, correctly and understandably, focuses on the patient and family after a serious error, caregivers also require empathy and attention. In a 2000 article, Albert Wu of Johns Hopkins coined the term "second victim" to describe how caregivers themselves are affected after they commit an error.[69] In a 2011 interview with me, he expanded on this concept:

> I think that there are two ways that healthcare workers are traumatized. The first are things we do to ourselves; these are self-inflicted wounds that result from internalized judgments .... we feel anxious, depressed, and demoralized. On the other hand, some healthcare workers are actively victimized by elements of the system or by other organizations. Those are people who work in places that still believe in shame-and-blame or crime-and-punishment, and they're sometimes official bodies like nursing boards and so forth. They actually punish people and, I think, add insult to those self-inflicted injuries .... Some people have persistent problems—the incidents go on to cause

lasting harm. Some people are so depressed that they need to be hospitalized; some people are suicidal. People quit medicine or nursing because of what they did …. In our hospital ... a boy with head trauma came in and was badly injured. He needed to be intubated, could not be intubated and could not be trached, and died in the emergency room. It was just a horrific incident and everyone felt unimaginably bad. But even though the emergency physician got some support, others were a little critical of his actions, and he quit clinical medicine within the year.[70]

Addressing the second victim issue is not easy. Colin West of the Mayo Clinic suggests that an opportunity be given to the caregiver to process the error, such as in an informal small group or a traditional M&M conference.[71–73] Whichever forum is chosen, it is critical that participants model the importance of error acknowledgment and open discussion. Emotional support provided by a trusted colleague or a professional counselor is also helpful; West recommends that this person should not be part of the clinician's performance evaluation team.

While such counseling can be obtained informally after an error, too often it is not, leaving caregivers to suffer in silence.[74,75] Because of this, some institutions have developed programs designed to sensitize all staff to the issues of second victims, including understanding that errors happen to every clinician and perfection is not an attainable goal. Such educational programs should arm clinicians with coping strategies, and caution against maladaptive strategies that are often employed.

A few programs go even further. One of the most advanced is the second victim support team (the *forYOU Team*) developed by Susan Scott and colleagues at the University of Missouri.[76,77] Based on interviews with clinicians after adverse events, the Missouri investigators identified six stages in the second victim recovery process: (i) chaos and accident response, (ii) intrusive reflections, (iii) restoring personal integrity, (iv) enduring the inquisition, (v) obtaining emotional first aid, and (vi) moving on.[78] To support caregivers through these stages, after a serious adverse event a trained supervisor or peer is immediately dispatched to offer support (such trained individuals are embedded on every high-risk service). The goal is to prevent clinicians from going home before they receive initial counseling. From there, referrals are made for additional support. Any investigation of the incident, including root cause analysis if appropriate, is conducted by different individuals than those on the support teams.

A few other institutions have instituted similar programs.[79–81] Early responses from clinicians to these programs are positive and the programs clearly fill an important gap. However, additional research is needed to determine the optimal structure, financing, and timing of second victim programs, and how to ensure that caregivers receive needed support while also allowing for rapid and effective incident investigations and responses (Chapter 14).

KEY POINTS

- Increasing attention is being paid to the importance of a well-trained, well-rested workforce to patient safety.
- In nursing, good studies have linked longer work hours, lower nurse-to-patient ratios, and higher patient turnover to poor outcomes.
- Many hospitals have organized specialized teams of caregivers available to respond to unexpected patient deteriorations (RRTs). While the concept has face validity, studies of this strategy have yielded mixed results.
- Although research has linked long hours and fatigue in physicians to errors, it has not yet led to widespread efforts to regulate physician staffing. The exception is in residency training programs, where regulations now limit weekly hours and shift lengths. These limits have improved house staff well-being, but the impact on safety or education is not yet clear.
- Attention is turning to the safety hazards of hospital care on nights and weekends, and to the risk of receiving care early in the training year in teaching hospitals.
- Clinicians involved in serious errors are deeply affected by the experience. Several programs designed to support such "second victims" have been launched.

REFERENCES

1. Aiken LH, Clarke SP, Sloane DM, et al. Hospital nurse staffing and patient mortality, nurse burnout, and job dissatisfaction. *JAMA* 2002;288:1987–1993.
2. Aiken LH, Clarke SP, Cheung RB, et al. Educational levels of hospital nurses and surgical patient mortality. *JAMA* 2003;290:1617–1623.
3. Rogers AE, Hwang WT, Scott LD, et al. The working hours of hospital staff nurses and patient safety. *Health Aff (Millwood)* 2004;23:202–212.
4. Hugonnet S, Chevrolet JC, Pittet D. The effect of workload on infection risk in critically ill patients. *Crit Care Med* 2007;35:76–81.
5. Needleman J, Buerhaus P, Pankratz VS, et al. Nurse staffing and inpatient hospital mortality. *N Engl J Med* 2011;364:1037–1045.

6. Buerhaus PI, Auerbach DI, Staiger DO. The recent surge in nurse employment: causes and implications. *Health Aff* 2009;28:w657–w668.

7. Rosenstein AH, O'Daniel M. Disruptive behavior and clinical outcomes: perceptions of nurses and physicians. *Am J Nurs* 2005;105:54–64 [quiz 64–65].

8. Rosenstein AH, O'Daniel M. Impact and implications of disruptive behavior in the perioperative arena. *J Am Coll Surg* 2006;203:96–105.

9. Walrath JM, Dang D, Nyberg D. Hospital RNs' experiences with disruptive behavior: a qualitative study. *J Nurs Care Qual* 2010;25:105–116.

10. Leape LL, Fromson JA. Problem doctors: is there a system-level solution? *Ann Intern Med* 2006;144:107–115.

11. The Joint Commission. *Sentinel event alert. Behaviors that Undermine a Culture of Safety*. July 9, 2008;(40):1–3.

12. Rich V. Nurse staffing ratios: the crucible of money, policy, research, and patient care. *AHRQ WebM&M* (serial online); August 2009. Available at: http://webmm.ahrq.gov/case.aspx?caseid=203.

13. Litvak E, Buerhaus PI, Davidoff F, et al. Managing unnecessary variability in patient demand to reduce nursing stress and improve patient safety. *Jt Comm J Qual Patient Saf* 2005;31:330–338.

14. Needleman J, Kurtzman ET, Kizer KW. Performance measurement of nursing care: state of the science and the current consensus. *Med Care Res Rev* 2007;64 (2 suppl):10S–43S.

15. Kurtzman ET, Buerhaus PI. New Medicare payment rules: danger or opportunity for nursing? *Am J Nursing* 2008;108:30–35.

16. Aiken LH, Havens DS, Sloane DM. The Magnet Nursing Services Recognition Program: a comparison of two groups of magnet hospitals. *J Nurs Adm* 2009;39:S5–S14.

17. Devita MA, Bellomo R, Hillman K, et al. Findings of the first consensus conference on medical emergency teams. *Crit Care Med* 2006;34:2463–2478.

18. Silber JH, Romano PS, Rosen AK, et al. Failure-to-rescue: comparing definitions to measure quality of care. *Med Care* 2007;45:918–925.

19. Jones DA, DeVita MA, Bellomo R. Rapid-response teams. *N Engl J Med* 2011;365:139–146.

20. Berwick DM, Calkins DR, McCannon CJ, et al. The 100,000 Lives Campaign: setting a goal and a deadline for improving health care quality. *JAMA* 2006;295:324–327.

21. Wachter RM, Pronovost PJ. The 100,000 Lives Campaign: a scientific and policy review. *Jt Comm J Qual Patient Saf* 2006;32:621–627.

22. Bellomo R, Goldsmith D, Uchino S, et al. A prospective before-and-after trial of a medical emergency team. *Med J Aust* 2003;179:283–287.

23. Sebat F, Musthafa AA, Johnson D, et al. Effect of a rapid response system for patients in shock on time to treatment and mortality during 5 years. *Crit Care Med* 2007;35:2568–2575.

24. Sharek PJ, Parast LM, Leong K, et al. Effect of a rapid response team on hospital-wide mortality and code rates outside the ICU in a children's hospital. *JAMA* 2007;298:2267–2274.

25. Hillman K, Chen J, Cretikos M, et al. Introduction of the medical emergency team (MET) system: a cluster-randomised controlled trial. *Lancet* 2005;365:2091–2097.

26. Chan PS, Jain R, Nallmothu BK, et al. Rapid response teams: a systematic review and meta-analysis. *Arch Intern Med* 2010;170:18–26.

27. McGaughey J, Alderdice F, Fowler R, et al. Outreach and early warning systems (EWS) for the prevention of intensive care admission and death of critically ill adult patients on general hospital wards. *Cochrane Database Syst Rev* 2007;3:CD005529–CD005529.

28. Jones D, Baldwin I, McIntyre T, et al. Nurses' attitudes to a medical emergency team service in a teaching hospital. *Qual Saf Health Care* 2006;15:427–432.

29. The Joint Commission. *2009 National Patient Safety Goals*. Available at: http://www.jointcommission.org/standards_information/npsgs.aspx.

30. Winters BD, Pham J, Pronovost PJ. Rapid response teams—walk, don't run. *JAMA* 2006;296:1645–1647.

31. Auerbach AD, Landefeld CS, Shojania KG. The tension between needing to improve care and knowing how to do it. *N Engl J Med* 2007;357:608–613.

32. Berwick DM. The science of improvement. *JAMA* 2008;299:1182–1184.

33. Drazen JM, Epstein AM. Rethinking medical training—the critical work ahead. *N Engl J Med* 2002;347:1271–1272.

34. Goitein L, Shanafelt TD, Wipf JE, et al. The effects of work-hour limitations on resident well-being, patient care, and education in an internal medicine residency program. *Arch Intern Med* 2005;165:2601–2606.

35. Lockley SW, Landrigan CP, Barger LK, et al. Harvard Work Hours Health and Safety Group. When policy meets physiology: the challenge of reducing resident work hours. *Clin Orthop Relat Res* 2006;449:116–127.

36. Hutter MM, Kellogg KC, Ferguson CM, et al. The impact of the 80-hour resident workweek on surgical residents and attending surgeons. *Ann Surg* 2006;243:864–871 [discussion 871–875].

37. Antiel RM, Thompson SM, Reed DA, et al. ACGME duty-hour recommendations—a national survey of residency program directors. *N Engl J Med* 2010;363:e12.

38. Dawson D, Reid K. Fatigue, alcohol and performance impairment. *Nature* 1997;388:235.

39. Linde L, Bergstrom M. The effect of one night without sleep on problem-solving and immediate recall. *Psychol Res* 1992;54:127–136.

40. Gaba DM, Howard SK. Patient safety: fatigue among clinicians and the safety of patients. *N Engl J Med* 2002;347:1249–1255.

41. Gordon JA, Alexander EK, Lockley SW, et al.; Harvard Work Hours, Health, and Safety Group (Boston, Massachusetts). Does simulator-based clinical performance correlate with actual hospital behavior? The effect of extended work hours on patient care provided by medical interns. *Acad Med* 2010;85:1583–1588.

42. Veasey S, Rosen R, Barzansky B, et al. Sleep loss and fatigue in residency training: a reappraisal. *JAMA* 2002;288:1116–1124.

43. Pastores SM, O'Connor MF, Kleinpell RM, et al. The Accreditation Council for Graduate Medical Education resident duty hour new standards: history, changes, and impact on staffing of intensive care units. *Crit Care Med* 2011;39:2540–2549.

44. Shetty KD, Bhattacharya J. Changes in hospital mortality associated with residency work-hour regulations. *Ann Intern Med* 2007;147:73–80.

45. Horwitz LI, Kosiborod M, Lin Z, Krumholz HM. Changes in outcomes for internal medicine inpatients after work-hour regulations. *Ann Intern Med* 2007;147:97–103.

46. Moonesinghe SR, Lowery J, Shahi N, et al. Impact of reduction in working hours for doctors in training on postgraduate medical education and patients' outcomes: systematic review. *BMJ* 2011;342:d1580.

47. Drolet BC, Spalluto LB, Fischer SA. Residents' perspectives on ACGME regulation of supervision and duty hours—a national survey. *N Engl J Med* 2010;363:e34.

48. Landrigan CP, Rothschild JM, Cronin JW, et al. Effect of reducing interns' work hours on serious medical errors in intensive care units. *N Engl J Med* 2004;351:1838–1848.

49. Ulmer C, Wolman DM, Johns MME, eds. Committee on Optimizing Graduate Medical Trainee (Resident) Hours and Work Schedule to Improve Patient Safety. *Resident Duty Hours: Enhancing Sleep, Supervision, and Safety.* Institute of Medicine. Washington, DC: National Academies Press; 2008.

50. Iglehart JK. The ACGME's final duty-hour standards—special PGY-1 limits and strategic napping. *N Engl J Med* 2010;363:1589–1591.

51. Nuckols TK, Escarce JJ. Cost implications of ACGME's 2011 changes to resident duty hours and the training environment. *J Gen Intern Med* July 21, 2011 [Epub ahead of print].

52. Landrigan CP, Barger LK, Cade BE, et al. Interns' compliance with Accreditation Council for Graduate Medical Education work-hour limits. *JAMA* 2006;296:1063–1070.

53. Carpenter RO, Spooner J, Arbogast PG, et al. Work hours restrictions as an ethical dilemma for residents: a descriptive survey of violation types and frequency. *Curr Surg* 2006;63:448–455.

54. Vaughan L, McAlister G, Bell D. 'August is always a nightmare': results of the Royal College of Physicians of Edinburgh and Society of Acute Medicine August transition survey. *Clin Med* 2011;11:322–326.

55. Young JQ, Ranji SR, Wachter RM, et al. "July Effect": impact of the academic year-end changeover on patient outcomes. A systematic review. *Ann Intern Med* 2011;155:309–315.

56. Young JQ, Wachter RM. Academic year-end transfers of outpatients from outgoing to incoming residents: an unaddressed patient safety issue. *JAMA* 2009;302:1327–1329.

57. Barach P, Philibert I. The July Effect: fertile ground for systems improvement. *Ann Intern Med* 2011;155:331–332.

58. Shulkin DJ. Like night and day—shedding light on off-hours care. *N Engl J Med* 2008;358:2091–2093.

59. Saposnik G, Baibergenova A, Bayer N, et al. Weekends: a dangerous time for having a stroke? *Stroke* 2007;38:1211–1215.

60. Bell CM, Redelmeier DA. Mortality among patients admitted to hospitals on weekends as compared with weekdays. *N Engl J Med* 2001;345:663–668.

61. Aylin P, Yunus A, Bottle A, Majeed A, et al. Weekend mortality for emergency admissions. A large, multicentre study. *Qual Saf Health Care* 2010;19:213–217.

62. Kostis WJ, Demissie K, Marcella SW, et al.; for the Myocardial Infarction Data Acquisition System (MIDAS 10) Study Group. Weekend versus weekday admission and mortality from myocardial infarction. *N Engl J Med* 2007;356:1099–1109.

63. Bendavid E, Kaganova Y, Needleman J, et al. Complication rates on weekends and weekdays in US hospitals. *Am J Med* 2007;120:422–428.

64. Peberdy MA, Ornato JP, Larkin GL, et al.; for National Registry of Cardiopulmonary Resuscitation Investigators. Survival from in-hospital cardiac arrest during nights and weekends. *JAMA* 2008;299:785–792.

65. Hendey GW, Barth BE, Soliz T. Overnight and postcall errors in medication orders. *Acad Emerg Med* 2005;12:629–634.

66. Cavallazzi R, Marik PE, Hirani A, et al. Association between time of admission to the ICU and mortality: a systematic review and metaanalysis. *Chest* 2010;138:68–75.

67. Mourad M, Adler J. Safe, high quality care around the clock: what will it take to get us there? *J Gen Intern Med* 2011;26:948–950.

68. McKinney JS, Deng Y, Kasner SE, et al.; Myocardial Infarction Data Acquisition System (MIDAS 15) Study Group. Comprehensive stroke centers overcome the weekend versus weekday gap in stroke treatment and mortality. *Stroke* 2011;42: 2403–2409.

69. Wu AW. Medical error: the second victim. *BMJ* 2000;320:726–727.

70. In conversation with ... Albert Wu, MD, MPH. *AHRQ WebM&M* (serial online); May 2011. Available at: http://www.webmm.ahrq.gov/perspective.aspx?perspectiveID=101.

71. West CP, Huschka MM, Novotny PJ, et al. Association of perceived medical errors with resident distress and empathy: a prospective longitudinal study. *JAMA* 2006;296:1071–1078.

72. West CP. How do providers recover from errors? *AHRQ WebM&M* (serial online); January 2008. Available at: http://webmm.ahrq.gov/case.aspx?caseID=167.

73. Orlander JD, Barber TW, Fincke BG. The morbidity and mortality conference: the delicate nature of learning from error. *Acad Med* 2002;77:1001–1006.

74. Waterman AD, Garbutt J, Hazel E, et al. The emotional impact of medical errors on practicing physicians in the United States and Canada. *Jt Comm J Qual Patient Saf* 2007;33:467–476.

75. Pollack C, Bayley C, Mendiola M, et al. Helping clinicians find resolution after a medical error. *Camb Q Healthc Ethics* 2003;12:203–207.

76. Scott SD, Hirschinger LE, Cox KR, et al. Caring for our own: deployment of a second victim rapid response system. *Jt Comm J Qual Patient Saf* 2010;36:233–240.

77. Scott SD. The second victim phenomenon: a harsh reality of health care professions. *AHRQ WebM&M* (serial online); May 2011. Available at: http://webmm.ahrq.gov/perspective.aspx?perspectiveID=102.

78. Scott SD, Hirschinger LE, Cox KR, et al. The natural history of recovery for the health care provider "second victim" after adverse patient events. *Qual Saf Health Care* 2009;18:325–330.

79. O'Reilly KB. New culture for coping: turning to peer support after medical errors. *American Medical News*. September 11, 2006 [professional issues section]. Available at: http://www.ama-assn.org/amednews/2006/09/11/prl20911.htm.

80. van Pelt F. Peer support: healthcare professionals supporting each other after adverse medical events. *Qual Saf Health Care* 2008;17:249–252.

81. McDonald TB, Helmchen LA, Smith KM, et al. Responding to patient safety incidents: the "seven pillars". *Qual Saf Health Care* 2010;19:e11.

ADDITIONAL READINGS

Christensen JF, Levinson W, Dunn PM. The heart of darkness: the impact of perceived mistakes on physicians. *J Gen Intern Med* 1992;7:424–431.

Fletcher KE, Underwood W 3rd, Davis SQ, et al. Effects of work hour reduction on residents' lives: a systematic review. *JAMA* 2005;294:1088–1100.

IOM (Institute of Medicine). *The Future of Nursing: Leading Change, Advancing Health.* Washington, DC: National Academies Press; 2011.

Needleman J, Buerhaus PI, Stewart M, et al. Nurse staffing in hospitals: is there a business case for quality? *Health Aff (Millwood)* 2006;25:204–211.

Page A, ed. *Keeping Patients Safe: Transforming the Work Environment of Nurses.* Committee on the Work Environment for Nurses and Patient Safety, Board on Health Care Services. Washington, DC: National Academy Press; 2004.

Ranji SR, Auerbach AD, Hurd CJ, et al. Effects of rapid response systems on clinical outcomes: systematic review and meta-analysis. *J Hosp Med* 2007;2:422–432.

Rothschild JM, Gandara E, Woolf S, et al. Single-parameter early warning criteria to predict life-threatening adverse events. *J Patient Saf* 2010;6:97–101.

Vidyarthi AR, Auerbach AD, Wachter RM, et al. The impact of duty hours on resident self reports of errors. *J Gen Intern Med* 2007;22:205–209.

Weissman JS, Rothschild JM, Bendavid E, et al. Hospital workload and adverse events. *Med Care* 2007;45:448–455.

West CP, Shanafelt TD, Kolars JC. Quality of life, burnout, educational debt, and medical knowledge among internal medicine residents. *JAMA* 2011;306:952–960.

Wylie CD. Sleep, science, and policy change. *N Engl J Med* 2005;352:196–197.

ADDITIONAL READINGS

EDUCATION AND TRAINING ISSUES | 17

OVERVIEW

Medicine has a unique problem when it comes to its trainees. Although all fields must allow trainees some opportunity to "practice" their craft before being granted a credential allowing them to work without supervision, legal, accounting, or architectural errors made by trainees generally have fewer consequences than medical errors do.

Moreover, the demands of medical practice (particularly the need for around-the-clock and weekend coverage; Chapter 16) have led to the use of trainees as cheap labor, placing them in situations in which they have too little supervision for their skill level and experience. Although this early independence has been justified pedagogically as the need to allow "trainees to learn from their mistakes" and hone their clinical instincts, in truth much of it flowed from economic imperatives.

Yet the solution is not obvious. One can envision a training environment in which patients are protected from trainees—after all, who would *not* want the senior surgeon, rather than the second-year resident, performing his or her cholecystectomy? While such an environment might be safer initially, the downstream result would be more poorly trained physicians who lack the real-world, supervised experience needed to transform them from novices into experienced professionals. The problem would be similar for nurses and other caregivers.

These two fundamental tensions form the backdrop of any discussion of training issues in the context of patient safety. First, what is the appropriate balance between autonomy and supervision? Second, are there ways for trainees to traverse their learning curves more quickly without necessarily "learning from their mistakes" on real patients? This chapter will address these issues, closing with a short discussion about teaching patient safety. Other important training-related issues, such as teamwork training and duty-hour restrictions for residents, are covered elsewhere (Chapters 15 and 16, respectively).

AUTONOMY VERSUS OVERSIGHT

The third-year medical student was sent in to "preround" on a patient, a 71-year-old man who had had a hip replacement a few days earlier. The patient complained of new shortness of breath, and on exam was anxious and perspiring, with rapid, shallow respirations. The student, on his first clinical rotation, listened to the man's lungs, expecting to hear the crackles of pulmonary edema or pneumonia or perhaps the wheezes of asthma, yet they were clear as a bell.

The student was confused, and asked the patient what he thought was going on. "It's really hot in here, doc," said the patient, and, in fact, it was. The student reassured himself that the patient was just over-heated, and resolved to discuss the case later that morning with his supervising resident. In his mind, calling the resident now would be both embarrassing and unnecessary—he had a good explanation for the patient's condition. An hour later, the patient was dead of a massive pulmonary embolism. The student never told anyone of his observations that morning, and felt shame about the case for decades afterwards.

In his terrific book, *Complications*, Harvard surgeon Atul Gawande describes the fundamental paradox of medical training:

> In medicine, we have long faced a conflict between the imperative to give patients the best possible care and the need to provide novices with experience. Residencies attempt to mitigate potential harm through supervision and graduated responsibility…. But there is still no getting around those first few unsteady times a young physician tries to put in a central line, remove a breast cancer, or sew together two segments of colon. No matter how many protections we put in place, on average, these cases go less well with the novice than with someone experienced.
>
> This is the uncomfortable truth about teaching. By traditional ethics and public insistence (not to mention court rulings), a patient's right to the best care possible must trump the objective of training novices. We want perfection without practice. Yet everyone is harmed if no one is trained for the future. So learning is hidden behind drapes and anesthesia and the elisions of language.[1]

Traditionally, supervisors in medicine erred on the side of autonomy, in the belief that trainees needed to learn by doing—giving rise to the iconic mantra of medical training, "see one, do one, teach one." We now recognize this paradigm as being both ethically troubling and one more slice of the proverbial Swiss cheese, a constant threat to patient safety (Chapter 2).

Supervising physicians (the issues also play out with other health professionals such as nurses, but the autonomy that trainees in other fields can exercise and the danger they can cause seem less than those of physicians) are terribly conflicted about all this. Supervisors know that they could do many things better and more safely, but also recognize that trainees truly do need to learn by doing. Moreover, providing the degree of supervision necessary to ensure that trainees never get into trouble would create job descriptions for supervising attendings that might not be compatible with career longevity.

On a scale that has, at one extreme, supervising physicians doing everything while trainees watch, and, at the other, trainees doing everything and calling their supervisors only when they are in trouble, until fairly recently most medical training systems were far too tilted toward autonomy. Prodded by some widely publicized cases of medical error that were due, at least in part, to inadequate supervision (the death of Libby Zion at New York Hospital in 1986 was the most vivid example[2]; Table 1-1), the traditional model of medical education—dominated by unfettered resident autonomy—is giving way to something safer. (As a side note, while the Libby Zion case is popularly attributed to long resident hours, the chair of the commission that investigated the case [Dr. Bertrand Bell] clearly saw the root cause more as inadequate supervision than sleepy residents.[3]) We now recognize that "learning from mistakes" is fundamentally unethical when it is built into the system, and that it is unreasonable to assume trainees will even know when they need help, particularly if they are thrust into the clinical arena with little or no practice and supervision.[4]

Our new appreciation of these issues has led not only to some system reforms (including the increased supervision requirements enacted by the Accreditation Council on Graduate Medical Education in 2011[5]; Table 16-2) but also to a crack in the dike of academic medical culture. For example, many attendings now stay late with their teams on admitting nights, a practice that would have been judged pathologically obsessive only 20 years ago (during my medical school days, one such attending picked up a nickname among the house staff of "the world's oldest intern").

In addition, the old culture of the "strong resident" or "strong student" (translated: one who never bothers his supervisors) is changing. Growing numbers of programs are building in expectations of oversight and creating structures to support it. For instance, around-the-clock attending presence (often with hospitalists and intensivists) to help supervise trainees at night is increasingly common. At UCSF Medical Center, for example, we now have hospitalists stay overnight with our residents. In addition to managing some patients independently, these faculty members supervise residents' care of critically ill patients and are available to help with more stable patients. I routinely tell faculty who take on these "nocturnist" roles that they should always ask the resident, "What would you be doing if I wasn't here?" before offering recommendations. I also ask these supervising physicians to emphasize to the residents that a call for help is a sign of strength and professionalism, not weakness.[6]

Ensuring appropriate communication is partly a cultural problem, but it also needs a scaffolding of thoughtfully developed guidelines. After analyzing a series of malpractice cases, the chiefs of surgical services at Harvard, working with the Harvard Risk Management Foundation, identified a series of "triggers" that should prompt direct communication between residents and attendings (Table 17-1).[7] A study at four of Harvard's teaching hospitals showed that, in one-third of cases, attendings were not notified after such trigger events.[8] The guidelines were subsequently codified, with promising results.[9]

Table 17-1   EXPECTED COMMUNICATION PRACTICES FOR PATIENTS ADMITTED TO SURGICAL SERVICES OF HARVARD TEACHING HOSPITALS

1. **For all critical changes in a patient's condition, the attending will be notified promptly (generally within one hour following evaluation). These include:**
   - Admission to the hospital
   - Transfer to the intensive care unit (ICU)
   - Unplanned intubation or ventilatory support
   - Cardiac arrest
   - Hemodynamic instability (including arrhythmias)
   - Code blue
   - Development of significant neurological changes (suspected cerebrovascular accident/seizure/new-onset paralysis)
   - Development of major wound complications (dehiscence, evisceration)
   - Medication or treatment errors requiring clinical intervention (invasive procedure(s), increased monitoring, new medications except Narcan)
   - First blood transfusion without prior attending knowledge or instruction (before or after operation)
   - Development of any clinical problem requiring an invasive procedure or operation for treatment

2. **The following will be discussed with and approved by the attending before they occur:**
   - Discharge from the hospital or from the emergency department
   - Transfer out of ICU

3. **The attending should also be contacted if:**
   - Any trainee feels that a situation is more complicated than he or she can manage
   - Nursing or physician staff, or the patient, request that the attending surgeon be contacted

Reproduced with permission from ElBardissi AW, Regenbogen SE, Greenberg CC, et al. Communication practices on 4 Harvard surgical services. *Ann Surg* 2009;250:861–865.

Oversight is not a monolithic construct. Supervisors must modulate their degree of oversight based on their comfort with the trainee's level and demonstrated competency with the task at hand. After over 200 hours of ethnographic observation, as well as interviews with emergency department and general medicine teams, Kennedy et al. documented four types of oversight, each of which might be appropriate in different situations (Table 17-2).[10]

The challenge going forward will be to find the very narrow sweet spot between unfettered trainee autonomy and stifling attending oversight, varying the level of supervision to ensure patient safety while also permitting the graded independence that trainees need to become independent practitioners.[11,12] Thankfully, we are now much closer to finding the correct balance than we were even a decade ago.

I appreciate the importance of this issue in a very personal way. You see, in the case that began this section, I was the third-year medical student who missed the fatal pulmonary embolism.[12]

SIMULATION TRAINING

Although many discussions about medical simulation emphasize the ability of simulators to create realistic situations in which participants "suspend disbelief" (including supporting role plays that focus on teamwork and communication skills; Chapter 15), another key use of simulation is to allow individuals to traverse their procedural learning curves without harming patients. Even if we tested for procedural aptitude, like the military, novices' first few operations or procedures would still be hazardous to patients' health. Recognizing this, new surgeons traditionally work under the close supervision of a veteran—but not for very long. The adage of "see one, do one, teach one" is not much of an exaggeration: after a couple of years' training, apprentice surgeons or other proceduralists are largely on their own for all but the most complex cases.

The problem does not end once formal training is completed. After the completion of residency or fellowship, practicing surgeons and other interventionalists are essentially left to their own devices to acquire new skills or keep up with the latest techniques. In *Complications*, Gawande writes that his father, a senior urologist in private practice, once estimated that three-quarters of the procedures he performed routinely did not exist when he was trained.[1] This means the issue of acquiring new skills safely is a lifelong challenge, not simply a trainee issue.

Consider the case of laparoscopic cholecystectomy, "lap choley" for short. Since being introduced more than two decades ago, this gallbladder removal technique has almost entirely replaced the much more invasive, and far more costly and risky, "open choley." Laparoscopic techniques have also

Theme	Definition	Representative Transcript Excerpt
Routine oversight	Clinical oversight activities that are planned in advance	"... each patient is always reviewed with the attending" (*a junior ED resident*) "At the end of the day we go over all the patients with either the senior resident or staff at some point, so we kind of go through what we have been doing so far … this happens on a daily basis" (*a junior general medicine resident*)
Responsive oversight	Clinical oversight activities that occur in response to trainee- or patient-specific issues (requested or not)	"I can recall working with a junior resident and, um, she had taken a history and there were a couple of things that were very important to confirm because it would affect your management, so I went back in and asked the patient the same questions. (I was) double-checking; I knew that she had asked them, she said she had asked them, but I needed to hear it myself to be sure" (*an ED attending physician*)
Direct patient care	Refers to instances when a supervisor moves beyond oversight to actively provide care for a trainee's patient	"If their patient is crashing I usually go there myself and do the acute management and I bring the clerk with me and I try to teach them how to observe …" (*a senior general medicine resident*)
Backstage oversight	Clinical oversight activities of which the trainee is not directly aware	"I go back to check the patients post-call when the students are not there" (*a general medicine attending physician*) "I read the nursing notes and I hear the nurses talking and so I know kind of what is going on. So in my mind I already have a picture of the patient" (*an ED attending physician*)

Table 17-2 FOUR THEMES DRAWN FROM OBSERVING THE OVERSIGHT ACTIVITIES OF SUPERVISORS

Reproduced with permission from Kennedy TJ, Lingard L, Baker GR, et al. Clinical oversight: conceptualizing the relationship between supervision and safety. *J Gen Intern Med* 2007;22:1080–1085.

revolutionalized other surgeries, including joint repair, hysterectomy, splenectomy, and even some open heart surgeries.

The problem is that few surgeons trained before 1990 learned laparoscopic technique during their supervised apprenticeship. Is that a problem? Well, yes. One early study of lap choleys showed that injuries to the common bile duct dropped almost 20-fold once surgeons had performed more than 12 cases. And the learning curve didn't end there: the rate of common bile duct injury on the 30th case was still 10 times higher than the rate after 50 cases.[13]

Until recently, the requirement that a surgeon certify his or her competency in any new procedure was nil—the system "trusted" that professionalism would ensure adequate training before physicians began practicing on patients. Adding to the problem, there were few training models in which surgeons or other operators could efficiently learn new techniques without putting patients at risk. I spoke earlier (Chapters 8, 9, and 15) about what healthcare can learn from aviation when it comes to teamwork and communication. Here is yet another area in which aviation's approach to this problem— how to efficiently and safely achieve competency in high-risk situations using new equipment and procedures—seems far safer than medicine's.

In both commercial and military aviation, pilots prepare to fly new planes by first undergoing considerable formal training (in classrooms and in highly realistic simulators), followed by extensive, hands-on experience in the real thing, with an instructor pilot seated next to the pilot-in-training, manning a dual set of controls. After that, pilots must pass both written and flight tests to qualify in the new machine, and they are continually evaluated with annual "check rides" administered by senior instructors. If a pilot flunks a check ride, he or she is put back on training status until the deficiencies are eradicated. When pilots fail several of these checks or are involved in a serious incident or accident, they are evaluated by what the Air Force calls a "Flight Evaluation Board," which has the power to clip their wings.

Contrast this with medicine's laissez-faire attitude toward recertification. Until relatively recently, there was no requirement for recertification in any specialty in American medicine, no requirement for demonstrated competency in new procedures, and no formal, required apprenticeship in new techniques (although some individual hospitals have enforced more rigorous criteria, and most states require some form of continuing education). This situation has improved in recent years: all major specialty boards now require recertification ("*Maintenance of Certification*" [MOC]; Table 20-1) and a number of specialty societies have set minimum volume thresholds before allowing independent practice. Moreover, accrediting bodies (including the Accreditation Council for Graduate Medical Education and the Joint Commission) are beginning to enforce more stringent requirements for competency-based credentialing of trainees and practicing physicians, respectively (Chapter 20).[14]

Even before these more rigorous requirements were enacted, many physicians *did* receive some training before beginning to perform new procedures, driven by both individual professional integrity and the malpractice system. But the data are sobering: a 1991 survey found that 55% of 165 practicing surgeons who had participated in a two-day course on laparoscopic cholecystectomy felt the workshop had left them inadequately trained to start performing the procedure. Yet 74% of these surgeons admitted that they began performing lap choleys immediately after completing the course[15] (Chapter 5).

Now that the patient safety movement has convinced most observers that learning on patients is unethical when there are practical, safer alternatives, healthcare is increasingly looking to simulation. Procedural simulators have been around for decades in other industries. Military fliers used them even before World War II, although these "Link Trainers" were only crude approximations of the real thing. Static aircraft simulators (in which the cockpit is fixed to the floor while instruments give the impression of flight) became more sophisticated during the jet age, allowing new pilots not only to learn and practice normal instrument procedures but also to handle a wide variety of airborne emergencies. By the age of jumbo jets, supersonic airliners, and space shuttles, "full motion" simulators that gave the illusion of true flight became available—pilots could actually look out the window and "take off" and "land" at any airport in the world. And the U.S. military now uses sophisticated training simulators, with 10-channel sound effects, voice recognition software (including the languages of potential enemies and allies), and "battle smells" (burnt charcoal) to prepare troops for war.

Such training and performance evaluation aids—in which trainees interact with other human beings as well as with machinery and virtual displays—may hold the highest potential for medical simulations, which, until a decade or two ago, were pretty primitive. During medical school in the 1980s, I practiced giving injections using oranges, and sutured pig's feet. A somewhat lifelike mannequin (nicknamed "Annie," for unknown reasons) has been used for years to teach cardiopulmonary resuscitation (CPR). Recently, however, these models have become far more realistic. Today's training mannequins allow students to deliver electric shocks with defibrillator paddles and note changes to heart rhythms, insert intravenous and intra-arterial lines, and perform intubations (Figure 17-1). Surgical simulators are now available to provide basic practice for medical students and residents and to help experienced surgeons learn new techniques. The major hurdle for these systems is simulating the feel of real flesh, but new technologies and materials are helping to overcome even that obstacle.

Until recently the link between improved dexterity from simulator training and fewer errors seemed intuitive but was not fully proven.[16,17] But modern studies have begun to demonstrate tangible improvements in meaningful outcomes. For example, one study found that giving surgical trainees standardized

Figure 17-1 ▪ A team practicing its skills on a modern high-fidelity simulator. (Photo courtesy of the UCSF Kanbar Center for Simulation and Clinical Skills.)

feedback on simulated laparoscopic surgeries resulted in lower error rates.[18] Another demonstrated that anesthesia residents who underwent high-fidelity simulation training were more adept at weaning their patients off cardiopulmonary bypass than colleagues who received standard classroom-based training.[19] A third found that surgical residents who underwent proficiency-based virtual reality training committed fewer technical errors during their first 10 laparoscopic cholecystectomies.[20]

A high-fidelity simulator program is expensive (some surgical simulators run over $100,000, and training practicing clinicians requires both paying for the instructors and covering provider "downtime") and logistically complex to administer. Salas et al. have identified 10 principles and tips for a successful simulation program (Table 17-3).[21] Because of this cost and complexity, the broad dissemination of simulator training will depend not only on evidence of effectiveness but also on regulatory requirements, cost sharing (e.g., some regions and professional societies have formed consortia to purchase simulators), and return-on-investment considerations. One study showed that, because novice surgeons are slower in the operating room (OR) and require substantial hand-holding by senior physicians, an average of $50,000 in precious OR time is "wasted" during each resident's four-year training period.[22] In the end, the arguments for simulator training may hinge as much on clinical efficiency as on safety.

Table 17-3 TEN PRINCIPLES FOR AN EFFECTIVE SIMULATOR-BASED TRAINING (SBT) PROGRAM

Principle	Related Tips
1. SBT should focus on reinforcing and promoting the needed competencies (i.e., knowledge/skills/attitudes)	▪ Train competencies, not tasks ▪ Conduct a training needs analysis ▪ Conduct a job/task analysis ▪ Conduct a cognitive task analysis to uncover cognitive aspects of the job ▪ Use Anesthesia Crisis Resource Management as a guide ▪ Develop learning outcomes that will serve as a guide
2. Adopt a systems approach	▪ Think about "before," "during," and "after" influences on SBT
3. Prepare the organization for SBT	▪ Pay attention to organizational factors ▪ Make sure you have top-level support ▪ Send positive messages about simulation ▪ Help employees see value of simulation ▪ Ensure key players are on board
4. Set up appropriate presimulation conditions	▪ Prepare trainees for training through preparatory information ▪ Set an appropriate presimulation climate
5. Ensure trainee motivation	▪ Show value of SBT ▪ Send positive messages about SBT
6. Apply sound instructional principles to the design of SBT	▪ Tailor instructional strategy to learning objectives ▪ Present relevant information ▪ Demonstrate skills to be learned ▪ Match fidelity of SBT to task (if possible) ▪ Provide guided hands-on practice ▪ Provide constructive and diagnostic feedback
7. Develop performance measures	▪ Create scenarios to elicit the desired knowledge/skills/attitudes ▪ Focus on process measurement
8. Set up the simulation environment	▪ Provide the appropriate training setting ▪ Provide resources ▪ Adequately train the instructors and observers
9. Prepare the transfer environment	▪ Create a continuous learning culture ▪ Show management support ▪ Create opportunities to practice what is learned ▪ Provide incentives ▪ Reinforce desired behaviors ▪ Keep sending positive signals
10. Determine training effectiveness	▪ Examine training objectives and link evaluation criteria to them ▪ Measure at multiple levels (reactions, learning, behavior, and results)

Reproduced with permission from Salas E, Wilson KA, Lazzara E, et al. Simulation-based training for patient safety: 10 principles that matter. *J Patient Saf* 2008;4:3–8.

Although one clever experiment showed that trainees improved as much on a urologic simulator costing less than a dollar (rubber tubes standing in for the urethra, styrofoam cup for the bladder) as on a high-tech version costing tens of thousands of dollars,[23] today's trend is clearly toward more realistic, technologically sophisticated simulators. Modern virtual reality simulators are beginning to input actual human data, such as those drawn from an extraordinarily detailed digitized cadaver model known as the "Visible Human." Other simulators are being developed that, rather than using generic anatomical data, use real patients' anatomy drawn from computed tomography (CT) or magnetic resonance imaging (MRI) scans. The day may come when surgeons will practice their patient's operation virtually (based on actual anatomy) before scrubbing in for a complex procedure.

While it is easy to get breathless about this futuristic technology, simulators are unlikely to completely replace having a well-prepared young learner observing, then doing, and then being corrected by a seasoned veteran. The line between learning and doing will be further blurred as simulations become more realistic and real surgeries become less invasive and more like the simulations. As more and more surgeries and procedures become "virtual," it will be important to remember that simulators can help augment trainees' technical competence, but are highly unlikely to fully replace the need for trainees to learn their craft—as safely as possible—with real patients.

TEACHING PATIENT SAFETY

Over the past few years, the central importance of teaching patient safety and its related competencies has come to be appreciated. Without high-quality and effective educational programs for health professionals, the progress we need to make in safety will be stunted. Of course, this book is one small part of many efforts to fill that gap.

While the needs are broad and encompass practicing clinicians as well as trainees in medicine, nursing, pharmacy, and healthcare administration, medical students have been a primary focus of efforts to transform education. In an influential 2010 white paper, the Lucian Leape Institute at the National Patient Safety Foundation offered a series of thoughtful and ambitious recommendations, including the need to modify medical student selection criteria, provide foundational knowledge in patient safety and associated areas through a core curriculum, and alter trainees' clinical experiences to reinforce safety-related competencies (Table 17-4).[24] Importantly, the latter recommendation takes heed of the informal "hidden curriculum," which is closely linked to the overall safety culture (Chapter 15) and whose lessons can easily trump those of even the most well-intended formal programs.[25] For example, educating

Table 17-4   THE LUCIAN LEAPE INSTITUTE'S RECOMMENDATIONS FOR IMPROVING PATIENT SAFETY EDUCATION

Recommendation 1. Medical school and teaching hospital leaders should place the highest priority on creating learning cultures that emphasize patient safety, model professionalism, enhance collaborative behavior, encourage transparency, and value the individual learner.

Recommendation 2. Medical school deans and teaching hospital CEOs should launch a broad effort to emphasize and promote the development and display of interpersonal skills, leadership, teamwork, and collaboration among faculty and staff.

Recommendation 3. As part of continuing education and ongoing performance improvement, medical school deans and teaching hospital CEOs should provide incentives and make available necessary resources to support the enhancement of faculty capabilities for teaching students how to diagnose patient safety problems, improve patient care processes, and deliver safe care.

Recommendation 4. The selection process for admission to medical school should place greater emphasis on selecting for attributes that reflect the concepts of professionalism and an orientation to patient safety.

Recommendation 5. Medical schools should conceptualize and treat patient safety as a science that encompasses knowledge of error causation and mitigation, human factors concepts, safety improvement science, systems theory and analysis, system design and redesign, teaming, and error disclosure and apology.

Recommendation 6. The medical school experience should emphasize the shaping of desired skills, attitudes, and behaviors in medical students that include, but are not limited to, the IOM and ACGME/ABMS core competencies—such as professionalism, interpersonal skills and communication, provision of patient-centered care, and working in interdisciplinary teams.

Recommendation 7. Medical schools, teaching hospitals, and residency training programs should ensure a coherent, continuing, and flexible educational experience that spans the four years of undergraduate medical education, residency and fellowship training, and lifelong continuing education.

Recommendation 8. The LCME should modify its accreditation standards to articulate expectations for the creation of learning cultures having the characteristics described in Recommendation 1, to establish patient safety education—having the characteristics described herein—as a curricular requirement, and to define specific terminal competencies for graduating medical students.

(continued)

Table 17-4 **THE LUCIAN LEAPE INSTITUTE'S RECOMMENDATIONS FOR IMPROVING PATIENT SAFETY EDUCATION** (*continued*)
Recommendation 9. The ACGME should expand its Common Program Requirements to articulate expectations for the creation of learning cultures having the characteristics described in Recommendation 1 and to emphasize the importance of patient safety–related behavioral traits.
Recommendation 10. The LCME and the ACGME should direct particular attention to the adequacy of the patient safety–related preparation of graduating medical students for entry into residency training.
Recommendation 11. A survey of medical schools should be developed to evaluate school educational priorities for patient safety, the creation of school and teaching hospital cultures that support patient safety, and school effectiveness in shaping desired student skills, attitudes, and behaviors.
Recommendation 12. Financial, academic, and other incentives should be utilized to leverage desired changes in medical schools and teaching hospitals that will improve medical education and make it more relevant to the real world of patient care.

Reproduced with permission from the Lucian Leape Institute at the National Patient Safety Foundation, *Unmet Needs: Teaching Physicians to Provide Safe Patient Care.* Boston, MA: Lucian Leape Institute at the National Patient Safety Foundation; March 2010.

ABMS, American Board of Medical Specialties; ACGME, Accreditation Council for Graduate Medical Education; CEO, chief executive officer; IOM, Institute of Medicine; LCME, Liaison Committee on Medical Education.

students about teamwork and professionalism in the classroom will mean little if they rotate onto the wards and see their supervising residents and attendings modeling noncollaborative and disrespectful behavior.

A number of key patient safety resources are listed in Appendix I. Individuals interested in learning more about patient safety can take advantage of many Web-based resources, such as *AHRQ WebM&M*,[26] a monthly case-based safety journal (Figure 14-1), and *AHRQ Patient Safety Network*,[27] a weekly update of studies, Web sites, conferences, and tools in patient safety (Figures 22-2 and 22-3). These free resources, along with additional sources of information for patient safety leaders, are described more fully in Chapter 22.

Many training programs have begun offering a wide variety of safety curricula, and several descriptive and empirical studies of these innovations have been published.[6,28–32] In addition, some larger organizations, such as the Institute for Healthcare Improvement (IHI), the VA's National Center for Patient Safety, and the Risk Management Foundation of the Harvard Medical Institutions, have made their curricula available.[33–35] As one measure of trainees' hunger for patient safety education, at this writing more than 65,000 students and residents are registered on www.IHI.org and thousands have taken courses through IHI's Open School for Health Professionals.[33]

Many other issues related to patient safety education, such as improving diagnostic reasoning (Chapter 6), computerized decision support (Chapter 13), teamwork training (Chapter 15), and using malpractice cases to teach patient safety (Chapter 18), are highlighted throughout this book.

KEY POINTS

- Medical training has always needed to balance autonomy and oversight, but has traditionally tipped this balance toward trainee autonomy, largely for economic reasons.
- Driven in large part by the patient safety movement, the scale is moving back toward oversight, reflected in more available and involved supervisors and efforts to encourage trainees to admit their limitations and call for help.
- Particularly in procedural fields, the use of simulation will help trainees—and practicing clinicians who need to learn new procedures—traverse their learning curves with fewer risks to patients. Emerging data support the logical premise that simulation training leads to fewer errors and improved efficiency.
- Training the next generation of health professionals in patient safety–related competencies is crucial, and many curricula and resources have been developed for this purpose. Such training will need not only to provide foundational knowledge but also to pay attention to the "hidden curriculum" that trainees experience during their clinical rotations.

REFERENCES

1. Gawande AA. *Complications: A Surgeon's Notes on an Imperfect Science.* New York, NY: Henry Holt and Company; 2002.
2. Robins N. *The Girl who Died Twice: Every Patient's Nightmare: The Libby Zion Case and the Hidden Hazards of Hospitals.* New York, NY: Delacorte Press; 1995.
3. Bell BM. Supervision, not regulation of hours, is the key to improving the quality of patient care. *JAMA* 1993;269:403–404.

4. Wu AW, Folkman S, McPhee SJ, et al. Do house officers learn from their mistakes? *JAMA* 1991;265:2089–2094.

5. Iglehart JK. The ACGME's final duty-hour standards—special PGY-1 limits and strategic napping. *N Engl J Med* 2010;363:1589–1591.

6. Ross PT, McMyler ET, Anderson SG, et al. Trainees' perceptions of patient safety practices: recounting failures of supervision. *Jt Comm J Qual Patient Saf* 2011;37:88–95.

7. Manuel BM, McCarthy JL, Berry W, et al. Risk management and patient safety. *AHRQ WebM&M* (serial online); December 2010. Available at: http://webmm.ahrq.gov/perspective.aspx?perspectiveID=96.

8. ElBardissi AW, Regenbogen SE, Greenberg CC, et al. Communication practices on 4 Harvard surgical services. *Ann Surg* 2009;250:861–865.

9. Arriaga AF, ElBardissi AW, Regenbogen SE, et al. A policy-based intervention for the reduction of communication breakdowns in inpatient surgical care: results from a Harvard surgical safety collaborative. *Ann Surg* 2011;253:849–854.

10. Kennedy TJ, Lingard L, Baker GR, et al. Clinical oversight: conceptualizing the relationship between supervision and safety. *J Gen Intern Med* 2007;22:1080–1085.

11. Shojania KG, Fletcher KE, Saint S. Graduate medical education and patient safety: a busy—and occasionally hazardous—intersection. *Ann Intern Med* 2006;145:592–598.

12. Wachter RM, Shojania KG. *Internal Bleeding: The Truth Behind America's Terrifying Epidemic of Medical Mistakes*. New York, NY: Rugged Land; 2004.

13. Moore MJ, Bennett CL. The learning curve for laparoscopic cholecystectomy. The Southern Surgeons Club. *Am J Surg* 1995;170:55–59.

14. Holmboe ES, Sherbino J, Long DM, et al. The role of assessment in competency-based medical education. *Med Teach* 2010;32:676–682.

15. Morino M, Festa V, Garrone C. Survey on Torino courses. The impact of a two-day practical course on apprenticeship and diffusion of laparoscopic cholecystectomy in Italy. *Surg Endosc* 1995;9:46–48.

16. Salas E, Wilson KA, Burke CS, et al. Using simulation-based training to improve patient safety: what does it take? *Jt Comm J Qual Patient Saf* 2005;31:363–371.

17. Sutherland LM, Middleton PF, Anthony A. Surgical simulation: a systematic review. *Ann Surg* 2006;243:291–300.

18. Boyle E, Al-Akash M, Gallagher AG, et al. Optimising surgical training: use of feedback to reduce errors during a simulated surgical procedure. *Postgrad Med J* 2011; 87:524–528.

19. Bruppacher HR, Alam SK, LeBlanc VR, et al. Simulation-based training improves physicians' performance in patient care in high-stakes clinical setting of cardiac surgery. *Anesthesiology* 2010;112:985–992.

20. Ahlberg G, Enochsson L, Gallagher AG, et al. Proficiency-based virtual reality training significantly reduces the error rate for residents during their first 10 laparoscopic cholecystectomies. *Am J Surg* 2007;193:797–804.

21. Salas E, Wilson KA, Lazzara E, et al. Simulation-based training for patient safety: 10 principles that matter. *J Patient Saf* 2008;4:3–8.

22. Bridges M, Diamond DL. The financial impact of teaching surgical residents in the operating room. *Am J Surg* 1999;177:28–32.

23. Matsumoto ED, Hamstra SJ, Radomski SB, et al. The effect of bench model fidelity on endourological skills: a randomized controlled study. *J Urol* 2002;167:2354–2357.

24. Lucian Leape Institute at the National Patient Safety Foundation. *Unmet Needs: Teaching Physicians to Provide Safe Patient Care*. Boston, MA: Lucian Leape Institute at the National Patient Safety Foundation; March 2010.

25. Pingleton SK, Davis DA, Dickler RM. Characteristics of quality and patient safety curricula in major teaching hospitals. *Am J Med Qual* 2010;25:305–311.

26. Available at: http://webmm.ahrq.gov.

27. Available at: http://psnet.ahrq.gov.

28. Galt KA, Paschal KA, O'Brien RL, et al. Description and evaluation of an interprofessional patient safety course for health professions and related sciences students. *J Patient Saf* 2006;2:207–216.

29. Thompson DA, Cowan J, Holzmueller C, et al. Planning and implementing a systems-based patient safety curriculum in medical education. *Am J Med Qual* 2008;23:271–278.

30. Bell SK, Moorman DW, Delbanco T. Improving the patient, family, and clinician experience after harmful events: the "when things go wrong" curriculum. *Acad Med* 2010;85:1010–1017.

31. Stahl K, Augenstein J, Schulman CI, et al. Assessing the impact of teaching patient safety principles to medical students during surgical clerkships. *J Surg Res* 2011;170:e29–e40.

32. Dudas RA, Bundy DG, Miller MR, et al. Can teaching medical students to investigate medication errors change their attitudes towards patient safety? *BMJ Qual Saf* 2011;20:319–325.

33. The IHI Open School. Institute for Healthcare Improvement. Available at: http://www.ihi.org/offerings/ihiopenschool/Pages/default.aspx.

34. U.S. Department of Veterans Affairs. *Patient Safety Curriculum*. Ann Arbor, MI: National Center for Patient Safety. Available at: http://www.patientsafety.gov/curriculum/.

35. *Core Curriculum for Patient Safety*. Risk Management Foundation of the Harvard Medical Institutions. Available at: http://www.rmf.harvard.edu/education-interventions/materials-for-instructors/index.aspx.

ADDITIONAL READINGS

Amalberti R, Auroy Y, Berwick D, et al. Five system barriers to achieving ultrasafe health care. *Ann Intern Med* 2005;142:756–764.

Bosk CL. *Forgive and Remember: Managing Medical Failure*. 2nd ed. Chicago, IL: University of Chicago Press; 2003.

Cooper JB, Singer SJ, Hayes J, et al. Design and evaluation of simulation scenarios for a program introducing patient safety, teamwork, safety leadership, and simulation to healthcare leaders and managers. *Simul Healthc* 2011;6:231–238.

Gawande A. Personal best. *New Yorker*. October 3, 2011:44–53.

Griner PF. Leadership strategies of medical school deans to promote quality and safety. *Jt Comm J Qual Patient Saf* 2007;33:63–72.

Howard JN. The missing link: dedicated patient safety education within top-ranked US nursing school curricula. *J Patient Saf* 2010;6:165–171.

Kachalia A, Johnson JK, Miller S, et al. The incorporation of patient safety into board certification examinations. *Acad Med* 2006;81:317–325.

Kneebone RL. Practice, rehearsal, and performance: an approach for simulation-based surgical and procedure training. *JAMA* 2009;302:1336–1338.

Moorthy K, Munz Y, Forrest D, et al. Surgical crisis management skills training and assessment: a simulation-based approach to enhancing operating room performance. *Ann Surg* 2006;244:139–147.

Voelker R. Medical simulation gets real. *JAMA* 2009;302:2190–2192.

Wong BM, Etchells EE, Kuper A, et al. Teaching quality improvement and patient safety to trainees: a systematic review. *Acad Med* 2010;85:1425–1439.

THE MALPRACTICE SYSTEM | 18

OVERVIEW

A middle-aged woman was admitted to the medical ward with a moderate case of pneumonia. After being started promptly on antibiotics and fluids, she stabilized for a few hours. But she deteriorated overnight, leading to symptoms and signs of severe hypoxemia and septic shock. The nurse paged a young physician working the overnight shift.

The doctor arrived within minutes. She found the patient confused, hypotensive, tachypnic, and hypoxic. Oxygen brought the patient's oxygen saturation up to the low 90s, and the doctor now had a difficult choice to make. The patient, confused and agitated, clearly had respiratory failure: the need for intubation and mechanical ventilation was obvious. But should the young doctor intubate the patient on the floor or quickly transport her to the ICU, a few floors below, where the experienced staff could perform the intubation more safely?

Part of this trade-off was the doctor's awareness of her own limitations. She had performed only a handful of intubations in her career, most under the guidance of an anesthesiologist in an unhurried setting, and the ward nurses also lacked experience in helping with the procedure. A third option was to call an ICU team to the ward, but that could take as long as transferring the patient downstairs.

After thinking about it for a moment, she made her decision: bring the patient promptly to the ICU. She called the unit to be ready. "In my mind it was a matter of what would be safest," she reflected later. And so the doctor, a floor nurse, and a respiratory therapist wheeled the patient's bed to the elevator, and then to the ICU.

Unfortunately, in the 10 minutes between notifying the ICU and arriving there, the patient's condition worsened markedly, and orders are often violated when compliance would cause unnecessary patient suffering, such as when a patient urgently requires analgesia). That is not to condone healthcare anarchy—*routine rule violations* (Chapter 15) should cause us to rethink the rule in question, and some rules (such as "clean your hands before touching a patient" or "sign your site") should virtually never be broken. But the malpractice system will seize upon evidence that a rule was broken when there is a bad outcome, ignoring the fact that some particular rules are broken by nearly everyone in the name of efficiency—or sometimes even quality and safety.

Tort law is fluid: every society must decide how to set the bar regarding fault and compensation. By marrying the recompense of the injured to the finding of fault, tort systems inevitably lower the fault-finding bar to allow for easier compensation of sympathetic victims. But this is not the only reason the bar tilts toward fault finding. Humans (particularly of the American variety) tend to be unsettled by vague "systems" explanations, and even more bothered by the possibility that a horrible outcome could have been "no one's fault." Moreover, the continuing erosion of professional privilege and a questioning of all things "expert" (driven by the media, the Internet, and more) have further tipped the balance between plaintiff and defendant. But it was already an unfair match: faced with the heart-wrenching story of an injured patient or grieving family, who can possibly swallow an explanation that "things like this just happen" and that no one is to blame, especially when the potential source of compensation is a "rich doctor," or a faceless insurance company?[5]

The role of the expert witness further tips the already lopsided scales of malpractice justice. Almost by definition, expert witnesses are particularly well informed about their areas of expertise, which makes it exceptionally difficult for them to assume the mindset of "the reasonable practitioner," especially as the case becomes confrontational and experts gravitate to more polarized positions.

Finally, adding to the confusion is the fact that doctors and nurses feel guilty for our errors (even when there was no true fault), often blaming ourselves because we failed to live up to our own expectation of perfection (Chapter 16). Just as naturally, what person would not instinctively lash out against a provider when faced with a brain-damaged child or spouse? It is to be expected that families or patients will blame the party holding the smoking gun, just as they would a driver who struck their child who ran into the street to chase a ball. Some bereaved families (and drivers and doctors) will ultimately move on to a deeper understanding that no one is to blame—that the tragedy is just that. But whether they do or do not, write Merry and McCall Smith, "It is essential that the law should do so."[2]

If the malpractice system unfairly assigns fault when there is none, what really is the harm, other than the payment of a few (or a few million) dollars by physicians, hospitals, or insurance companies to injured patients and families? I believe that there *is* harm, particularly as we try to engage rank-and-file clinicians in patient safety efforts. A 2011 study found that the vast majority of physicians are sued at some point in their careers, and nearly one in five physicians in the highest-risk fields (neurosurgery and cardiac surgery) is sued *each year* (Figure 18-1).[6] Physicians, particularly in these fields, often

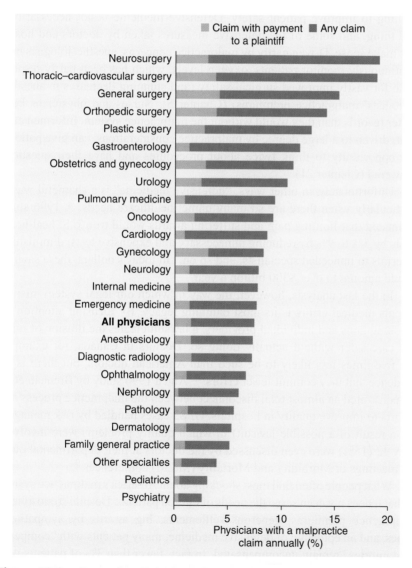

Figure 18-1 ■ Proportion of physicians facing a malpractice claim annually, according to specialty. (Reprinted with permission from Jena AB, Seabury S, Lakdawalla D, et al. Malpractice risk according to physician specialty. *N Engl J Med* 2011;365:629–636.)

become demoralized, and depressed providers are not likely to be enthusiastic patient safety leaders. Tort law is adversarial by nature, while a culture of safety is collaborative (Chapter 15). In a safety-conscious culture, doctors and nurses willingly report their mistakes as opportunities to make themselves and the system better (Chapter 14), something they are unlikely to do in a litigious environment.

This is not to say—as some do—that the malpractice system has done nothing to improve patient safety. Defensive medicine is not necessarily a bad thing, and some of the defensive measures taken by doctors and hospitals make sense. Driven partly by malpractice concerns, anesthesiologists now continuously monitor patients' oxygen levels, which has been partly responsible for vastly improved surgical safety (and stunning decreases in anesthesiologists' malpractice premiums) (Chapter 5). Nurses and physicians keep better records than they would without the malpractice system. Informed consent, driven to a large degree by malpractice considerations, can give patients the opportunity to think twice about procedures and have their questions answered (Chapter 21).

Unfortunately, in other ways, "defensive medicine" is a shameful waste, particularly when there are so many unmet healthcare needs. A 1996 study estimated that limiting pain and suffering awards would trim U.S. healthcare costs by 5% to 9% by reducing unnecessary and expensive tests, diminishing referrals to unneeded specialists, and so on.[7] In today's dollars, these savings would amount to over $300 billion a year.

In the last analysis, however, the way in which our legal system misrepresents medical errors is its most damning legacy. By focusing attention on smoking guns and individual providers, a lawsuit creates the illusion of making care safer without actually doing so. Doctors in Canada, for example, are five times less likely to be sued than American doctors, but there is no evidence that they commit fewer errors.[1,8] And a 1990 study by Brennan et al. demonstrated an almost total disconnect between the malpractice process and efforts to improve quality in hospitals. Of 82 cases handled by risk managers (as a result of a possible lawsuit) in which quality problems were involved, only 12 (15%) were even discussed by the doctors at their departmental quality meetings or Morbidity and Mortality (M&M) conferences.[9]

What people often find most shocking about America's malpractice system is that it does not even serve the needs of injured patients. Despite stratospheric malpractice premiums, generous settlements, big awards by sympathetic juries, and an epidemic of defensive medicine, many patients with "compensable injuries" remain uncompensated. In fact, fewer than 3% of patients who experience injuries associated with negligent care file claims. The reasons for this are varied, and include patients' unawareness that an error occurred, the fact that most cases are taken by attorneys on contingency (and thus will not be brought if the attorneys think that their investment in preparing the case is unlikely to be recouped), and the fact that many of the uncompensated or undercompensated claimants are on government assistance and lack the resources, personal initiative, or social clout to seek redress. Thus, some worthy malpractice claims go begging while others go forward for a host of reasons that have nothing to do with the presence or degree of negligence.

Even when injured patients' cases do make it through the malpractice system to a trial or settlement, it is remarkable how little money actually ends up in the hands of the victims and their families. After deducting legal fees and expenses, the average plaintiff sees about 40 cents of every dollar paid by the defendant. If the intent of the award is to help families care for a permanently disabled relative or to replace a deceased breadwinner's earnings, this 60% overhead makes the malpractice system a uniquely wasteful business.

ERROR DISCLOSURE, APOLOGIES, AND MALPRACTICE

For generations, physicians and health systems responded with silence after a medical error. This was a natural outgrowth of the shame that most providers feel after errors (driven, in part, by the traditional view of errors as stemming from individual failures rather than system problems) and by a malpractice system that nurtures confrontation and leads providers to worry that an apology will be taken as an admission of guilt, only to be used against them later.

The cycle played out time and time again: patients who believed they had possibly been victims of medical errors wanted to learn what really happened, but their caregivers and healthcare organizations frequently responded with defensiveness, sometimes even stonewalling. This, in turn, made patients and families angry, frustrated, and even more convinced that they were on the receiving end of a terrible mistake. Hickson et al. found that nearly half the families who sued their providers after perinatal injuries were motivated by their suspicion of a cover-up or a desire for revenge.[10]

But could this cycle be broken? Until the patient safety field began, most observers would have said no. Each side, after all, appeared to be acting in its own interests: patients seeking information and ultimately redress, and providers and hospitals trying to avoid painful conversations and payouts. Yet the results were so damaging to everyone that some began wondering whether there was a better way. Since the patient safety movement emphasized the role of improving systems, could a change in the system, and mental model, alter the toxic dynamics of malpractice?

After losing two large malpractice cases in the late 1980s, the Veterans Affairs Medical Center in Lexington, Kentucky, decided to adopt a policy of disclosure, apology, and early offer of a reasonable settlement, a policy it called "extreme honesty." Perhaps surprisingly, they found that their overall malpractice payouts were lower than those of comparable VA institutions.[11,12] While the study caught people's attention, the fact that it is challenging to sue a VA hospital (it *is* the federal government, after all) led many to question the generalizability of these results.

In 2007, Studdert et al. modeled the likely impact of policies to promote fuller disclosure. Full disclosure reveals errors to patients who knew or strongly suspected that they were victims of mistakes, and also to patients who did not suspect they were harmed by an error (and therefore had not considered suing). Because of this, Studdert et al.'s analysis revealed that even if fuller disclosure prevented some patients from suing, it would generate far *more* lawsuits overall because of new lawsuits filed by those patients previously unaware of an error. While affirming that from an ethical standpoint disclosure is "the right thing to do," Studdert et al. concluded that policies promoting it would be "an improbable risk management strategy."[13]

These concerns were put to rest, at least to a degree, in 2010, when the University of Michigan reported the results of its medical disclosure policy built on the same principles as the Lexington VA's: rapid disclosure of adverse events, apologies, and prompt and fair settlement offers when internal review found evidence of culpability.[14,15] (Importantly, the university vigorously defends cases when it believes there was no negligence.) While overall rates of malpractice payouts have been declining in the United States over the past 5 years (for reasons that are not entirely understood), Michigan's improvements far exceeded the secular trends: a 65% decrease in the rate of lawsuits, a 40% decrease in the time between a claim being made and its resolution, and a 60% decrease in total payouts (Figure 18-2).

It is important to acknowledge that the Michigan and Lexington findings do not entirely trump Studdert's argument. In the medical literature, we often find early studies—conducted at atypical institutions with highly motivated leaders and investigators—that show breathtakingly positive effects that were not matched when the intervention was rolled out to other settings (I already discussed a similar experience with computerized provider order entry; Chapter 13). But this new approach does open the door to a broad rethinking of both the ethical and pragmatic implications of disclosure. The field of risk management has taken note, unquestionably moving toward a more pro-disclosure stance in the past few years.[16]

Patients generally favor disclosure of all harmful errors, accompanied by an explanation of why the error occurred, how the error's impact will be minimized (in their own care), and steps the physician and organization will take to prevent its recurrence (in their own care and that of other patients) (Table 18-1).[17–20] Physicians favor disclosure as well, at least in theory, but they "choose their words carefully."[21] In responding to a variety of scenarios,

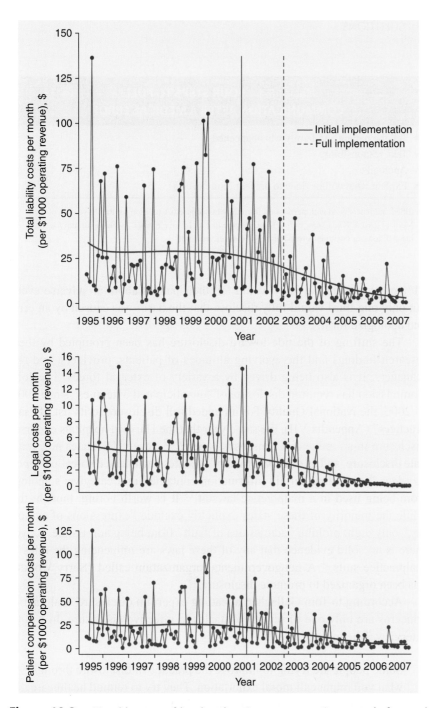

Figure 18-2 ▪ Monthly rates of legal and patient compensation costs before and after implementation of the University of Michigan Health System's disclosure-with-offer program. (Reprinted with permission from Kachalia A, Kaufman SR, Boothman R, et al. Liability claims and costs before and after implementation of a medical error disclosure program. *Ann Intern Med* 2010;153:213–221. © 2010 by American College of Physicians.)

Table 18-1   FOUR STEPS TO FULL COMMUNICATION AFTER A MEDICAL ERROR
■ Tell the patient and family what happened ■ Take responsibility ■ Apologize ■ Explain what will be done to prevent future events

Modified and reproduced with permission from the Massachusetts Coalition for the Prevention of Medical Errors. *When Things Go Wrong: Responding to Adverse Events.* Available at: http://www.macoalition.org/documents/respondingToAdverseEvents.pdf.

61% of physicians say they would tell their patient about an adverse event, but only one-third would fully disclose that the harm was caused by an error and apologize for it.[21]

The shifting of the tide toward disclosure has been prompted by these research findings and the evolving attitudes of patients, providers, and risk managers. It is also being driven by a variety of external forces. The Joint Commission has required disclosure of "unanticipated outcomes" since 2001. In 2006, the National Quality Forum added full disclosure to its list of "safe practices" (Appendix VII), the same year that the Harvard hospitals endorsed disclosure in an influential consensus paper.[20,22] Seven U.S. states now mandate disclosure, and as of 2008 a total of 36 states had enacted so-called "*apology laws*," excluding certain information contained in a caregiver's apology from being used in a malpractice lawsuit.[23] It is worth noting, though, that while the majority of these states explicitly exclude "expressions of sympathy," only eight prohibit "admissions of fault" from being admissible. As yet, there is no solid evidence that any of these laws are influencing the rates of malpractice suits.[24] A nongovernmental organization called "Sorry Works!" has been organized to promote disclosure.[25]

According to Tom Gallagher, a leading expert on disclosure, malpractice concerns are only one of several obstacles to effective disclosure. In a 2009 interview,[26] he told me:

> Some people are trying to improve the practice of disclosure through what you might call moral exhortation. They try to remind healthcare workers that this is a professional and ethical duty, and then the implication is that we need to up our quotient of moral courage and just go do what we know is the right thing to do. But when you talk with healthcare workers … they really endorse the concept of disclosure, but struggle with its implementation. Among the key barriers we have encountered, one is clearly worry about the impact of disclosure on

litigation. But that was not the only barrier, and for many clinicians it was not the most important barrier. Lots of clinicians really struggle with the concern that sometimes disclosure may not be beneficial to the patient …. The other barrier is the challenge of how awkward and uncomfortable these conversations are. Most physicians have told us that they haven't had any formal training in disclosure and are uncertain of just what to say.

Gallagher believes that the best disclosure training programs will combine some foundational knowledge, scenario-based training (probably using simulation; Chapter 17), and just-in-time coaching provided by experienced and trained medical directors or risk managers. Rathert and Phillips argue that training in disclosure will have additional benefits for organizations, in that it provides tangible evidence of an organization's "value-based ethics."[27] Some model language for telling a patient about a medication error is shown in Box 18-1.[20]

Box 18-1 MODEL LANGUAGE FOR TELLING A PATIENT ABOUT A MEDICATION ERROR

"Let me tell you what happened. We gave you a chemotherapeutic agent, carboplatin, instead of the pamidronate you were supposed to receive.

I want to discuss with you what this means for your health, but first I'd like to apologize.

I'm sorry. This shouldn't have happened. Right now, I don't know exactly how this happened, but I promise you that we're going to find out what happened and do everything we can to make sure that it doesn't happen again. I will share with you what we find as soon as I know, but it may take some time to get to the bottom of it all.

Once again, let me say how sorry I am that this happened.

Now, what does this mean for your health? You received only a fraction of the usual dose of carboplatin, so it is unlikely you will have any adverse effects from the infusion. However, I would like to monitor you closely over the next weeks. In patients who receive a full dose, the side effects we expect include …. We usually monitor patients for these side effects by …. We treat these side effects by …. I want to see you in my clinic tomorrow so we can …"

Modified and reproduced with permission from the Massachusetts Coalition for the Prevention of Medical Errors, November 18, 2011. *When Things Go Wrong: Responding to Adverse Events.* Available at: http://www.macoalition.org/documents/respondingToAdverseEvents.pdf.

Clearly, the approach to patients after an error or an adverse event is evolving rapidly, after many years of stasis. The breadth of the rethinking—involving ethical imperatives, practical implications, training models, and laws and policies—is impressive, and ensures that this area will continue to change in coming years. McDonald et al., who have developed another widely praised disclosure program at the University of Illinois, describe seven pillars of an effective and comprehensive system of responding to adverse events in Table 18-2.[29]

NO-FAULT SYSTEMS AND "HEALTH COURTS": AN ALTERNATIVE TO TORT-BASED MALPRACTICE

A U.S. physician has a more than 1-in-100 chance of being sued after a patient has an adverse event, even when the doctor has done nothing wrong.[30,31] Although this may not sound like an excessive "risk" of a lawsuit, when you consider all the patients who suffer adverse events, this rate adds up to a lot of lawsuits. As noted earlier, recent research has shown that nearly all doctors will be sued at least once over the course of their career, and many will be sued multiple times.[6]

What types of cases trigger the most malpractice suits and yield the biggest awards? In past studies, the magnitude of the patient's disability was by far a better predictor of victory and award size than was proof of a breach of "standard of care." In other words, the American malpractice system distributes compensation based on the degree of injury, not the degree of malpractice.

This is not altogether surprising, because malpractice cases are generally heard by juries composed of ordinary citizens who can see themselves in the plaintiff's shoes. "In a case like this," said the attorney who represented the physician in the case that began this chapter, "involving a patient who was already in the hospital, who has an arrest and anoxic [brain damage], one of the very significant perceptual issues we have to consider … is the fact that there was a catastrophic outcome, and to some jurors, catastrophic outcomes may equate with 'somebody must have messed up.'"[1] And so, despite expert testimony that the doctor's decision to postpone intubation was medically sound, the attorney advised his client to settle out of court, which she did. The frequency of this outcome—even when the physician believes she was anything but negligent—provides an incentive for more lawsuits.

Given the problems in the American malpractice system, *pain-and-suffering caps* (first implemented in California after a malpractice crisis in the 1980s) have been touted as a way of at least moderating insurance premiums and keeping doctors in business.[32] However, such caps are politically charged, and at least one U.S. state (Illinois) has ruled them

Table 18-2 **THE "SEVEN PILLARS" OF AN EFFECTIVE, COMPREHENSIVE SYSTEM OF RESPONDING TO ADVERSE EVENTS WITHIN A HEALTHCARE DELIVERY ORGANIZATION**	
"Pillar"	**Explanation**
1. Patient safety reporting system	Reports are "applauded"; can be made by phone, handwritten, online, or in person; clinical departments are penalized financially for failing to report incidents involving patient harm
2. Investigation	Risk manager performs preliminary investigation to ascertain harm. If yes, investigation and root cause analysis are commissioned. RCA to be completed within 72 hours of incident, including determination of whether "care was reasonable," using Reason's algorithm of unsafe acts (Chapter 19)[4,28]
3. Communication and disclosure	The "centerpiece of the process": ongoing communication with patient/family throughout process, including findings of "reasonableness" (#2). Third-party review offered if no consensus on whether care was reasonable. If "unreasonable," then full disclosure and apology follow— but this is "a process" that plays out over time and avoids premature disclosure before clear conclusions. A "Patient Communications Consult Service" is available to aid in disclosure process; a member of the service is present at all disclosures
4. Apology and remediation	Combines saying "we are sorry" with offer of a remedy, with rapid remediation (including waiving hospital bills) and early offer of compensation, if warranted
5. System improvement	Even after apology, the investigation continues to identify and implement system improvements. Patients and families are invited to participate in these efforts
6. Data tracking and performance evaluation	Data regarding all aspects of this process are tracked and fed back into system for subsequent improvements
7. Education and training	Staff required to participate in initial and continuing training requirement on this process, including disclosure practices. In addition, providers are made aware of availability of a caregiver support program ("second patient") for use after errors

Reproduced with permission from McDonald TB, Helmchen LA, Smith KM, et al. Responding to patient safety incidents: the "seven pillars". *Qual Saf Health Care* 2010;19:e11.

unconstitutional.[33,34] Moreover, they don't solve the fundamental problem. Physicians worry more about the costs—both financial and psychic—of the process than the costs of the settlement. If a patient comes in with a headache and, after a conscientious workup, we conclude it is almost certainly not a brain tumor, we reassure the patient and look for other diagnoses. However, if one out of every 5000 times a patient *does* have a brain tumor and we skipped the computed tomography (CT) scan, we can count on being sued. In that case, the expense and emotional costs—time lost to depositions, hand-wringing and demoralization, sleepless nights, and suppressed anger over the unfairness of it all—are essentially the same for the physician, whether the payout is $400,000 or $2 million. As doctors, our decision making is driven more by the potential for being sued than by the cost of losing a judgment.

A decade ago, Studdert, Brennan, and colleagues made a strong case for replacing the adversarial tort-based malpractice approach with a *no-fault system* modeled on workers' compensation.[1,35] It would work this way: a no-fault pool would be created from insurance premiums, from which awards would be made following the simple establishment of healthcare-associated harm. There would be no need to prove that the caregiver was negligent or the care was substandard. The proposed advantages of the system include more rapid adjudication of cases and far lower overhead (to lawyers, expert witnesses, and so on). In most no-fault proposals, institutions would be "experience rated" (i.e., their premiums would be set based on their payout histories), providing an incentive to create and maintain safe systems of care.

There are many concerns about the viability and political feasibility of a no-fault system in the United States, and setting the bar for compensation will be challenging. For instance, setting a low bar (such as compensation for a gastrointestinal bleed after appropriate use of a nonsteroidal anti-inflammatory agent) would cause the compensation pool to go broke. Then again, if compensation goes to only those patients who are the victims of horrible and dramatic events such as wrong-site surgery, then too many people suffering significant harm go uncompensated. Some experts also worry that a compensation pool approach would cause healthcare professionals to slacken their safety efforts. However, evidence supporting a deterrent effect of the current malpractice system is quite limited.[1]

In part because of political objections to the concept of—even the very words—"no fault," the discussion in recent years has tilted to so-called "*health courts*."[34,36] These build on the disclosure trend discussed earlier, but go further by informing patients at the time of disclosure that they can file a compensation claim. Such claims are heard by a panel of experts, which determines "avoidability" (a somewhat lower bar than negligence) and recommends a settlement: full recompense for economic losses and a pain and suffering award based on a predetermined compensation schedule that hinges on the severity of the injury. Enthusiasm for this model is growing, and some federal funding has been made available for pilot experiments.

The reports from other countries that have tried no-fault or health court systems have been mixed but generally favorable. New Zealand, for example, switched to a no-fault system for *all* personal injuries, including healthcare related ones, in 1972. The no-fault system is seen as a partial success, although there has been agitation for a more fault-based system to deal with egregious errors.[2,37] The Swedish no-fault system remains effective and popular after more than two decades. Sweden limits compensable events to medical injuries that were "avoidable," and eligible patients must have spent at least 10 days in the hospital or endured at least 30 sick days.[2,35,36]

These early experiences and international comparisons are helpful. Yet if there is one thing about the malpractice system that is clear, it is that the debate about the best way to handle patient injuries is driven more by political realities than policy arguments and data. So for now, the American malpractice system remains highly unpopular, with few people believing that it fairly assesses blame or compensates victims.[38] From the standpoint of patient safety, the system's main problems are that it promotes an adversarial environment that encourages secrecy rather than the openness necessary for problem solving, and that it tends to point fingers at people rather than focus on system defects. In the past five years, we have seen some impressive institutionally based innovations, particularly around disclosure. But there seems little hope that the larger American malpractice system will give way to a better alternative any time in the foreseeable future, particularly if such a shift requires the passage of new federal legislation.

MEDICAL MALPRACTICE CASES AS A SOURCE OF SAFETY LESSONS

Before concluding our discussion of the malpractice system, it is worth recalling that it was a study of malpractice—the Harvard Medical Practice Study—that inspired the patient safety movement by generating the estimate of 44,000 to 98,000 yearly deaths from errors used by the Institute of Medicine in *To Err is Human*.[39–41] Malpractice claims databases offer an important way of viewing patient safety, illustrating, for example, a far higher frequency of diagnostic errors (Chapter 6) than do other safety "lenses" such as incident reporting systems or administrative databases.[42] Many important safety insights have come from so-called *closed claim analyses*—analyses of malpractice cases that have already been settled.[43–48]

In addition, malpractice cases are a rich source of information for teaching about both patient safety content areas and the malpractice system itself. Hochberg et al. recently reported on a training intervention that used data from their own hospital's malpractice experience to educate surgical residents about both safety and malpractice.[49]

The fact that this intervention is considered an innovation points to yet another maddening aspect of the malpractice system: it is so politically charged that its potential as a rich font of patient safety knowledge and wisdom generally goes untapped. We live in a world of ever-increasing transparency, in which a hospital's mortality rates, readmission rates, financial health, and even what patients think of the food are all a click away on the Web. Yet information about malpractice cases remains the most cloistered in healthcare. As Alper and I wrote in response to the Hochberg article, it is time to begin tearing down this particular wall.[50] As we do, it will be vital for clinician-leaders, educators, and researchers to use this information prudently and effectively in the service of improving safety.

KEY POINTS

- The medical malpractice system in the United States is governed by the rules of tort law, which compensates injury victims with the resources of at-fault providers.
- Among the criticisms of the malpractice system are its arbitrariness, its high administrative costs, and its tendency to assign individual blame rather than seek system solutions. The latter issue in particular often places the malpractice system in conflict with the goals of the patient safety movement.
- An important recent trend has been to promote disclosure of adverse events and errors to patients. Emerging evidence is that disclosure and apology, when accompanied by rapid settlement offers where appropriate, may lower overall malpractice costs. Many states have passed laws protecting some portions of disclosures and accompanying apologies from being used in court.
- Pain and suffering award caps can help limit the size of awards and decrease the propensity of attorneys to accept cases on contingency, but do not improve the fundamental flaws in the system.
- Recently, no-fault or health court systems, in which patients are compensated based on their injuries without the need to assign fault, have been promoted in the United States. Early international experiences with such systems have been generally positive.

REFERENCES

1. Brennan TA, Mello MM. Patient safety and medical malpractice: a case study. *Ann Intern Med* 2003;139:267–273.
2. Merry A, McCall Smith A. *Errors, Medicine, and the Law*. Cambridge, England: Cambridge University Press; 2001.
3. Johnston N. Do blame and punishment have a role in organizational risk management? *Flight Deck* 1995;Spring:33–36.
4. Reason JT. *Managing the Risks of Organizational Accidents*. Aldershot, Hampshire, England: Ashgate Publishing Limited; 1997.
5. Wachter RM, Shojania KG. *Internal Bleeding: The Truth Behind America's Terrifying Epidemic of Medical Mistakes*. New York, NY: Rugged Land; 2004.
6. Jena AB, Seabury S, Lakdawalla D, et al. Malpractice risk according to physician specialty. *N Engl J Med* 2011;365:629–636.
7. Kessler DP, McClellan M. Do doctors practice defensive medicine? *Q J Econ* 1996; 111:353–390.
8. Blendon RJ, Schoen C, DesRoches CM, et al. Confronting competing demands to improve quality: a five-country hospital survey. *Health Aff (Millwood)* 2004;23:119–135.
9. Brennan TA, Localio AR, Leape LL, et al. Identification of adverse events occurring during hospitalization. A cross-sectional study of litigation, quality assurance, and medical records at two teaching hospitals. *Ann Intern Med* 1990;112:221–226.
10. Hickson GB, Clayton EW, Githens PB, et al. Factors that prompted families to file medical malpractice claims following perinatal injuries. *JAMA* 1992; 267:1359–1363.
11. Kraman SS, Hamm G. Risk management: extreme honesty may be the best policy. *Ann Intern Med* 1999;131:963–967.
12. Kraman SS, Cranfill L, Hamm G, et al. John M. Eisenberg Patient Safety Awards. Advocacy: the Lexington Veterans Affairs Medical Center. *Jt Comm J Qual Improv* 2002;28:646–650.
13. Studdert DM, Mello MM, Gawande AA, et al. Disclosure of medical injury to patients: an improbable risk management strategy. *Health Aff (Millwood)* 2007;26:215–226.
14. Kachalia A, Kaufman SR, Boothman R, et al. Liability claims and costs before and after implementation of a medical error disclosure program. *Ann Intern Med* 2010;153:213–221.
15. Boothman RC, Blackwell AC, Campbell DA, et al. A better approach to medical malpractice claims? The University of Michigan experience. *J Health Life Sci Law* 2009;2:125–159.
16. Loren DJ, Garbutt J, Dunagan WC, et al. Risk managers, physicians, and disclosure of harmful medical errors. *Jt Comm J Qual Patient Saf* 2010;36:101–108.
17. Gallagher TH, Waterman AD, Ebers AG, et al. Patients' and physicians' attitudes regarding the disclosure of medical errors. *JAMA* 2003;289:1001–1007.
18. Mazor KM, Reed GW, Yood RA, et al. Disclosure of medical errors: what factors influence how patients respond? *J Gen Intern Med* 2006;21:704–710.
19. Helmchen LA, Richards MR, McDonald TB. How does routine disclosure of medical error affect patients' propensity to sue and their assessment of provider quality? Evidence from survey data. *Med Care* 2010;48:955–961.

20. *When Things Go Wrong: Responding to Adverse Events. A Consensus Statement of the Harvard Hospitals*. Burlington: Massachusetts Coalition for the Prevention of Medical Errors; 2006.

21. Gallagher TH, Garbutt JM, Waterman AD, et al. Choosing your words carefully: how physicians would disclose harmful medical errors to patients. *Arch Intern Med* 2006;166:1585–1593.

22. National Quality Forum. *Safe Practices for Better Healthcare: 2006 Update*. Washington, DC: National Quality Forum; 2007.

23. McDonnell WM, Guenther E. Narrative review: do state laws make it easier to say "I'm sorry?" *Ann Intern Med* 2008;149:811–815.

24. Perez B, DiDona T. Assessing legislative potential to institute error transparency: a state comparison of malpractice claims rates. *J Healthc Qual* 2010;32:36–41.

25. Available at: http://www.sorryworks.net/.

26. In Conversation with … Thomas H. Gallagher, MD. *AHRQ WebM&M* (serial online); January 2009. Available at: http://psnet.ahrq.gov/resource.aspx?resourceID=269.

27. Rathert C, Phillips W. Medical error disclosure training: evidence for values-based ethical environments. *J Bus Ethics* 2010;97:491–503.

28. Reason J. Human errors: models and management. *BMJ* 2000;320:768–770.

29. McDonald TB, Helmchen LA, Smith KM, et al. Responding to patient safety incidents: the "seven pillars". *Qual Saf Health Care* 2010;19:e11.

30. Localio AR, Lawthers AG, Brennan TA, et al. Relation between malpractice claims and adverse events due to negligence. Results of the Harvard Medical Practice Study III. *N Engl J Med* 1991;325:245–251.

31. Studdert DM, Thomas EJ, Burstin HR, et al. Negligent care and malpractice claiming behavior in Utah and Colorado. *Med Care* 2000;38:250–260.

32. Hellinger FJ, Encinosa WE. The impact of state laws limiting malpractice damage awards on health care expenditures. *Am J Public Health* 2006;96:1375–1381.

33. Mello MM, Brennan TA. The role of medical liability reform in federal health care reform. *N Engl J Med* 2009;361:1–3.

34. Mello MM, Gallagher TH. Malpractice reform—opportunities for leadership by health care institutions and liability insurers. *N Engl J Med* 2010;362:1353–1356.

35. Studdert DM, Brennan TA. No-fault compensation for medical injuries: the prospect for error prevention. *JAMA* 2001;286:217–223.

36. Mello MM, Studdert DM, Kachalia AB, et al. "Health courts" and accountability for patient safety. *Milbank Q* 2006;84:459–492.

37. Bismark MM, Brennan TA, Patterson RJ, et al. Relationship between complaints and quality of care in New Zealand: a descriptive analysis of complainants and non-complainants following adverse events. *Qual Saf Health Care* 2006;15:17–22.

38. Gawande AA. The malpractice mess. *New Yorker*. 2005:62–71.

39. Brennan TA, Leape LL, Laird NM, et al. Incidence of adverse events and negligence in hospitalized patients. Results of the Harvard Medical Practice Study I. *N Engl J Med* 1991;324:370–376.

40. Leape LL, Brennan TA, Laird N, et al. The nature of adverse events and negligence in hospitalized patients. Results of the Harvard Medical Practice Study II. *N Engl J Med* 1991;324:377–384.

41. Kohn L, Corrigan J, Donaldson M, eds. *To Err is Human: Building a Safer Health System*. Committee on Quality of Health Care in America, Institute of Medicine. Washington, DC: National Academy Press; 2000.

42. Levtzion-Korach O, Frankel A, Alcalai H, et al. Integrating incident data from five reporting systems to assess patient safety: making sense of the elephant. *Jt Comm J Qual Patient Saf* 2010;36:402–410.

43. Bhananker SM, Posner KL, Cheney FW, et al. Injury and liability associated with monitored anesthesia care: a closed claims analysis. *Anesthesiology* 2006;104:228–234.

44. Gandhi TK, Kachalia A, Thomas EJ, et al. Missed and delayed diagnoses in the ambulatory setting: a study of closed malpractice claims. *Ann Intern Med* 2006;145:488–496.

45. Manuel BM, Greenwald LM. Using medical malpractice claims data to reduce surgical risk and improve patient safety. *Bull Am Coll Surg* 2007;92:27–30.

46. Singh H, Thomas EJ, Petersen LA, et al. Medical errors involving trainees: a study of closed malpractice claims from 5 insurers. *Arch Intern Med* 2007;167:2030–2036.

47. Katz HP, Kaltsounis D, Halloran L, et al. Patient safety and telephone medicine: some lessons from closed claim case review. *J Gen Intern Med* 2008;23:517–522.

48. Bishop TF, Ryan AK, Casalino LP. Paid malpractice claims for adverse events in the inpatient and outpatient settings. *JAMA* 2011;305:2427–2431.

49. Hochberg MS, Seib CD, Berman RS, et al. Perspective: malpractice in an academic medical center: a frequently overlooked aspect of professionalism education. *Acad Med* 2011;86:365–368.

50. Alper EJ, Wachter RM. Commentary: medical malpractice and patient safety: tear down that wall. *Acad Med* 2011;86:282–284.

ADDITIONAL READINGS

Gallagher TH. A 62-year-old woman with skin cancer who experienced wrong-site surgery: review of medical error. *JAMA* 2009;302:669–677.

Gallagher TH, Studdert D, Levinson W. Disclosing harmful medical errors to patients. *N Engl J Med* 2007;356:2713–2719.

Gawande A. *Complications: A Surgeon's Notes on an Imperfect Science*. New York, NY: Metropolitan Books; 2002.

O'Reilly KB. "I'm sorry": why is that so hard for doctors to say? *American Medical News*. February 1, 2010.

Roland M, Rao SR, Sibbald B, et al. Professional values and reported behaviours of doctors in the USA and UK: quantitative survey. *BMJ Qual Saf* 2011;20:515–521.

Studdert DM, Mello MM, Gawande AA, et al. Claims, errors, and compensation payments in medical malpractice litigation. *N Engl J Med* 2006;354:2024–2033.

Thomas MO, Quinn CJ, Donohue GM. *Practicing Medicine in Difficult Times: Protecting Physicians from Malpractice Litigation*. Sudbury, MA: Jones Bartlett; 2009.

Wachter RM. Patient safety at ten: unmistakable progress, troubling gaps. *Health Aff (Millwood)* 2010;29:165–173.

Youngberg BJ, ed. *Principles of Risk Management and Patient Safety*. Sudbury, MA: Jones Bartlett; 2011.

ACCOUNTABILITY | 19

OVERVIEW

As I have emphasized throughout this book, the fundamental underpinning of the modern patient safety field is "systems thinking"—the notion that most errors are made by competent, caring people, and that safe care therefore depends on embedding providers in systems that anticipate errors and block them from causing harm. That is an attractive viewpoint, and undoubtedly correct in the main. But it risks causing us to avert our eyes from those providers or institutions who, for a variety of reasons, are not competent, or worse.

After last chapter's discussion of the malpractice system—the most visible, but often dysfunctional, incarnation of accountability in healthcare—this chapter focuses on more subtle issues, including "Just Culture," dealing with disruptive providers, and the role of the media in patient safety. At its heart, the chapter aims to address one of the most challenging questions in patient safety: can our desire for a "no blame" culture, with all its benefits, be reconciled with the need for accountability?

ACCOUNTABILITY

Scott Torrence, a 36-year-old insurance broker, was struck in the head while going up for a rebound during his weekend basketball game. Over the next few hours, a mild headache escalated into a thunderclap, and he became lethargic and vertiginous. His girlfriend called an ambulance to take him to the emergency room in his local rural hospital, which lacked a CT or MRI scanner.

The ER physician, Dr. Jane Benamy, worried about brain bleeding, called neurologist Dr. Roy Jones at the regional referral hospital (a few hundred miles away) requesting that Torrence be transferred. Jones refused, reassuring Benamy that the case sounded like "benign positional vertigo." Benamy worried, but had no recourse. She sent Torrence home with medications for vertigo and headache.

The next morning, Benamy reevaluated Torrence, and he was markedly worse, with more headache and vertigo, now accompanied by vomiting and photophobia (bright lights hurt his eyes). She called neurologist Jones again, who again refused the request for transfer. Completely frustrated, she hospitalized Torrence for intravenous pain medications and close observation.

The next day, the patient was even worse. Literally begging, Benamy found another physician (an internist named Soloway) at Regional Medical Center to accept the transfer, and Torrence was sent there by air ambulance. The CT scan at Regional was read as unrevealing (in retrospect, a subtle but crucial abnormality was overlooked), and Soloway managed Torrence's symptoms with more pain medicines and sedation. Overnight, however, the patient deteriorated even further—"awake, moaning, yelling," according to the nursing notes—and needed to be physically restrained. Soloway called the neurologist, Dr. Jones, at home, who told him that he "was familiar with the case and . . . the non-focal neurological exam and the normal CT scan made urgent clinical problems unlikely." He went on to say that "he would evaluate the patient the next morning."

But by the next morning, Torrence was dead. An autopsy revealed that the head trauma had torn a small cerebellar artery, which led to a cerebellar stroke (an area of the brain poorly imaged by CT scan). Ultimately, the stroke caused enough swelling to trigger brainstem herniation—extrusion of the brain through one of the holes in the base of the skull, like toothpaste squeezing through a tube. This cascade of falling dominoes could have been stopped at any stage, but that would have required the expert neurologist to see the patient, recognize the signs of the cerebellar artery dissection, take a closer look at the CT scan, and order an MRI.[1]

Cases like this one—specifically Dr. Jones's refusal to personally evaluate a challenging and rapidly deteriorating patient when asked repeatedly by concerned colleagues to do so—demonstrate the tension between the "no-fault" stance embraced by the patient safety field and the importance of establishing and enforcing standards. That such cases occur should not surprise anyone. Despite years of training, doctors are as vulnerable as anyone to all the maladies that can beset professionals in high-demand, rapidly changing professions: not keeping up, drug and alcohol abuse, depression, burnout, or just failing to care enough.

But how can we reconcile the need for accountability with our desire to abandon our traditional "blame and shame" approach and embrace a new focus on system safety? As Dr. Lucian Leape, the Harvard surgeon and father of the modern patient safety movement, once told me:

> There is no accountability. When we identify doctors who harm patients, we need to try to be compassionate and help them. But in the end, if they are a danger to patients, they shouldn't be caring for them. A fundamental principle has to be the development and then the enforcement of procedures and standards. We can't make real progress without them. When a doctor doesn't follow them, something has to happen. Today, nothing does, and you have a vicious cycle in which people have no real incentive to follow the rules because they know there are no consequences if they don't. So there *are* bad doctors and bad nurses, but the fact that we tolerate them is just another systems problem.[1]

One of the definitions of a profession is that it is self-policing: it sets its own standards and enforces them with its members ("*peer review*"). Despite this responsibility, it is undeniable that doctors and hospitals tend to protect their own, sometimes at the expense of patients. Hospital credentials committees, which certify and periodically recertify individual doctors, rarely limit a provider's privileges, even when there is stark evidence of failure to meet a reasonable standard of care. If alcohol or drug abuse is the problem, a physician may be ordered to enter a "diversion" program, a noble idea, but one that sometimes errs on the side of protecting the interests of the dangerous provider over an unwitting public. A recent survey found that 70% of physicians believe it is their professional responsibility to report an impaired or incompetent colleague. However, of physicians familiar with just such a colleague, one-third admitted that they failed to report him or her to a relevant authority.[2]

Why has healthcare not lived up to its ethical mandate to self-regulate? One reason is that it is difficult to sanction one's own peers, especially when the evidence of substandard practice is anecdotal and sometimes concerns issues of personality (i.e., the disruptive physician [an issue I'll return to below], or the physician who appears to be insufficiently responsive) rather than "hard outcomes." A second issue is more practical: given the length of time that it takes to train physicians, credentials committees and licensing bodies are understandably reluctant to remove a physician's privileges after the community has invested so much money and effort in training.

A final reason is that physicians tend not to be strong organizational managers. Unlike fields like law and business, in which conflict and competition are commonplace, physicians are generally not accustomed to confronting colleagues, let alone managing the regulatory and legal consequences of such confrontations. This final point is important: because litigation often follows any challenges to a physician's clinical competence (and credentials committee members are only partially shielded from lawsuits), many physicians understandably will do backflips to avoid confrontation.

Unfortunately, the evidence that there *are* bad apples—and that they are not dealt with effectively—is reasonably strong. For example, from 1990 to 2002, just 5% of U.S. doctors were involved in 54% of the payouts reported to the National Practitioner Data Bank, the confidential log of malpractice cases maintained by the federal government. Of the 35,000 doctors with two or more payouts, only 8% were disciplined by state boards. And among the 2774 doctors who had made payments in five or more cases, only 463 (just one out of six) had been disciplined. One Pennsylvania doctor paid a whopping 24 claims totaling $8 million between 1993 and 2001, including a wrong-site surgery and a retained instrument case, yet had been neither stripped of his clinical credentials nor disciplined by the state licensing board.[3]

Of course, in this group of oft-sued doctors[4] are some very busy obstetricians and neurosurgeons who take on tough cases (probably accompanied by poor bedside manner—there is a striking correlation between the number of patient complaints about a physician's personal style and the probability of lawsuits[5]). But this group undoubtedly also includes some very dangerous doctors. We simply must find better ways to measure whether doctors are meeting the relevant professional standards—the increasing computerization of practice should help by making it easier to tell whether doctors are practicing high-quality, evidence-based medicine. Moreover, efforts at remediation (and discipline, if necessary) must begin early: one study found that evidence of unprofessional behavior in medical school was a powerful predictor of subsequent disciplinary action by medical boards, often decades later.[6]

While the above discussion has emphasized the quality of physician care, similar issues arise with other health professionals. In these other fields, however, there has been a stronger tradition of accountability, in part because nurses often work for institutions such as hospitals (and therefore can be more easily fired or disciplined) and because they have less power. But these judgments can also be arbitrary and ineffective, and the disparity with physicians creates its own problems. The bar for competence and performance should be set high for all healthcare professionals, and the consequences of failing to meet standards should be similar.[7] Nothing undermines an institution's claim to be committed to safety more than for frontline workers to see that there is one set of standards for nurses and a wholly different one for physicians.

In this regard, a major change over the past few years has been the development of critical safety rules and standards (see also Chapter 15). Whereas concerns about professional performance in the past largely centered on clinical competence (i.e., frequent diagnostic errors, poor surgical skill), they increasingly relate to failure to adhere to standards and regulations. For example, what should be done about the physician who chooses not to perform a "time out" prior to surgery (Chapter 5)? Or the nurse who habitually fails to clean her hands before patient contact (Chapter 10)? In the end, healthcare organizations must find the strength to enforce these rules and standards, recognizing that there is no conflict between this tough love stance and the "systems approach" to patient safety. As safety expert James Reason says of habitual rule benders:

> Seeing them get away with it on a daily basis does little for morale or for the credibility of the disciplinary system. Watching them getting their "come-uppance" is not only satisfying, it also serves to reinforce where the boundaries of acceptable behavior lie ... Justice works two ways. Severe sanctions for the few can protect the innocence of the many.[8]

Moreover, there are cases of such egregious deviations from professional norms that the perpetrators *must* be held accountable in the name of justice and patient protection. Take the case of the Saskatchewan anesthetist convicted of criminal negligence for leaving the operating room to make a phone call (after disconnecting the ventilator alarms), leading to permanent brain injury in a 17-year-old patient,[9] or the Boston surgeon who left his patient anesthetized on the table with a gaping incision in his back to go cash a check at his local bank.[10] And even these cases pale in comparison to those of psychopathic serial killers such as Dr. Michael Swango and Dr. Harold Shipman.[11,12] These cases cry out for justice and accountability, but they are overwhelmingly the exception, which is what makes the issue of exercising appropriate accountability so vexing. The more pressing issue is how to create and enforce a system of accountability in more common situations, such as when caregivers' behavior gets in the way of good patient care.

| DISRUPTIVE PROVIDERS

Although TV physicians of yesteryear were usually kind, grandfatherly types (exemplified most famously by Robert Young as Marcus Welby, MD), today's version is Dr. Gregory House: a brilliant diagnostician who is virtually impossible to work with. This stereotype, though both dramatic and amusing, can obscure the fact that disruptive and unprofessional behavior by clinicians is relatively common and can compromise patient safety.

While only 2% to 4% of caregivers regularly engage in disruptive behavior, those who do cause substantial problems.[13] In a 2008 survey of nearly 5000 nurses and physicians, 77% reported witnessing physicians engage in *intervention*, including termination of privileges or employment and appropriate reporting to outside entities such as state licensing boards.[21]

| THE "JUST CULTURE"

The balancing act is a tricky one—in our zeal to hold the habitual rule-breaker or disruptive caregiver appropriately accountable, we need to guard against creating overly punitive and aggressive licensing boards and credentials committees. After all, the fundamental underpinning of patient safety remains trust on the part of caregivers that raising concerns about dysfunctional systems— through open disclosure of errors and near misses—will lead to improvements (Chapter 14). An overly punitive system will diminish this kind of open dialogue and exchange, and ultimately harm safety efforts.

How then to reconcile the tension between "no blame" and "blame?" In his classic book, *Managing the Risks of Organizational Accidents*, James Reason introduced the concept of Just Culture this way:

> A 'no-blame' culture is neither feasible nor desirable. A small proportion of human unsafe acts are egregious...and warrant sanctions, severe ones in some cases. A blanket amnesty on all unsafe acts would lack credibility in the eyes of the workforce. More importantly, it would be seen to oppose natural justice. What is needed is a *just culture*, an atmosphere of trust in which people are encouraged, even rewarded, for providing essential safety-related information—but in which they are also clear about where the line must be drawn between acceptable and unacceptable behavior.[8]

David Marx, an attorney and engineer, has popularized this concept over the past decade by helping to articulate where these behavioral boundaries lie. In Marx's model, Just Culture distinguishes between "human error," "at-risk behavior," and "reckless behavior." Only the latter category, defined as "acting in conscious disregard of substantial and unjustifiable risk," is blameworthy.[23,24] A simplified version of Marx's model is shown in Table 19-1.

The UK's National Patient Safety Agency (NPSA) has refined this concept and produced a more complex "Incident Decision Tree," backed up by 60 pages of supporting documentation.[25,26] It can all become a bit overwhelming, so I am attracted to an algorithm developed by safety expert Allan Frankel, which combines several of the elements from Reason's, Marx's, and the NPSA's models (Figure 19-2).[27] Before approaching it in the context of a safety incident, Frankel asks us to reflect on several questions:

- Was the individual knowingly impaired?
- Did the individual consciously decide to engage in an unsafe act?

Table 19-1	SIMPLIFIED VERSION OF MARX'S JUST CULTURE MODEL	
Mechanisms of Breach in Duty to Patient	Description	Appropriate Response by the System*
Human error	An inadvertent act by a caregiver (a "slip" or "mistake")	Console the provider
At-risk behavior	Taking shortcuts: conscious drift away from safe behaviors; caregiver violates a safety rule but doesn't perceive it as likely to cause harm (the equivalent of rolling through a stop sign)	Coach the provider
Reckless behavior	Conscious choice by caregiver to engage in behavior that he or she knows poses significant risk; ignoring required safety steps	Discipline the provider

*Importantly, Marx notes that these responses should be independent of the actual patient outcome.
Adapted from Marx D. Patient safety and the "just culture": a primer for health care executives, April 17, 2001. Available at: http://www.mers-tm.org/support/Marx_Primer.pdf; Marx D. *Whack-a-Mole: The Price We Pay for Expecting Perfection*. Plano, TX: By Your Side Studios; 2009.

- Did the caregiver make a mistake that individuals of similar experience and training would be likely to make under the same circumstances ("substitution test")?
- Does the individual have a history of unsafe acts?

After having considered the answers to these questions, the algorithm guides the user through a series of steps, ultimately identifying the appropriate response for a given unsafe act.

RECONCILING "NO BLAME" AND ACCOUNTABILITY

I once heard a prominent physician-executive give a lecture in which he quipped that he had three boxes on his corporate desk: his Inbox, his Outbox, and his "TooHard" box. During the first few years of the safety movement, I believe that our enthusiasm for the "no blame" model led us to file the vital question of balancing "no blame" and accountability in our own TooHard box. The recent interest in these Just Culture models tells me that we have finally dropped this issue into our collective Inboxes, where it belongs. Organizational leaders should study these models and then educate their providers and managers about the overall concept and at least one of the models.

1. Choose the column that best describes the caregiver's action. Read down the column for recommended responses.				
The caregiver's thinking was impaired by illegal or legal substances, cognitive impairment, or severe psychosocial stressors.	The caregiver wanted to cause harm.	The caregiver knowingly violated a rule and/or made a dangerous or unsafe choice. The decision appears to have been made with little or no concern about risk.	The caregiver made a potentially unsafe choice. Faulty or self-serving decision-making may be evident.	The caregiver makes or participates in an error while working appropriately and in the patient's best interest.
IMPAIRED JUDGEMENT	**MALICIOUS ACTION**	**RECKLESS ACTION**	**RISKY ACTION**	**UNINTENTIONAL ERROR**
• Discipline is warranted if illegal substances were used. • The caregiver's performance should be evaluated to determine whether a temporary work suspension would be helpful. • Help should be actively offered to the caregiver.	• Discipline and/or legal proceedings are warranted. • The caregiver's duties should be suspended immediately.	• Discipline may be warranted. • The caregiver is accountable and needs re-training. • The caregiver should participate in teaching others the lessons learned.	• The caregiver is accountable and should receive coaching. • The caregiver should participate in teaching others the lessons learned.	• The caregiver is not accountable. • The caregiver should participate in investigating why the error occured and teach others about the results of the investigation.

2. If three other caregivers with similar skills and knowledge would do the same in similar circumstances:		
The system supports reckless action and requires fixing. The caregiver is probably less accountable for the action, and system leaders share in the accountability.	The system supports risky action and requires fixing. The caregiver is probably less accountable for the action, and system leaders share in the accountability.	The system supports errors and requires fixing. The system's leaders are accountable and should apply error-proofing improvements.

3. If the caregiver has a history of repeatedly making mistakes, the caregiver may be in the wrong position. Evaluation is warranted, and coaching, transfer or termination should be considered. The corrective actions above should be modified accordingly.

Figure 19-2 ■ Frankel's algorithm for analyzing caregivers' actions and recommended responses in analyzing risks. (Reproduced with permission from Leonard MW, Frankel A. The path to safe and reliable healthcare. *Patient Educ Couns* 2010;80:288–292.)

Peter Pronovost and I explored this issue more fully in a 2009 *New England Journal of Medicine* article, focusing specifically on the need to include physicians in an accountability framework—one that does not shy away from blame and even penalties for those who fail to follow important evidence-based safety rules.[28] We used the example of hand hygiene to highlight a number of prerequisites that should be met before an accountability approach is applied (Table 19-2), and our recommended actions once such conditions are met. We concluded the article this way:

Part of the reason we must do this is that if we do not, other stake-holders, such as regulators and state legislatures, are likely to judge the

Table 19-2 **PREREQUISITES FOR MAKING THE CHOICE TO PUNISH PROVIDERS FOR NOT ADHERING TO A PATIENT SAFETY PRACTICE, USING THE EXAMPLE OF HAND HYGIENE**

Prerequisite	Example of Hand Hygiene
The patient safety problem that is being addressed is important	Rates of healthcare-associated infections are unacceptably high, resulting in serious morbidity and mortality
The literature or expert consensus strongly supports adherence to the practice as an effective strategy to decrease the probability of harm	Many studies and long-standing expert consensus support the value of hand hygiene, and healthcare-associated infections are now reported publicly and are subject to "no pay" initiatives*
Clinicians have been educated about the importance of the practice and the evidence supporting it	Lectures, reminder systems, academic detailing, dissemination of literature, and other steps to educate caregivers have been completed
The system has been modified, if necessary, to make it as easy as possible to adhere to the practice without disrupting other crucial work or creating unanticipated negative consequences; concerns by providers regarding barriers to compliance have been addressed†	Hand gel dispensers have been placed in convenient locations throughout the building; dispensers are never empty and work well (e.g., they do not squirt gel onto providers' clothes)
Physicians, other providers, and leaders have reached a consensus on the value of the practice and the process by which it will be measured; physicians understand the behaviors for which they will be held accountable	Meetings have been held with relevant provider groups, including medical staff, to review the evidence behind hand hygiene, the rates of hospital-acquired infections, and the steps that have been taken to optimize the system
A fair and transparent auditing system has been developed, and clinicians are aware of its existence	Providers know that observers will periodically audit hand-hygiene practices; observers can determine whether providers adhere to the practices, even if hands are cleaned inside patients' rooms (including the use of video or systems that sound an alarm when providers approach patients' beds without using nearby hand-cleaning dispensers)

(*continued*)

Table 19-2	PREREQUISITES FOR MAKING THE CHOICE TO PUNISH PROVIDERS FOR NOT ADHERING TO A PATIENT SAFETY PRACTICE, USING THE EXAMPLE OF HAND HYGIENE *(continued)*
Prerequisite	**Example of Hand Hygiene**
Clinicians who do not adhere to the practice once or perhaps twice have been counseled about the importance of the practice, about the steps that have been taken to make it easy to adhere, and about the fact that further transgressions will result in punishment; the consequences of failure to adhere have been described	A physician, for example, might receive a warning note or be counseled by a departmental chair after the first or second observed transgression
The penalties for infractions are understood and applied fairly	Chronic failure to clean hands will result in a 1-week suspension from clinical practice, accompanied by completion of a 2-hour online educational module on infection prevention

*Because of the vigorous regulatory and reporting environment in patient safety, it is likely that if the first two criteria are met, the practice will be one that is mandated by an accrediting organization (such as the Joint Commission) or that adherence to the practice, or instances of the patient safety problem it addresses, are being publicly reported or are the subject of financial penalties (e.g., through Medicare's "no pay for errors" initiative). However, we do not believe that such external pressures should be the sole reason that a practice reaches the level of punishment, since some regulated or publicly reported safety standards are flawed. On the other hand, some safety practices may meet the first two criteria before they are regulated or reported publicly, and such practices should be candidates for the above approach.

†In light of the complexities of the healthcare workplace, it is important that staff members with training in systems engineering and human factors be involved in the creation of new systems of care wherever possible.

Reproduced with permission from Wachter RM, Pronovost PJ. Balancing "no blame" with accountability in patient safety. *N Engl J Med* 2009;361:1401–1406.

reflexive invocation of the "no blame" approach as an example of guild behavior—of the medical profession circling its wagons to avoid confronting harsh realities, rather than as a thoughtful strategy for attacking the root causes of most errors. With that as their conclusion, they will be predisposed to further intrude on the practice of medicine, using the blunt and often politicized sticks of the legal, regulatory, and payment systems.

Having our own profession unblinkingly deem some behaviors as unacceptable, with clear consequences, will serve as a vivid example of our professionalism and thus represent our best protection against such outside intrusions. But the main reason to find the right balance between "no blame" and individual accountability is that doing so will save lives.[28]

Before leaving the topic of accountability, it is worthwhile connecting the dots between the issues explored in this chapter and those highlighted in Chapter 2, when I discussed sharp-end and blunt-end errors. The kind of accountability that I've discussed in this chapter largely relates to sharp-end providers: the clinician who makes the diagnosis of aortic dissection, cuts out the lung tumor, reads the pathology specimen, or hangs the bag of dobutamine. Bell et al. emphasize the importance of *collective accountability*—accountability at the level of the individual clinician, the healthcare team, *and the institution*.[29] The increasing emphasis on public reporting (Chapter 14), disclosure of adverse events (Chapter 18), and regulatory and accreditation solutions (Chapter 20) are ways of promoting collective accountability. As you can see, even if we reach consensus that accountability and even blame are appropriate at times, trying to fairly identify the target for this accountability is yet another issue that has been in our "TooHard" box until recently. It will require a lot of thoughtful analysis and discussion to get this balance right as well.

Other issues surrounding safety and culture are covered, from a somewhat different angle, in Chapter 15.

THE ROLE OF THE MEDIA

Many people look to the media to shine a light on the problem of patient safety and to ensure accountability. The thinking goes that such transparency (sometimes driven by mandated public reporting of errors; see Chapters 3 and 14) will create a powerful business case for safety, drive hospitals and providers toward enforcing rules and standards, and generate the resources needed to catalyze needed systems change. And there is no doubt that such scrutiny can have precisely this effect—it is difficult to find hospitals or health systems as energized to improve safety as those that have been the subject of widespread media coverage after a major error (Table 1-1).

But while the patient safety efforts at institutions such as Johns Hopkins, Duke, Cedars-Sinai, and Dana-Farber were clearly turbocharged by mediagenic errors, media scrutiny can also tap into institutional and individual fear of public disclosure and spur an atmosphere of silence. Such a response increases the chance that providers and organizations will fail to discuss and learn from their own errors. Although this response is usually a reflection of organizational culture and leadership (Chapters 15 and 22), the way the media chooses to handle errors also influences the way organizations respond to the prospect of media attention. The more distorted the coverage (e.g., emphasizing bad apples over systems), the more harmful the effect is likely to be.[30] Over the past decade, media reports of medical errors have increasingly (though far from uniformly) reflected a more sophisticated understanding of the issues, which increases the probability that such reports will help more than harm.[31,32]

KEY POINTS

- Although the systems focus is the (correct) underpinning of the modern patient safety movement, incompetent or dangerous providers and institutions must also be held accountable.
- Healthcare tends to "protect its own," which undermines public trust in the medical professions.
- Some clinicians' behavior is sufficiently disruptive to create a patient safety risk. Organizations need a strategy to manage such behavior, which sabotages teamwork, communication, and job satisfaction among colleagues.
- Vehicles to determine and enforce accountability can be local (such as hospital credentials committees) or outside organizations (such as state licensing boards or national professional organizations).
- In recent years, several Just Culture algorithms have emerged to help organizations and managers determine which acts represent human errors, "at-risk" behaviors, or examples of negligence. Only the latter should lead to punishment.
- The media can play an important role in ensuring accountability, especially if reporting on errors is seen as fair and reflective of our modern understanding of patient safety.

| REFERENCES

1. Wachter RM, Shojania KG. *Internal Bleeding: The Truth Behind America's Terrifying Epidemic of Medical Mistakes*. New York, NY: Rugged Land; 2004.
2. DesRoches CM, Rao SR, Fromson JA, et al. Physicians' perceptions, preparedness for reporting, and experiences related to impaired and incompetent colleagues. *JAMA* 2010;304:187–193.
3. Wolfe SM. Bad doctors get a free ride. *NY Times* (Print). 2003:A27.

4. Jena AB, Seabury S, Lakdawalla D, et al. Malpractice risk according to physician specialty. *N Engl J Med* 2011;365:629–636.

5. Hickson GB, Federspiel CF, Pichert JW, et al. Patient complaints and malpractice risk. *JAMA* 2002;287:2951–2957.

6. Papadakis MA, Teherani A, Banach MA, et al. Disciplinary action by medical boards and prior behavior in medical school. *N Engl J Med* 2005;353:2673–2682.

7. Johnstone MJ, Kanitsaki O. Processes for disciplining nurses for unprofessional conduct of a serious nature: a critique. *J Adv Nurs* 2005;50:363–371.

8. Reason JT. *Managing the Risks of Organizational Accidents*. Aldershot, Hampshire, England: Ashgate Publishing Limited; 1997.

9. Williams LS. Anesthetist receives jail sentence after patient left in vegetative state. *CMAJ* 1995;153:619–620.

10. Anonymous. Surgeon who left an operation to run an errand is suspended. *NY Times* (Print). 2002:A13.

11. Stewart J. *Blind Eye: The Terrifying Story of a Doctor who Got Away with Murder*. New York, NY: Simon and Schuster; 2000.

12. O'Neill B. Doctor as murderer. Death certification needs tightening up, but it still might not have stopped Shipman. *BMJ* 2000;320:329–330.

13. Rosenstein AH, O'Daniel M. Invited article: managing disruptive physician behavior: impact on staff relationships and patient care. *Neurology* 2008;70:1564–1570.

14. Rosenstein AH, O'Daniel M. A survey of the impact of disruptive behaviors and communication defects on patient safety. *Jt Comm J Qual Patient Saf* 2008:34; 464–471.

15. Saxton R, Hines T, Enriquez M. The negative impact of nurse–physician disruptive behavior on patient safety: a review of the literature. *J Patient Saf* 2009;5:180–183.

16. Lingard L, Espin S, Whyte S, et al. Communication failures in the operating room: an observational classification of recurrent types and effects. *Qual Saf Health Care* 2004;13:330–334.

17. The Joint Commission. *Sentinel event alert. Behaviors that undermine a culture of safety*. July 9, 2008;(40):1–3.

18. Leape LL, Fromson JA. Problem doctors: is there a system-level solution? *Ann Intern Med* 2006;144:107–115.

19. Rosenstein AH, O'Daniel M. How to identify and manage problem behaviors. *AHRQ WebM&M* (serial online); December 2009. Available at: http://webMM.ahrq.gov/perspective.aspx?perspectiveID=82.

20. ABIM Foundation, ACP-ASIM Foundation, European Federation of Internal Medicine. Medical professionalism in the new millennium: a physician charter. *Ann Intern Med* 2002;136:243–246.

21. Hickson GB, Pichert JW, Webb LE, et al. A complementary approach to promoting professionalism: identifying, measuring, and addressing unprofessional behaviors. *Acad Med* 2007;82:1040–1048.

22. In conversation with ... Gerald Hickson. *AHRQ WebM&M* (serial online); December 2009. Available at: http://webmm.ahrq.gov/perspective.aspx?perspectiveID=81.

23. Marx D. *Patient Safety and the "Just Culture": A Primer for Health Care Executives*; April 17, 2001. Available at: http://www.mers-tm.org/support/Marx_Primer.pdf.

24. Marx D. *Whack-a-Mole: The Price We Pay for Expecting Perfection*. Plano, TX: By Your Side Studios; 2009.

25. Meadows S, Baker K, Butler J. The incident decision tree. *Clin Risk* 2005;11:66–68.

26. National Patient Safety Agency. *The Incident Decision Tree. Information and Advice on Use*. National Patient Safety Agency, National Health Service; 2003. Available at: http://www.chpso.org/just/IDTadvice2003.pdf.

27. Leonard MW, Frankel A. The path to safe and reliable healthcare. *Patient Educ Couns* 2010;80:288–292.

28. Wachter RM, Pronovost PJ. Balancing "no blame" with accountability in patient safety. *N Engl J Med* 2009;361:1401–1406.

29. Bell SK, Delbanco T, Anderson-Shaw L, et al. Accountability for medical error: moving beyond blame to advocacy. *Chest* 2011;140:519–526.

30. Dentzer S. Media mistakes in coverage of the Institute of Medicine's error report. *Eff Clin Pract* 2000;3:305–308.

31. Millenson ML. Pushing the profession: how the news media turned patient safety into a priority. *Qual Saf Health Care* 2002;11:57–63.

32. Emanuel EJ. What cannot be said on television about health care. *JAMA* 2007;297:2131–2133.

ADDITIONAL READINGS

Bosk CL. *Forgive and Remember: Managing Medical Failure*. 2nd ed. Chicago, IL: University of Chicago Press; 2003.

Dekker S. *Just Culture: Balancing Safety and Accountability*. Aldershot, Hampshire, England: Ashgate Publishing Limited; 2007.

Dekker SWA. Just culture: who gets to draw the line? *Cogn Technol Work* 2009;11:177–185.

Goldmann D. System failure versus personal accountability—the case for clean hands. *N Engl J Med* 2006;355:121–123.

Lee TH, Meyer GS, Brennan TA. A middle ground on public accountability. *N Engl J Med* 2004;350:2409–2412.

McLaren K, Lord J, Murray S. Perspective: delivering effective and engaging continuing medical education on physicians' disruptive behavior. *Acad Med* 2011;86:612–617.

Pettker CM, Funai EF. Getting it right when things go wrong. *JAMA* 2010;303:977–978.

Satava RM. The nature of surgical error: a cautionary tale and a call to reason. *Surg Endosc* 2005;19:1014–1016.

Wachter RM. Patient safety at ten: unmistakable progress, troubling gaps. *Health Aff (Millwood)* 2010;29:165–173.

Whittemore AD. The competent surgeon: individual accountability in the era of "systems" failure. *Ann Surg* 2009;250:357–362.

ACCREDITATION AND REGULATIONS | 20

OVERVIEW

One might hope that professionalism and concern for patients would be sufficient incentive to motivate safe behaviors on the part of providers, as well as institutional investments in system safety. Sadly, experience has taught us that this is not the case. There are simply too many competing pressures for attention and resources, and the nature of safety is that individuals and organizations can often get away with bad behavior for long periods of time. Moreover, it is unlikely that all providers and institutions will or can keep up with best practices, given a rapidly evolving research base and the never-ending need to keep at least one eye on the bottom line.

These realities create a need for more prescriptive solutions to safety: standards set by external organizations, such as accreditors, regulatory bodies, payer representatives, and government. This chapter will examine some of these solutions, beginning with regulations and accreditation.

ACCREDITATION

Regulation is "an authoritative rule," while accreditation is a process by which an authoritative body formally recognizes that an organization or a person is competent to carry out specific tasks. Much of what we tend to call regulation is actually accreditation, but takes place in an environment in which a lack of accreditation has nearly the impact of failing to adhere to a regulatory mandate. For example, the *Accreditation Council for Graduate Medical Education* (ACGME), the body that blesses U.S. residency and fellowship programs, is not a regulator but an accreditor. Nevertheless, when the ACGME mandated that residents work less than 80 hours per week in 2003 and proscribed traditional overnight call shifts for first-year residents in 2011 (Chapter 16), these directives had the force of regulation, because ACGME has the power to shut down training programs for noncompliance.[1]

The most important accreditor in the patient safety field (in the United States) is *the Joint Commission* (formerly the Joint Commission on Accreditation of Healthcare Organizations [JCAHO]). The Joint Commission, which began in 1951 as a joint program of the American College of Surgeons (which launched the first hospital inspections in 1918), the American College of Physicians, the American Hospital Association, the American Medical Association, and the Canadian Medical Association, has become an increasingly powerful force over the last decade by more aggressively exercising its mandate to improve the safety of American hospitals (and now, through its Joint Commission International subsidiary, hospitals around the world). A list of Joint Commission *National Patient Safety Goals*, one of the organization's key mechanisms for endorsing practices, highlighting safety problems, and generating action, is shown in Appendix IV.

Until the mid-2000s, Joint Commission visits to hospitals were announced years in advance and focused on hospitals' adherence to various policies and procedures. In 2006, the process became far more robust: the accreditor's visits now come unannounced (in my own hospital, it is now a staff member's job to check the Joint Commission's Web site at 7 AM every Monday to see if there will be inspectors in our lobby a half-hour later), and much of the visit centers around the "*Tracer Methodology*," a process by which the inspectors follow a given patient's course throughout the hospital, checking documentation of care and speaking to caregivers about their actions and their understanding of safety principles and regulations. In my judgment, this more vigorous approach to safety enforcement has been an important force for improving safety.[2,3]

Beginning soon after Medicare was founded in 1965, the Joint Commission was granted an exclusive arrangement by the Centers for Medicare & Medicaid Services (CMS) to act as its inspection arm. Known as a *deeming authority*, CMS made the presumption that a hospital that passed a Joint Commission inspection was also in compliance with the CMS *Conditions of Participation*. In essence, this is what gives a Joint Commission inspection its teeth: failure puts an organization at risk of losing its Medicare payments, a significant portion of most U.S. hospitals' revenue. After a few high profile cases in which Joint Commission-accredited hospitals were later revealed to have major safety problems, in 2008 CMS announced that it would extend deeming authority to other organizations that met its requirements.[4] As of this writing (late 2011), only one other entity (DNV Healthcare) has been granted such authority; it now accredits a few hundred U.S. hospitals (vs. several thousand for the Joint Commission).[5]

Although the Joint Commission does regulate some physicians' offices and ambulatory sites (such as surgery centers), most such sites are either unaccredited or accredited by another organization, such as the American Association for the Accreditation of Ambulatory Surgical Facilities (AAAASF).[6] In recent years, concerns have been raised about the safety of ambulatory surgery, in particular, and an increasingly forceful set of accreditation standards has been implemented in these environments. Despite this change, the ambulatory environment continues to be affected far less by the pressures of regulation and accreditation, one of the key differences between patient safety in inpatient and office settings (Chapter 12).

Physicians are subject to both regulation and accreditation standards as well. In the United States, physicians require a license to practice; such licenses are issued by the individual states, and are not specialty specific. While physicians can lose their licenses for problems that include substance abuse, criminal convictions, and incompetence, they rarely do (Chapter 19). The process of license renewal has traditionally been relatively benign, often involving proving attendance at a certain number of continuing education conferences rather than showing evidence of ongoing competence. The Federation of State Medical Boards has announced its intention to implement *Maintenance of Licensure* (MOL) requirements, in which physicians will need to demonstrate ongoing competency and commitment to professional development. The specifics of this program are still being worked out, and it is likely that specialty board *Maintenance of Certification* (MOC) activities (see below) will be accepted as meeting MOL requirements.[7]

A higher bar for physicians is *board certification*, a voluntary process through which doctors participate in activities designed to show that they are currently competent in their own specialty (truth in advertising: I have long served on the largest specialty board, the American Board of Internal Medicine). While board certification differs from licensure in many ways, a key difference is that board certification *is* specialty specific: one is board certified, for example, as an internist or a pediatric cardiologist, whereas licensure has traditionally been specialty agnostic. To become board certified, physicians complete training programs (either residencies, for initial training in areas such as internal medicine, surgery, or pediatrics, or fellowships, for specialized fields such as endocrinology or interventional radiology). They then "sit for the boards" to obtain their initial board certification. Approximately 750,000 U.S. physicians are board certified in at least one of 147 specialties and subspecialties. There is good evidence that board certification is associated with higher quality of care.[8–11]

Until the late 1980s, initial board certification lasted for an entire career for the vast majority of medical specialists. However, given healthcare's breakneck pace of change, the fact that other professionals (e.g., pilots and teachers) have to recertify every few years, and the evidence that older physicians may, in fact, deliver lower quality care,[12] the *American Board of Medical Specialties* (the umbrella organization for all 24 specialty boards) now

Table 20-1   **THE STRUCTURE OF MAINTENANCE OF CERTIFICATION (MOC) PROGRAMS***
Part I: Licensure and Professional Standing—Medical specialists must hold a valid, unrestricted medical license in at least one (1) state or jurisdiction in the United States, its territories, or Canada.
Part II: Lifelong Learning and Self-Assessment—Specialists participate in educational and self-assessment programs that meet specialty-specific standards that are set by their member board.
Part III: Cognitive Expertise—Specialists demonstrate, through formalized examination, that they have the fundamental, practice-related and practice environment–related knowledge to provide quality care in their specialty.
Part IV: Practice Performance Assessment—Specialists are evaluated in their clinical practice according to specialty-specific standards for patient care. They are asked to demonstrate that they can assess the quality of care they provide compared to peers and national benchmarks, and then apply the best evidence or consensus recommendations to improve that care using follow-up assessments.

*Source: American Board of Medical Specialties. The individual "member boards" (such as the American Board of Internal Medicine) vary somewhat in how they apply these requirements. Most have traditionally required physicians to provide evidence of meeting the Part I requirement at the same time that they took the secure examination (Part III), approximately every 10 years. Diplomates were required to perform self-assessment (Part II) and complete a Practice Improvement Module (Part IV) periodically, perhaps every 5 to 10 years. As of 2012, all of the boards are moving to a program of *Continuous MOC*, which will require more frequent activity. It is likely that some MOC activity (probably self-assessment [Part II] and quality improvement [Part IV]) will be required every 2 to 5 years, while the exam (Part III) will remain less frequent.

requires that its diplomates participate in MOC programs.[13] The requirements for MOC include not only passing a specialty-specific test (Part III) but also engaging in activities to measure the quality of care in one's own practice, and demonstrating a commitment to improving quality and safety (Table 20-1). As of 2011, more than 300,000 U.S. physicians were participating in at least one MOC program, although a similar number finished their training prior to recertification requirements ("grandfathers"). The size of this latter group, of course, will rapidly fall over the next several years, and by 2020, the vast majority of board certified physicians will be enrolled in MOC, an important development in efforts to promote patient safety.

While there are many other ways of measuring physician competence,[14] and a variety of other stakeholders (such as insurance companies and consumer-oriented Web sites) are trying to do so, the boards have some unique attributes. First, board certification is a voluntary process organized by the medical profession itself, giving it higher credibility among physicians than measures created by outside organizations. Second, because of the challenges in measuring diagnostic acumen (Chapter 6), the boards have a singular role in assessing physicians' knowledge and diagnostic abilities. Patients generally put a significant amount of stock in knowing that their doctor is board certified, rating it among their most highly valued measures of quality.[8] Increasingly, insurers and hospitals are requiring that their physicians be board certified and actively participate in MOC, although many gaps remain.[15]

REGULATIONS

Regulation is more potent than accreditation, in that compliance is mandatory (no hospital *has* to be accredited by the Joint Commission and no doctor *has* to be board certified, though the vast majority of both hospitals and physicians choose to be) and failure to comply generally carries stiff penalties. Today, the main U.S. regulatory authorities relevant to patient safety are state governments, although there are a few federal regulations and a handful of counties and cities have safety-related regulations. Unlike countries with national health systems (such as the UK's National Health Service[16]), in the United States there is no single entity with the authority and mandate to regulate patient safety, which explains why this function has largely been left to states. (Medicare is increasingly assuming this role, a point I'll return to a little later.)

For example, 15 states, including California, now regulate nurse-to-patient ratios (Chapter 16), 26 states now require reporting of certain types of errors to a state entity (Chapter 14), seven states have passed laws mandating error disclosure (Chapter 18), and 10 states require that patients admitted to hospitals be screened for methicillin-resistant *Staphylococcus aureus* (Chapter 10). Pennsylvania and Virginia have even added requirements for a certain number of hours of patient safety–specific content within their overall continuing education requirements for license renewal.

OTHER LEVERS TO PROMOTE SAFETY

One of the most important organizations in the patient safety world is not a regulator or an accreditor, but rather a Washington, DC–based nonprofit organization called the *National Quality Forum* (NQF). The NQF was established in 1999 with a three-part mission: to set goals for performance improvement, to endorse standards for measuring and reporting on performance, and to promote educational and outreach programs. In the quality world (Chapter 3), the NQF is best known for its endorsement process: many organizations that are in the business of selecting measures for public reporting or payment changes now insist on using NQF-endorsed measures. Measures that receive such endorsement have survived a rigorous and multistakeholder process focusing on the strength of the evidence.

In the patient safety world, NQF has made two other major contributions. In 2002, the NQF published a list of serious adverse events, which NQF founding president Ken Kizer famously dubbed the *Never Events* list (Kizer described the items on the list as "things that should never happen" in healthcare).[17] While early items on the list included dramatic and iconic adverse events such as wrong-site surgery and retained foreign objects after surgery (Chapter 5), the list has grown (now to 29 items) and matured over the years (Appendix VI). Because many items are not known to be fully preventable even with perfect care, the name "Never Events" is now a misnomer (the list's actual name is *Serious Reportable Events*), though it is still frequently referred to by its original, evocative name.[18] The SRE list has assumed great importance over the years, as it now provides a basis for several key safety policies, including Medicare's "no pay for errors" initiative and a wide variety of state-based adverse event reporting programs.[19,20]

In addition to the SRE list, NQF also endorses another list of "safe practices" (Appendix VII), originally based on the *Making Healthcare Safer* report that my colleagues and I produced for the U.S. Agency for Healthcare Research and Quality.[21] The safe practices list is updated regularly (it now contains 34 items) and it is used by many stakeholders to focus their safety efforts.

Healthcare payers also have tremendous leverage to move the system, though they have not wielded it in the safety arena very aggressively. One exception has been the *Leapfrog Group*, a healthcare arm of many of America's largest employers (and thus the source of a significant amount of hospital and doctor payments), which was founded in 2000 in part to catalyze patient safety activities. Leapfrog uses its contracting power to promote safe practices, either through simple transparency or by steering patients toward institutions it deems to be better performers. In 2001, it recommended three "safe practices" (computerized provider order entry [CPOE], favoring high-volume providers when there was evidence linking higher volume to better outcomes [Table 5-1], and having full-time intensivists provide critical care). In 2006, Leapfrog endorsed the NQF list of serious reportable events (Appendix VI). While there is some evidence that Leapfrog's activities have led to more widespread implementation of the endorsed practices,[22,23] the evidence that Leapfrog scores are associated with other measures of quality and safety is mixed.[24,25]

Even softer influence has been exercised by professional societies and nonprofit safety-oriented organizations. For example, several professional physician and nursing societies have led campaigns to improve hand hygiene (Chapter 10) and discharge coordination (Chapter 8). In 2005, the *Institute for Healthcare Improvement* (IHI), a nonprofit support and consulting organization, launched a "campaign to save 100,000 lives" by promoting a set of six safety-oriented practices in American hospitals.[26] Although IHI lacks regulatory authority and is not a payer, its campaign succeeded in enrolling more than half the hospitals in the United States. This tremendous response was followed in late 2006 by another campaign to "prevent 5 million cases of harm" through six additional practices (Table 20-2).[27] Given the various forces promoting safety in American hospitals, it is difficult to isolate the effect of the IHI campaigns, but there is no doubt that they captured the attention of the American healthcare system and generated significant change.[28,29]

It is worth adding that funders—particularly the *Agency for Healthcare Research and Quality* (AHRQ) but including foundations and other agencies in the United States and worldwide—have had a critical influence on safety extending well beyond the dollars they distribute. AHRQ, for example, has promoted education, disseminated best practices, commissioned evidence reviews, convened stakeholders, and engaged in myriad other activities that have made it an indispensable safety leader.

Table 20-2 THE "PLANKS" IN THE IHI'S 2005–2006 "100,000 LIVES CAMPAIGN" AND ITS 2006–2007 "CAMPAIGN TO PROTECT 5 MILLION LIVES FROM HARM"	
100,000 Lives Campaign	**5 Million Lives Campaign**
Prevent ventilator-associated pneumonia	Prevent pressure ulcers
Prevent catheter-related bloodstream infections	Reduce the incidence of methicillin-resistant *Staphylococcus aureus* (MRSA) infection
Prevent surgical site infections	Prevent harm from high-alert medications such as anticoagulants, sedatives, and insulins
Improve care for acute myocardial infarction	Reduce surgical complications
Prevent adverse drug reactions with medication reconciliation	Deliver reliable, evidence-based care for patients with heart failure
Deploy rapid response teams	Get healthcare system "boards on board"

Increasingly, the U.S. healthcare system—led by CMS—is embracing transparency (e.g., public reporting of performance) and differential payments for better performance ("pay for performance" and "no pay for errors").[19,30–33] The idea behind these efforts is to create a *business case for quality and safety*—a set of incentives generated by patients choosing better and safer providers, or by providers receiving higher payments for better performance. These initiatives (such as *value-based purchasing* and "*no pay for errors*") may ultimately become more important than both regulation and accreditation in driving safety efforts. They are described in considerable detail in Chapter 3. In 2011, CMS announced a billion dollar campaign (the "Partnership for Patients") to promote patient safety.[34] The fact that it drew many of its themes and strategies from the two IHI campaigns should have come as no great surprise: Dr. Don Berwick, the founding head of the IHI, became CMS director the prior year (he stepped down in December, 2011).

Finally, while patient-oriented and consumer groups have added an important voice to the patient safety field, they remain relatively small. None are influential enough yet to drive the national safety agenda by themselves, but they have made important contributions by working with more powerful organizations such as the IHI, the National Patient Safety Foundation, and AHRQ (Chapter 21).

PROBLEMS WITH REGULATORY, ACCREDITATION, AND OTHER PRESCRIPTIVE SOLUTIONS

Since regulators and accreditors have the power to mandate change, why not use these levers more aggressively? Given the toll of medical errors, wouldn't we want to use our biggest, most prescriptive guns?

Perhaps, but regulation, accreditation, and laws are what policy experts call "blunt tools," because of their highly limited ability to take into account local circumstances or institutional culture and calibrate their mandates accordingly. Therefore, they are best used for "low-hanging fruit"—areas amenable to one-size-fits-all solutions, usually because they are not particularly complex and tend not to vary from institution to institution. Examples of such areas might be "sign-your-site" (Chapter 5) and abolition of high-risk abbreviations (Chapter 4): these standards are as applicable in a 600-bed academic medical center as in an 80-bed rural hospital.

But as regulation and accreditation inch into areas that are more nuanced and dependent on cultural changes, the risk of unforeseen consequences increases. For example, the Joint Commission's 2005 requirement for medication reconciliation, though based on legitimate concerns about medication errors at points of transition (Chapters 4 and 8), vexed hospitals around the United States because of implementation problems and the absence of established best practices.[35] Leapfrog's 2001 mandate that hospitals have CPOE seemed reasonable, but it was based on the experiences of only a few, highly atypical hospitals and it proved difficult for the coalition to distinguish between effective and ineffective CPOE (Chapter 13). ACGME's duty-hour limits (Chapter 16) have allowed residents to sleep but also created collateral damage by increasing handoffs (Chapter 8). And some nurses have complained that mandatory nurse-to-patient ratios have not enhanced safety, because some hospitals have replaced clerical staff or lifting teams to meet the ratios, leaving nurses with no more direct patient care time than they had before the law (Chapter 16).

Despite these limitations, regulation is vital in certain areas, particularly when providers and institutions fail to voluntarily adopt reasonable safety standards. For example, many take-out restaurants have long read back take-out orders to ensure accurate communication (by the way, they did this without a regulatory mandate—the business case to get your take-out order right is powerful enough to motivate the practice), but no healthcare organization required this practice until the Joint Commission did so in 2003 (Chapter 8).[36]

Regulation can also standardize practices that should be standardized. Prior to the Joint Commission regulations regarding "sign-your-site," many orthopedic surgeons had taken it upon themselves to begin signing limbs in an effort to prevent wrong-site surgery. The problem: some well-meaning surgeons marked the leg *to be operated on* with an X (as in, "cut here"), while others put an X on the leg *not to be operated on* (as in, "don't cut here").[36] Obviously, without a standard system for signing the site (the Joint Commission now mandates signing the site *to be operated on*), the opportunity for misunderstanding and errors is great (Chapter 5).

This chapter's discussion mostly pertains to the United States, where the relatively limited influence of regulations reflects the decentralized structure of the healthcare system and America's traditional discomfort with central authority. In more centralized healthcare systems, the role of national regulators tends to be more important. For example, early in the patient safety movement Britain created a *National Patient Safety Agency* (NPSA), charged with assessing the state of patient safety, conducting investigations, and issuing recommendations and regulations.[16] While such agencies have the virtue of efficiency, too much central control can hamper grassroots efforts and be insufficiently responsive to local circumstances. (The Cameron government will dismantle the NPSA sometime in 2012–2013.)

The lessons of complex adaptive systems (Chapter 3) are worth heeding: one-size-fits-all solutions imposed by outside entities on frontline units in complex organizations are often surprisingly ineffective. With Medicare now demonstrating increased interest in using its vast market share to act more like a regulator of safety and quality than a "dumb payer," it will be important for the United States to learn what it can from other countries and organizations with long histories of centralized control.

In the end, prescriptive tools such as regulations, accreditation standards, and laws play an important role in ensuring patient safety. It is vital that they be used and enforced when they are the right instruments for the job, and that other vehicles (transparency, payment changes, market forces and competition, social marketing, changes in training, and appeals to professionalism) be employed when they are the more appropriate tools. A law or regulation can easily seem like the most straightforward way to fix an important safety problem, but we should never make the mistake of underestimating the messiness and complexity of our world.

KEY POINTS

- Regulation and accreditation are powerful tools to promote patient safety in that they can mandate (or nearly mandate) certain practices. In the United States, much of the regulation is state based, whereas other nations have more federally-based regulatory models. Medicare, though, is beginning to exert more central authority through its dual position as regulator and dominant payer.
- Accreditation of hospitals (such as by the Joint Commission), physicians (through board certification), and training programs (via the ACGME) has been an extremely important vehicle for patient safety change.
- Other organizations that lack regulatory or accreditation authority can also catalyze significant change, using levers such as the establishment of standards (the NQF), changing the payment system (the Leapfrog Group and other payers), promoting research (AHRQ), or taking advantage of well-established credibility and moral authority among caregivers and delivery organizations (the IHI).
- Regulation and accreditation are "blunt tools" that are best used for "low-hanging fruit": simple and relatively standardized processes whose effectiveness is independent of organizational size, complexity, and culture. They can be problematic when applied to more complex targets such as provider communication, leadership, computerization, and medication reconciliation.

REFERENCES

1. Pastores SM, O'Connor MF, Kleinpell RM, et al. The Accreditation Council for Graduate Medical Education resident duty hour new standards: history, changes, and impact on staffing of intensive care units. *Crit Care Med* 2011;39:2540–2549.

2. Wachter RM. The end of the beginning: patient safety five years after "To Err is Human." *Health Aff (Millwood)* 2004;(suppl W4):534–545.

3. Wachter RM. Patient safety at ten: unmistakable progress, troubling gaps. *Health Aff (Millwood)* 2010;29:165–173.

4. Gaul G. Accreditors blamed for overlooking problems. *The Washington Post*. July 25, 2005:A01.

5. DerGurahian J. DNV setting new standard. *Modern Healthcare*. October 27, 2008:3–4.

6. Yates JA. Liposuction gone awry. *AHRQ WebM&M* (serial online); March 2006. Available at: http://www.webmm.ahrq.gov/case.aspx?caseID=119.

7. Chaudhry H. Federation of State Medical Boards: maintenance of licensure and health IT. *Health Affairs Blog*. August 5, 2010. Available at: http://healthaffairs.org/blog/2010/08/05/fed-of-state-medical-boards-maintenance-of-licensure-and-health-it/.

8. Brennan TA, Horwitz RI, Duffy FD, et al. The role of physician specialty board certification status in the quality movement. *JAMA* 2004;292:1038–1043.

9. Norcini JJ, Lipner RS, Kimball HR. Certifying examination performance and patient outcomes following acute myocardial infarction. *Med Educ* 2002;36:853–859.

10. Holmboe ES, Wang Y, Meehan TP, et al. Association between maintenance of certification examination scores and quality of care for Medicare beneficiaries. *Arch Intern Med* 2008;168:1396–1403.

11. Chen J, Rathore SS, Wang Y, et al. Physician board certification and the care and outcomes of elderly patients with acute myocardial infarction. *J Gen Intern Med* 2006;21:238–244.

12. Choudhry NK, Fletcher RH, Soumerai SB. Systematic review: the relationship between clinical experience and quality of health care. *Ann Intern Med* 2005;142:260–273.

13. Weiss KB. Future of board certification in a new era of public accountability. *J Am Board Fam Med* 2010;23(suppl 1):S32–S39.

14. Landon BE, Normand SL, Blumenthal D, et al. Physician clinical performance assessment: prospects and barriers. *JAMA* 2003;290:1183–1189.

15. Freed GL, Dunham KM, Singer D. Use of board certification and recertification in hospital privileging: policies for general surgeons, surgical specialists, and nonsurgical subspecialists. *Arch Surg* 2009;144:746–752.

16. Lewis RQ, Fletcher M. Implementing a national strategy for patient safety: lessons from the National Health Service in England. *Qual Saf Health Care* 2005;14:135–139.

17. Vastag B. Kenneth W. Kizer, MD, MPH: health care quality evangelist. *JAMA* 2001;285:869–871.

18. Wachter RM. Never say never (events). *Wachter's World*. June 30, 2011. Available at: http://community.the-hospitalist.org/2011/06/30/never-say-never-events/.

19. Wachter RM, Foster NE, Dudley RA. Medicare's decision to withhold payment for hospital errors: the devil is in the details. *Jt Comm J Qual Patient Saf* 2008;34: 116–123.

20. Levinson DR. *Adverse Events in Hospitals: State Reporting Systems*. Washington, DC: US Department of Health and Human Services, Office of the Inspector General; December 2008. Report No. OEI-06-07-00471.

21. Shojania KG, Duncan BW, McDonald KM, et al., eds. *Making Health Care Safer: A Critical Analysis of Patient Safety Practices*. Evidence Report/Technology Assessment No. 43, AHRQ Publication No. 01-E058. Rockville, MD: Agency for Healthcare Research and Quality; July 2001.

22. Galvin RS, Delbanco S. Why employers need to rethink how they buy health care. *Health Aff (Millwood)* 2005;24:1549–1553.

23. Scanlon DP, Lindrooth RC, Christianson JB. Steering patients to safer hospitals? The effect of a tiered hospital network on hospital admissions. *Health Serv Res* 2008;43:1849–1868.

24. Kernisan LP, Lee SJ, Boscardin WJ, et al. Association between hospital-reported Leapfrog safe practices scores and inpatient mortality. *JAMA* 2009;301: 1341–1348.

25. Jha AK, Orav EJ, Ridgway AB, et al. Does the Leapfrog program help identify high-quality hospitals? *Jt Comm J Qual Patient Saf* 2008;34:318–325.

26. Berwick DM, Calkins DR, McCannon CJ, et al. The 100,000 Lives Campaign: setting a goal and a deadline for improving health care quality. *JAMA* 2006;295: 324–327.

27. McCannon CJ, Hackbarth AD, Griffin FA. Miles to go: an introduction to the 5 Million Lives Campaign. *Jt Comm J Qual Patient Saf* 2007;33:477–484.

28. Wachter RM, Pronovost PJ. The 100,000 Lives Campaign: a scientific and policy review. *Jt Comm J Qual Patient Saf* 2006;32:621–627, 631–633.

29. Berwick DM, Hackbarth AD, McCannon CJ. IHI replies to "The 100,000 Lives Campaign: a scientific and policy review". *Jt Comm J Qual Patient Saf* 2006;32:628–630 [discussion 631–633].

30. Lindenauer PK, Remus D, Roman S, et al. Public reporting and pay for performance in hospital quality improvement. *N Engl J Med* 2007;356:486–496.

31. Ferman JH. Value-based purchasing program here to stay: payments will be based on performance. *Health Exec* 2011;26:76, 78.

32. Ferris TG, Torchiana DF. Public release of clinical outcomes data—online CABG report cards. *N Engl J Med* 2010;363:1593–1595.

33. Berwick DM, James B, Coye MJ. Connections between quality measurement and improvement. *Med Care* 2003;41:I-30–I-38.

34. McCannon J, Berwick DM. A new frontier in patient safety. *JAMA* 2011;305: 2221–2222.

35. Anonymous. Practitioners agree on medication reconciliation value, but frustration and difficulties abound. *Institute for Safe Medication Practices Newsletter*. July 13, 2006. Available at: http://www.ismp.org/Newsletters/acutecare/articles/20060713.asp.

36. Wachter RM, Shojania KG. *Internal Bleeding: The Truth Behind America's Terrifying Epidemic of Medical Mistakes*. New York, NY: Rugged Land; 2004.

ADDITIONAL READINGS

Brennan TA, Gawande A, Thomas E, et al. Accidental deaths, saved lives, and improved quality. *N Engl J Med* 2005;353:1405–1409.

Devers KJ, Pham HH, Liu G. What is driving hospitals' patient-safety efforts? *Health Aff (Millwood)* 2004;23:103–115.

The Joint Commission. *National Patient Safety Goals.* Available at: http://www.jointcommission.org/PatientSafety/NationalPatientSafetyGoals/.

Langley GJ, Moen R, Nolan KM, et al. *The Improvement Guide: A Practical Approach to Enhancing Organizational Performance.* 2nd ed. San Francisco, CA: Jossey-Bass; 2009.

McClellan M, McKethan AN, Lewis JL, et al. A national strategy to put accountable care into practice. *Health Aff (Millwood)* 2010;29:982–990.

Plesk P. Redesigning health care with insights from the science of complex adaptive systems. Appendix B. In: *Crossing the Quality Chasm: A New Health System for the 21st Century.* Committee on Quality Health Care in America, Institute of Medicine. Washington, DC: National Academy Press; 2001:309–322.

Rozovsky FA, Woods JR Jr, eds. *The Handbook of Patient Safety Compliance: A Practical Guide for Health Care Organizations.* San Francisco, CA: Jossey-Bass; 2005.

THE ROLE OF PATIENTS | 21

OVERVIEW

With increasing public attention to patient safety have come calls for more participation by patients and their advocates in the search for solutions. Some of these calls have focused on individual healthcare organizations, such as efforts to include patients on hospital safety committees.[1] Most, however, have involved enlisting patients in efforts to improve their own individual safety—often framed as a version of the question: "What can patients do to protect themselves?" This chapter will explore some of the opportunities and challenges surrounding patient engagement in their own safety, including errors caused by patients themselves. The issues surrounding disclosure of errors to patients are covered in Chapter 18.

PATIENTS WITH LIMITED ENGLISH PROFICIENCY

A previously healthy 10-month-old girl was taken to a pediatrician's office by her monolingual Spanish-speaking parents, worried about their daughter's generalized weakness. The infant was diagnosed with iron-deficiency anemia. At the time of the clinic visit, no Spanish-speaking staff or interpreters were available. One of the nurses spoke broken Spanish and in general terms was able to explain that the girl had "low blood" and needed to take a medication. The parents nodded in understanding. The pediatrician wrote the following prescription in English:

Fer-Gen-Sol iron, 15 mg per 0.6 mL, 1.2 mL daily (3.5 mg/kg)

The parents took the prescription to the pharmacy. The local pharmacy did not have a Spanish-speaking pharmacist on staff, nor did they obtain an interpreter. The pharmacist attempted to demonstrate proper dosing and administration using the medication dropper and the parents nodded their understanding. The prescription label on the bottle was written in English.

The parents administered the medication at home and, within 15 minutes, the baby vomited twice and appeared ill. They took her to the nearest emergency department, where the serum iron level one hour after ingestion was found to be 365 mcg/dL, twice the upper therapeutic limit. She was admitted to the hospital for intravenous hydration and observation. On questioning, the parents stated that they had given their child a tablespoon of the medication, a 12.5-fold overdose. Luckily, the baby rapidly improved and was discharged the next day.[2]

Any discussion of patient engagement needs to start from square one—do patients understand their care and the benefits and risks of various diagnostic and therapeutic strategies (i.e., *informed consent*)? If patients cannot understand the basics of their clinical care, it seems unlikely that they can advocate for themselves when it comes to safety.

Unfortunately, many patients are in no position to understand even the basics of their care, let alone serve as bulwarks against errors. First of all, nearly 60 million Americans (20% of the population) speak a primary language other than English at home, and 25 million have limited English proficiency.[3] Both of these populations nearly doubled in the United States between 1980 and 2009 (Figure 21-1). Few hospitals have adequate translation services[4]—translation frequently takes place on an ad hoc basis, often by untrained clerical personnel or even family members.[5] In one case, an 11-year-old sibling interpreter made 58 interpretation errors, 84% of which had potential clinical consequences.[6]

Language barriers increase the chances of adverse events.[7] One UCSF study found that non-English-speaking patients had a 30% higher odds of 30-day readmission to the hospital than did English speakers.[8] Other studies have documented poorer adherence to treatment and follow-up, decreased satisfaction with care, decreased comprehension of diagnosis and treatment plans, and more adverse drug events.[9–12] The use of professional interpreters is associated with fewer communication errors, better patient comprehension, higher patient satisfaction, and improved clinical outcomes.[13]

Although state and federal legislation requires that adequate interpreting services be made available to limited English proficiency patients, the costs and scarcity of trained interpreters have made it difficult to ensure universal access to these services.[14] The increasingly widespread use of new communication technologies, including telephonic (Figure 21-2) and video interpreter services and even Web-based voice recognition and translation services, represents a hopeful trend.[15,16]

Figure 21-1 ▪ Growth in U.S. populations (adults and children over age 4) who speak languages other than English at home, or who have limited English proficiency, 1980 to 2009. (Reproduced with permission from U.S. Census Bureau data.)

PATIENTS WITH LOW HEALTH LITERACY

Even when patients do speak English well, many are at risk because of low "health literacy," which is defined as "the degree to which individuals have the capacity to obtain, process, and understand basic health information and services needed to make appropriate health decisions."[17] It includes the skills that patients need to communicate with providers, read medical information, make decisions about treatments, carry out care regimens, and decide when and how to seek help.

In 2003, approximately 80 million U.S. adults (36%) had limited health literacy[18] (Figure 21-3); the problems are greater in patients with lower income, less education, and lower English language proficiency. Low health literacy is associated with poor communication between patients and clinicians and worse health outcomes.[18–20] Medication errors are a particular problem: studies have

Figure 21-2 ▪ The use of telephonic interpretation services in the care of hospitalized patients. (Original image from http://main.uab.edu/Sites/reporter/photos/41843.jpg.)

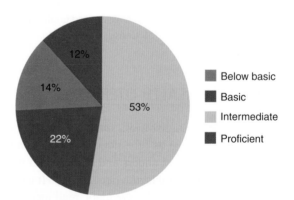

Figure 21-3 ▪ Health literacy of adults in the United States. *Below basic*: circle date on doctor's appointment slip. *Basic*: give two reasons a person with no symptoms should get tested for cancer based on a clearly written pamphlet. *Intermediate*: determine what time to take Rx medicine based on label. *Proficient*: calculate employee share of health insurance costs using table. (Reproduced with permission from National Assessment of Adult Literacy, National Center for Educational Statistics, U.S. Department of Education, 2003.)

shown that patients with poor health literacy frequently misunderstand common dosing regimens ("Take one tablet by mouth twice daily") and auxiliary warnings (e.g., *Do not chew or crush; For external use only*).[21]

A number of strategies have been employed to mitigate the effects of low health literacy on safety. Many of them have focused on identifying patients with low literacy,[22,23] and then providing them with simplified health materials (such as brochures and medication labels), Web sites, and interactive videos.[24] Newer interventions focus on training providers to interact with low health literacy patients in appropriate ways. For example, the use of the "*teach back*" (patients are asked to restate to the provider their understanding of their condition or treatment plan) can help ensure that patients truly comprehend their situation (Figure 21-4).[25,26] An alternative strategy is the "*Ask Me 3*," which prompts patients to ask their providers three questions: What is my main problem? What do I need to do? Why is it important for me to do this?[27] Patients who appear not to understand their care plan receive additional help.

In addition to these targeted interventions at the point of care, it will be important to embed education about health literacy into the training of physicians, nurses, and pharmacists. For example, a number of the newer competencies for residents involve issues of doctor–patient communication and improving physicians' sensitivity to patients' varying communication styles and needs. Because so many of the problems surrounding health literacy revolve around medications,[18,20,24,28] the involvement of trained pharmacists can be crucial.[29]

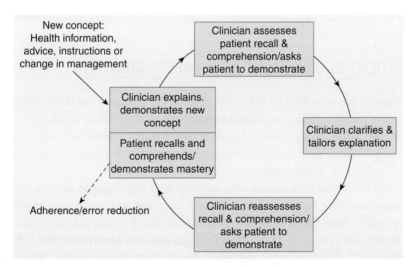

Figure 21-4 ■ Example of a "teach back." (Reproduced with permission from Schillinger D, Piette J, Grumbach K, et al. Closing the loop: physician communication with diabetic patients who have low health literacy. *Arch Intern Med* 2003;163:83–90.)

ERRORS CAUSED BY PATIENTS THEMSELVES

Even when low health literacy or language differences are not at issue, patients may contribute to errors in their care. The causes are usually similar to those leading to provider-related errors: generally competent humans interacting with a staggeringly complex system, sometime engaging in unsafe acts or violating safety rules. One group of New Zealand–based researchers divided patient errors into two groups: *action errors* (errors of patient behavior such as failing to attend an appointment or taking a medication with alcohol despite being advised not to do so) and *mental errors* (errors that involve patients' thought processes, such as "assuming I must OK because I'm feeling good").[30] One study conducted within a large health maintenance organization found that nearly one in four adverse drug events (Chapter 4) was caused by patient error, such as the failure to take the medication at the proper dose or follow medication use instructions.[31]

The solutions to patient-generated errors are likely similar to those that address errors caused by clinicians: better communication and teamwork, more robust information systems, identification of at-risk individuals (such as those on multiple medications, and those with low health literacy and language differences) to trigger tailored interventions, and learning from past mistakes and experiences. The recognition that some errors are caused by patients is not an occasion to assign blame, since in the vast majority of circumstances the errors simply prove that the patients are humans who, as we know, err. The task for clinicians and healthcare systems will be to better understand these human frailties and design systems and approaches that make them less likely to cause harm.

PATIENT ENGAGEMENT AS A SAFETY STRATEGY

Obviously, patients who do not speak English (or whatever the dominant language is) or who have poor health literacy are in no position to advocate for their own safety, and are limited in their ability to participate meaningfully in clinical decision making and informed consent. This is a problem that needs to be tackled on its own merits.

But what about the patient who *is* competent and engaged, or who brings a family member to the clinical encounter able and willing to play an advocacy role? I have listed a number of questions that I would ask of my doctor or healthcare system in an effort to keep myself or a family member safe in Appendix IX. Responding to the public demand for answers to the "What can I do to stay safe?" question, several advocacy groups and professional organizations have launched campaigns— such as the Joint Commission's "Speak Up" campaign) (Table 21-1)[32]—to address this issue.

Table 21-1 **THE JOINT COMMISSION'S "SPEAK UP" CAMPAIGN**
Speak up if you have questions or concerns. If you still don't understand, ask again. It's your body and you have a right to know.
Pay attention to the care you get. Always make sure you're getting the right treatments and medicines by the right healthcare professionals. Don't assume anything.
Educate yourself about your illness. Learn about the medical tests you get, and your treatment plan.
Ask a trusted family member or friend to be your advocate (advisor or supporter).
Know what medicines you take and why you take them. Medicine errors are the most common healthcare mistakes.
Use a hospital, clinic, surgery center, or other type of healthcare organization that has been carefully checked out. For example, the Joint Commission visits hospitals to see if they are meeting Joint Commission quality standards.
Participate in all decisions about your treatment. You are the center of the healthcare team.

Reproduced with permission from http://www.jointcommission.org/facts_about_speak_up_initiatives/.

However, as any healthcare provider who has been ill or has had a sick family member can attest, there are limits to what a layperson can do to protect against medical mistakes. These limitations were illustrated most vividly by Dr. Don Berwick, the founder of the Institute for Healthcare Improvement and former director of the U.S. Centers for Medicare & Medicaid Services. Berwick's poignant tale of his wife's series of hospitalizations (at several Harvard hospitals) for an obscure neurologic disease demonstrates the limitations of depending on patients or their families—even those with highly informed and engaged family members—to prevent medical errors:

The errors were not rare; they were the norm. During one admission, the neurologist told us in the morning, "By no means should you be getting anticholinergic agents [a medication that can cause neurological and muscle changes]," and a medication with profound anticholinergic side effects was given that afternoon. The attending neurologist in another admission told us by phone that a crucial and potentially toxic drug should be started immediately. He said, "Time is of the essence." That was on Thursday morning at 10:00 AM. The first dose was given 60 hours later—Saturday night at 10:00 PM. Nothing I could do, nothing I did, nothing I could think of made any difference.

It nearly drove me mad. Colace [a stool softener] was discontinued by a physician's order on Day 1, and was nonetheless brought by the nurse every single evening throughout a 14-day admission. Ann was supposed to receive five intravenous doses of a very toxic chemotherapy agent, but dose #3 was labeled as "dose #2." For half a day, no record could be found that dose #2 had ever been given, even though I had watched it drip in myself. I tell you from my personal observation, no day passed—not one—without a medication error.[33]

Before addressing the issue of patient engagement as a safety strategy, let's begin with core principles. The ethical virtues of an informed and participatory patient or family are unassailable, and the importance of patient engagement has been emphasized by groups ranging from the Joint Commission to the Institute of Medicine, often under the broad umbrella of *patient-centered care*. And, shifting to a patient safety perspective, an extra set of eyes primed to notice hazards and empowered to point them out probably *will* prevent medical errors from time to time. Asking for proof that patient/family engagement works might seem like seeking proof of the value of parachutes, the subject of a *BMJ* satirical shiv aimed at the heart of evidence-based medicine zealots several years ago.[34]

Parachutes notwithstanding, I have several reservations about the premise that patients and families can and should be central players in efforts to prevent medical mistakes.

The first is that it might not work, or might even hurt. In the early days of "sign your site," before the process was standardized (Chapter 5), patients sometimes tried to be helpful by marking their own limbs before they dozed off from their anesthetic. Unfortunately, some patients marked the limb *to be operated on*, while others marked the limb *to be avoided*. As you might imagine, this kind of anarchy introduces new error possibilities.

Second, even if a well-informed, alert patient or loved one can help prevent some errors, too many patients don't have the resources to act as advocates for their own safety. Particularly in the hospital, many patients lack involved family members, are confused, anxious, or sedated, or—as we've seen—have language differences or problems with health literacy. All of this means that relying on a strategy of patient engagement introduces an element of uncertainty. As British safety engineer Melinda Lyons observed:

> … in safety engineering terms, … patients are unlikely to provide a consistent and reliable contribution to the safety of the process of their own care. In a domain with a safety problem that is moving towards advocating the "systems approach," it seems nonsensical to also advocate a solution with apparently decreased reliability.[35]

Third, some patients and families, focused on doing what they can to prevent errors, will cross the thin line that separates being empowered and appropriately skeptical from being bellicose and confrontational. The latter attitude may lead providers to adopt a defensive stance or even generate outright avoidance (I've seen it happen on the wards). Such a situation is not likely to promote safety.

Finally, we need to consider the sobering observation that patients and families often feel guilty about medical errors, which means that an emphasis on patients protecting themselves might amplify this guilt.[36] As a family member of a sickle cell patient who became critically ill after a medication error recalled:

> The feeling was impotence, because you can't stay with a patient 24 hours a day. That's why you rely on hospitals—you rely on nurses. You feel like you failed your family in terms of 'I should have been there.' That's a guilt that everyone shares.[36]

Even with these caveats, certain patient engagement strategies may be helpful. One study showed that patients were willing to help monitor their providers' compliance with hand hygiene, were able to do so accurately, and did not feel that this would compromise the relationship with their caregivers.[37] (I should quickly add that another survey of Pennsylvania adults found that they were quite reluctant to challenge their providers.[38]) Researchers also found that patients often observe (and can report) errors that are missed through other ascertainment methods (Chapter 14).[39]

Turning our attention to the policy sphere, the involvement of patients and their families has been a major force for change, as has been vividly illustrated by those patients and families that have channeled their sorrow over a devastating medical error into helping the system improve. For example, Sorrel King's grief over her daughter's death at Johns Hopkins Hospital was a major impetus for Hopkins' seminal contributions to the safety field.[40–42] And patient engagement at the organizational level, such as by having patients serve on key committees, seems to help keep systems focused and honest.[1]

As I've reflected over the years on my own ambivalence regarding the role of patients in protecting themselves from mistakes, I've discovered that it flows partly from my lingering doubts about whether this strategy really works. But I've also come to realize that it stems from a more fundamental rejection of the premise itself: why *should* it fall to patients and family members to ensure their own safety?[43] When I board an airplane, I know that there is nothing I can do to keep myself safe. This allows me to relax (mostly), because my feelings of impotence are outweighed by my trust that the airlines and their regulators have done all they can to ensure my safety.

Patients encountering the healthcare system lack this trust, which makes relaxation and passivity seem maladaptive, sometimes even near-suicidal. That patients and families would want to do whatever they can to improve their odds of emerging unscathed is completely understandable. I'm just not sure how well this strategy works or how to apply it most effectively. Clearly, this should be the subject of ongoing research.

In the meantime, while we should support efforts by patients and families to participate in their own safety when feasible, our primary focus should be on making such hypervigilance unnecessary. In my judgment, this problem is ours to fix, not theirs.

KEY POINTS

- Many patients have limited language proficiency and/or health literacy, which increases the risk that they will be victims of medical errors.
- Patients can cause errors in their own care; the solutions are likely to parallel those used for other kinds of errors.
- Patients and families can help participate in their own safety, but (a) there are limitations to this strategy's effectiveness and (b) the responsibility to provide safe care should primarily be borne by providers, healthcare organizations, and policymakers, not patients.

REFERENCES

1. Conway JB, Weingart SN. Organizational change in the face of highly public errors I. The Dana-Farber Cancer Institute experience. *AHRQ WebM&M* (serial online); May 2005. Available at: http://www.webmm.ahrq.gov/perspective.aspx?perspectiveID=3.
2. Flores G. Language barrier. *AHRQ WebM&M* (serial online); April 2006. Available at: http://www.webmm.ahrq.gov/case.aspx?caseID=123.
3. U.S. Census Bureau. *Selected social characteristics: 2009*. Available at: http://factfinder.census.gov/servlet/ADPTable?_bm=y&-qr_name=ACS_2009_1YR_G00_DP2&-geo_id=01000US&-ds_name=ACS_2009_1YR_G00_&-_lang=en.
4. Baker DW, Parker RM, Williams MV, et al. Use and effectiveness of interpreters in an emergency department. *JAMA* 1996;275:783–788.
5. Diamond LC, Schenker Y, Curry L, et al. Getting by: underuse of interpreters by resident physicians. *J Gen Intern Med* 2009;24:256–262.
6. Flores G, Laws MB, Mayo SJ, et al. Errors in medical interpretation and their potential clinical consequences in pediatric encounters. *Pediatrics* 2003;111:6–14.

7. Divi C, Koss RG, Schmaltz SP, et al. Language proficiency and adverse events in US hospitals: a pilot study. *Int J Qual Health Care* 2007;19:60–67.

8. Karliner LS, Kim SE, Meltzer DO, et al. Influence of language barriers on outcomes of hospital care for general medicine inpatients. *J Hosp Med* 2010;5:276–282.

9. Manson A. Language concordance as a determinant of patient compliance and emergency room use in patients with asthma. *Med Care* 1988;26:1119–1128.

10. Carrasquillo O, Orav EJ, Brennan TA, et al. Impact of language barriers on patient satisfaction in an emergency department. *J Gen Intern Med* 1999;14:82–87.

11. Crane JA. Patient comprehension of doctor–patient communication on discharge from the emergency department. *J Emerg Med* 1997;16:1–7.

12. Gandhi TK, Burstin HR, Cook EF, et al. Drug complications in outpatients. *J Gen Intern Med* 2000;15:149–154.

13. Karliner LS, Jacobs EA, Chen AH. Do professional interpreters improve clinical care for patients with limited English proficiency? A systematic review of the literature. *Health Serv Res* 2007;42:727–754.

14. Ku L, Flores G. Pay now or pay later: providing interpreter services in health care. *Health Aff (Millwood)* 2005;24:435–444.

15. Masland MC, Lou C, Snowden L. Use of communication technologies to cost-effectively increase the availability of interpretation services in healthcare settings. *Telemed J E Health* 2010;16:739–745.

16. Standiford CJ, Nolan E, Harris M, et al. Improving the provision of language services at an academic medical center: ensuring high-quality health communication for limited-English-proficient patients. *Acad Med* 2009;84:1693–1697.

17. Institute of Medicine. *Health Literacy: A Prescription to End Confusion.* Washington, DC: National Academy Press; 2004.

18. Berkman ND, Sheridan SL, Donahue KE, et al. *Health Literacy Interventions and Outcomes: An Updated Systematic Review.* Evidence Report/Technology Assessment: Number 199. Rockville, MD: Agency for Healthcare Research and Quality; March 2011. AHRQ Publication No. 11-E006.

19. Kripalani S, Jacobson TA, Mugalla IC, et al. Health literacy and the quality of physician–patient communication during hospitalization. *J Hosp Med* 2010;5: 269–275.

20. Yin HS, Mendelsohn AL, Wolf MS, et al. Parents' medication administration errors: role of dosing instruments and health literacy. *Arch Pediatr Adolesc Med* 2010; 164:181–186.

21. Wolf MS, Bailey SC. The role of health literacy in patient safety. *AHRQ WebM&M* (serial online); Feb/Mar 2009. Available at: http://webmm.ahrq.gov/perspective.aspx?perspectiveID=72.

22. Davis TC, Long SW, Jackson RH, et al. Rapid estimate of adult literacy in medicine: a shortened screening instrument. *Fam Med* 1993;25:391–395.

23. Parker RM, Baker DW, Williams MV, et al. The test of functional health literacy in adults: a new instrument for measuring patients' literacy skills. *J Gen Intern Med* 1995;10:537–541.

24. Wolf MS, Curtis LM, Waite K, et al. Helping patients simplify and safely use complex prescription regimens. *Arch Intern Med* 2011;171:300–305.

25. Schillinger D, Piette J, Grumbach K, et al. Closing the loop: physician communication with diabetic patients who have low health literacy. *Arch Intern Med* 2003; 163:83–90.

26. Schwartzberg JG, Cowett A, VanGeest J, et al. Communication techniques for patients with low health literacy: a survey of physicians, nurses, and pharmacists. *Am J Health Behav* 2007;31:S96–S104.

27. Available at: http://www.npsf.org/askme3/.

28. Davis TC, Wolf MS, Bass PF III, et al. Literacy and misunderstanding prescription drug labels. *Ann Intern Med* 2006;145:887–894.

29. Youmans SL, Schillinger D. Functional health literacy and medication use: the pharmacist's role. *Ann Pharmacother* 2003;37:1726–1729.

30. Buetow S, Kiata L, Liew T, et al. Patient error: a preliminary taxonomy. *Ann Fam Med* 2009;7:223–231.

31. Field TS, Mazor KM, Briesacher B, et al. Adverse drug events resulting from patient errors in older adults. *J Am Geriatr Soc* 2007;55:271–276.

32. Available at: http://www.jointcommission.org/facts_about_speak_up_initiatives/.

33. Berwick DM. *Escape Fire: Lessons for the Future of Health Care.* New York, NY: The Commonwealth Fund; 2002.

34. Smith GCS, Pell JP. Parachute use to prevent death and major trauma related to gravitational challenge: systematic review of randomised controlled trials. *BMJ* 2003;327: 1459–1461.

35. Lyons M. Should patients have a role in patient safety? A safety engineering view. *Qual Saf Health Care* 2007;16:140–142.

36. Delbanco T, Bell SK. Guilty, afraid, and alone—struggling with medical error. *N Engl J Med* 2007;357:1682–1683.

37. Bittle MJ, LaMarche S. Engaging the patient as observer to promote hand hygiene compliance in ambulatory care. *Jt Comm J Qual Patient Saf* 2009;35:519–525, AP1–AP3.

38. Marella WM, Finley E, Thomas AD, et al. Health care consumers' inclination to engage in selected patient safety practices: a survey of adults in Pennsylvania. *J Patient Saf* 2007;3:184–189.

39. Weingart SN, Pagovich O, Sands DZ, et al. What can hospitalized patients tell us about adverse events? Learning from patient-reported incidents. *J Gen Intern Med* 2005;20:830–836.

40. In conversation with … Sorrel King. *AHRQ WebM&M* (serial online); March 2007. Available at: http://webmm.ahrq.gov/perspective.aspx?perspectiveID=39.

41. King S. *Josie's Story: A Mother's Inspiring Crusade to Make Medical Care Safe.* New York, NY: Atlantic Monthly Press; 2009.

42. Pronovost P, Vohr E. *Safe Patients, Smart Hospitals: How One Doctor's Checklist can Help Us Change Health Care from the Inside Out.* New York, NY: Hudson Street Press; 2010.

43. Entwistle VA, Mello MM, Brennan TA. Advising patients about patient safety: current initiatives risk shifting responsibility. *Jt Comm J Qual Patient Saf* 2005;31: 483–494.

ADDITIONAL READINGS

Flores G. Language barriers to health care in the United States. *N Engl J Med* 2006;355: 229–231.

Ring DC, Herndon JH, Meyer GS. Case 34-2010: a 65-year-old woman with an incorrect operation on the left hand. *N Engl J Med* 2010;363:1950–1957.

Saha S, Fernandez A. Language barriers in health care. *J Gen Intern Med* 2007;22 (suppl 2): 281–282.

Schillinger D. Misunderstanding prescription labels: the genie is out of the bottle. *Ann Intern Med* 2006;145:926–928.

Vincent CA, Coulter A. Patient safety: what about the patient? *Qual Saf Health Care* 2002; 11:76–80.

Wu HW, Nishimi RY, Page-Lopez CM, et al. *Improving Patient Safety through Informed Consent for Patients with Limited Health Literacy*. Washington, DC: National Quality Forum; 2005.

ADDITIONAL READINGS

(Bibliographic entries on this page are faded and illegible.)

ORGANIZING A SAFETY PROGRAM | 22

OVERVIEW

As the pressure to improve patient safety has grown, healthcare organizations, particularly hospitals but also larger healthcare systems, have struggled to create effective structures for their safety efforts. Although there are few studies comparing various organizational models, best practices for promoting organizational safety have begun to emerge.[1–6] This chapter will explore some of these issues. The organization of safety programs in ambulatory care is discussed in Chapter 12, and, of course, myriad issues relevant to organizing an effective safety program are addressed throughout this book.

STRUCTURE AND FUNCTION

Before the year 2000, few organizations had patient safety committees or officers. If there was any institutional focus on safety (in most institutions, there wasn't), it generally lived under the organization's top physician (sometimes a Vice President for Medical Affairs or Chief Medical Officer [CMO], or perhaps the elected Chief of the Medical Staff) or nurse (Chief Nursing Officer). In academic medical centers, safety issues were usually handled through the academic departmental structure (e.g., chair of the department of medicine or surgery), promoting a fragmented, siloed approach. When an institutional nonphysician leader *did* become involved in safety issues, it was usually a hospital risk manager, whose primary role was to protect the institution from liability.[7] Although many risk managers considered preventing future errors to be part of their role, they rarely had the institutional clout or resources to make durable changes in processes, information technology, or culture. Larger institutions with quality committees or quality officers sometimes subsumed patient safety under these individuals or groups.

The latter structure is still common in small institutions that lack the resources to have independent safety operations, but many larger organizations have recognized the value of a separate structure and staff to focus on safety. The responsibilities of safety personnel include: monitoring and responding to the incident reporting system, educating providers and others about new safety practices (driven by the experience of others and the literature), measuring safety outcomes and developing programs to improve them, and supervising the approach to serious events (e.g., organizing root cause analyses [RCAs]) and to preventing future errors (e.g., implementing action plans after RCAs, performing failure mode and effects analyses [FMEA]) (Chapter 14).[8] In addition, such personnel must work collaboratively with other departments and personnel, such as those in information technology, quality, compliance, and risk management.

▌MANAGING THE INCIDENT REPORTING SYSTEM

An organization interested in improving the quality of care (as opposed to patient safety) might not spend a huge amount of time and effort promoting reporting by caregivers to central administration. Why? To the extent that the quality issues of interest can be ascertained through outcome (e.g., mortality rates in patients with acute myocardial infarction, postoperative infection rates, readmission rates for patients with pneumonia) or process measures (did every patient with myocardial infarction for whom it was indicated receive a beta-blocker and aspirin?) (Chapter 3), performance assessment does not depend on the direct involvement of nurses and doctors. Instead, these data can be collected through chart review or, increasingly, by tapping into electronic data streams created in the course of care (Chapter 13). Obviously, when a quality leader identifies a "hot spot" through these measures, he or she cannot proceed without convening the relevant personnel to develop a complete understanding of the process and an action plan, but collecting the data can often be accomplished without provider participation.

Safety is different. In most cases, a safety officer or CMO will have no way of discovering errors or risky situations without receiving this information from frontline workers. Although other mechanisms (direct observation of practice, trigger tools) can identify some problems, the providers are the best repository of the knowledge and wisdom needed to understand safety hazards, near misses, and true errors, and thus to create the system changes to prevent them. As described in Chapter 14, the institutional incident reporting system is the usual, albeit imperfect, vehicle for tapping this rich vein of experience.

The *patient safety officer* will generally be charged with managing the incident reporting system. At small institutions, he or she will likely review every report, aggregate the data into meaningful categories (e.g., medication errors, falls), and triage the reports for further action. Based on the severity of the incidents, some reports will be simply noted, others will generate a limited analysis or an inquiry to a frontline manager, while still others will lead to a full-blown RCA. Many larger institutions have subdivided this task, selecting "category managers" to review incidents in a given domain (a pharmacist for medication errors, a nurse-leader for falls, the CMO for reports of unprofessional physician behavior; Table 14-2). The category managers are expected to review incidents within their categories, take appropriate action, and triage cases to the safety officer (or someone even higher in the organization) when the error is particularly serious or falls within an area that has regulatory or legal repercussions.

As with much of patient safety, results and culture are more important than structure. A technologically sophisticated incident reporting system will create little value if the frontline workers consider the approach to reports overly punitive, or if they see no evidence that reports are taken seriously or generate action.[9] So the safety officer is well advised to invest time and energy in making clear to caregivers that their reports result in important changes. Such an investment is every bit as important as one made in purchasing and maintaining a system that collects data and produces sophisticated pie charts. I described the RCA process in Chapter 14, including some of the changes we made at University of California, San Francisco (UCSF) Medical Center that markedly improved its value (Table 14-4).

DEALING WITH DATA

Although the safety officer will generally not be as data driven as the quality officer (for the reasons described above), he or she *will* have a steady stream of inputs that can be important sources of understanding and action. Some of these will be generated by the incident reporting system; here, it is important to use the information effectively while recognizing that voluntary reports capture only a small (and nonrandom) subset of errors, and that they cannot be used to determine rates of errors or harm.[10,11] An additional problem with incident reports is that nurses submit them far more frequently than physicians do, so they tend to underemphasize issues that physicians see (such as diagnostic errors, Chapter 6) and overemphasize nursing-related harms (e.g., falls).[12,13] Malpractice claims are an even more serendipitous source of safety concerns (Chapter 18). Several recent studies have illuminated an important point: there is no one "right" way to view an organization's safety, and the safety leader must look at a dashboard with multiple "dials."[14–16] In my judgment, to gain a complete view of the "elephant of patient safety,"[15] a hospital safety leader should regularly review at least a dozen sources of data (Table 22-1).

Table 22-1 **EXAMPLES OF TYPES OF INSTITUTIONAL DATA THAT SHOULD BE REGULARLY REVIEWED BY PATIENT SAFETY OFFICERS**

1. Data from the voluntary incident report system
2. Data drawn from trigger tools (and results of subsequent chart reviews)
3. Data drawn from real-time surveillance systems, such as those for certain healthcare-associated infections
4. Key outcome data such as risk-adjusted mortality and readmission rates
5. Key process and structural data (e.g., hand hygiene rates, appropriate use of checklists, use of computerized order entry, door-to-balloon time for patients with ST-segment elevation myocardial infarction)
6. Safety-related administrative and claims data, such as those used to produce the AHRQ Patient Safety Indicators (Appendix V)
7. Cases that qualify as National Quality Forum serious reportable events (Appendix VI)
8. Cases related to a Joint Commission National Patient Safety Goal (Appendix IV), or involve areas highlighted as concerns on a prior Joint Commission (or other important accreditation) local survey
9. Malpractice claims and payouts
10. Serious patient complaints
11. Data drawn from Executive Walk Rounds or other caregiver focus groups
12. Data drawn from Morbidity and Mortality conferences (or other sources of data from physicians)
13. Results of safety culture surveys completed by clinicians and managers
14. Results of patient experience surveys

For safety problems that *can* be measured as rates (such as hospital-acquired infections, Chapter 10), the role of the safety officer (assuming this is his or her domain; in large institutions, an infection preventionist may be charged with this task) becomes more like the quality officer: studying the data to see when rates have spiked above prior baselines or above local, regional, or national norms ("*benchmarks*"). In these circumstances, the safety officer will complete an in-depth analysis of the problem and develop an action plan designed to improve the outcomes.

Increasingly, safety officers will need to audit areas that have been the subject of regulatory requirements or new institutional policies. Such audits are best done through direct observation, and backsliding should be expected. In fact, the safety officer should be skeptical if an audit six months after implementation of a new policy demonstrates 100% compliance with the practice: there is an excellent chance that these are biased data and more should be done to get a true snapshot of what is really happening.

Finally, as medical records become electronic (Chapter 13), innovative methods for screening caregiver notes, lab results and medication orders (such as via trigger tools, Chapter 14), operative reports, and discharge summaries will generate new and useful safety information.[17–19] More and more of this work will involve real-time surveillance systems, with automatic "just-in-time" feedback to providers rather than the traditional process of (retrospective) audit and (markedly delayed) feedback.[20]

Some of the most important safety data will be the results of *patient safety culture surveys*. There are several well-constructed, validated surveys that can be used for this purpose; a few have been used at hundreds, or even thousands, of institutions, meaning that an institution's results can be compared with those from like institutions or units (e.g., other academic medical centers, or other intensive care units [ICUs]).[21,22] As I mentioned in Chapter 15, although it is appealing (after all, humans like simple explanations, even when they're wrong) to think of institutions (such as hospitals or large healthcare delivery systems) as having organization-wide safety cultures, work by Pronovost, Sexton, and others has demonstrated that safety culture tends to be local: even within a single hospital, there will often be huge variations in culture between units down the hall from one another.[23,24]

The safety officer's job, then, is to ensure administration of the surveys and a reasonable response rate, that the results are thoughtfully analyzed, and—as always—that the data are converted into meaningful action. For clinical units with poor safety culture, it is critical to determine the nature of the problem. Is it poor leadership, and, if so, is leadership training or a new leader required? Is it poor teamwork, and, if so, should we consider a crew resource management or other teamwork training program (Chapter 15)? And is there something to be learned from units with excellent culture that can be used to inform or stimulate change in the more problematic units?[25]

Finally, there is the challenge of integration and prioritization. The patient safety officer who monitors all of these data sources will have far more safety targets than he or she can possibly address in a year. This means that one crucial job is to help an organization prioritize among many worthwhile goals. It is natural that such prioritization will tend to elevate items required by regulators or accreditors over those that are not, measurable targets over softer ones, and efforts to change processes and structures over efforts to change culture and attitudes. The effective (and durably employed!) safety officer lives in the real world and addresses what needs to be addressed, but also works to counteract these biases when that is best for patients. For example, implementing a teamwork training initiative or an institution-wide program to prevent diagnostic errors may not be required, and their payoffs may be years away and hard to measure. The safety officer who believes that these activities are important for patients will—somehow—find the money, time, and political will to place them on the organization's agenda.

STRATEGIES TO CONNECT SENIOR LEADERSHIP WITH FRONTLINE PERSONNEL

Recognizing that an effective safety program depends on connecting the senior leadership (who control major resources and policies) with what is truly happening on the clinical units, and further appreciating that incident reporting systems paint a terribly incomplete picture of this frontline activity, many healthcare organizations have developed strategies to connect senior leaders with caregivers. The two most popular ways of accomplishing this are Executive Walk Rounds and "Adopt-a-Unit."

Executive Walk Rounds are the healthcare version of the old business leadership strategy of "Managing by Walking Around" (MBWA).[26–29] At some interval (some institutions do Walk Rounds weekly, others monthly), the safety officer will accompany another member of the senior leadership team (e.g., CEO, COO, CMO) to a clinical unit—a medical floor, the emergency department, the labor and delivery suite, or perhaps an operating room. The visits are usually preannounced. Although the unit manager is generally present for the visit, the most important outcome is a frank discussion (with senior leadership spending more time listening than talking) about the problems and errors on the unit, and brainstorming solutions to these problems. Some institutions have formalized these visits with a script; a sample one is shown in Box 22-1.

Another strategy (not mutually exclusive, but institutions tend to favor one or the other) is *"Adopt-a-Unit."*[30] Here, rather than executives visiting a variety of clinical areas around the hospital to get a broad picture of safety problems, one senior leader adopts a single unit and attends relevant meetings with staff there (perhaps monthly) for a long period (6–12 months). This method, pioneered at Johns Hopkins, has the advantage of more sustained engagement and automatic follow-through, and the disadvantage of providing each leader a more narrow view of the entire institution. Given that there are only so many senior leaders to go around, the Adopt-a-Unit strategy will generally mean that certain units will be neglected. For this reason, it is less popular than Executive Walk Rounds. However, for units experiencing important safety challenges or showing evidence of poor culture, this method, with its sustained focus, may have real value.

Whichever method is chosen, these efforts will be most useful if providers sense that senior leadership takes their concerns seriously, leaders demonstrate interest while being unafraid to show their ignorance about how things really work on the floor, and the frontline workers later learn about how their input led to meaningful changes.

Box 22-1 SELECTED SCRIPTS FOR PATIENT SAFETY EXECUTIVE WALK ROUNDS

Opening statements:

"We are moving as an organization to open communication and a blame-free environment because we believe that by doing so we can make your work environment safer for you and your patients"

"We're interested in focusing on the system and not individuals (no names are necessary)"

"The questions are very general. To help you think of areas to which the questions might apply, consider medication errors, miscommunication between individuals (including arguments), distractions, inefficiencies, invasive treatments, falls, protocols not followed, and so on"

Questions to ask:

"Can you think of any events in the past day or few days that have resulted in prolonged hospitalization for a patient?"

Examples:

Appointments made but missed

Miscommunications

Delayed or omitted medications

"Have there been any near misses that almost caused patient harm but didn't?"

Examples:

Selecting a drug dose from the medications cart or pharmacy to administer to a patient and then realizing it's incorrect

Misprogramming a pump, but having an alert warn you

Incorrect orders by physicians or others caught by nurses or other staff

"What aspects of the environment are likely to lead to the next patient harm?"

Examples:

Consider all aspects of admission, hospital stay, and discharge

Consider movement within the hospital

Consider communication

Consider informatics and computer issues

"Is there anything we could do to prevent the next adverse event?"

Examples:

What information would be helpful to you?

Consider alterations in the interaction between clinicians

Consider teamwork

Consider environment and workflow

"What specific intervention from leadership would make the work you do safer for patients?"

Examples:

Organize interdisciplinary groups to evaluate a specific problem

Assist in changing the attitude of a particular group

Facilitate interaction between two specific groups

"How are we actively promoting a blame-free culture and working on the development of a blame-free reporting policy?"

Examples:

We do not penalize individuals for inadvertent errors

The institution grants immunity to individuals who report adverse events in a timely fashion (where criminal behavior is not an issue)

Closing comment:

"We're going to work on the information you've given us. In return, we would like you to tell two other people you work with about the concepts we've discussed in this conversation"

Reproduced with permission from Frankel A. *Patient Safety Leadership Walkrounds*. Institute for Healthcare Improvement (IHI); 2004. Available at: http://www.ihi.org/knowledge/Pages/Tools/PatientSafetyLeadership WalkRounds.aspx.

STRATEGIES TO GENERATE FRONTLINE ACTIVITY TO IMPROVE SAFETY

Although connecting providers to senior leadership is vitally important, units must also have the capacity to act on their own. One of the dangers of an organizational "safety program" can be that individual clinical units will not be sufficiently active and independent—sharing stories of errors, problem solving, and doing the daily work of making care safer. Because many such efforts do not require major changes in policies or large infusions of resources, safety officers and programs need to create an environment and culture in which such unit-based problem solving is the norm, not the exception.

While some units will instinctively move in this direction (often as an outgrowth of strong local leadership and culture), others will need help. Many of the programs discussed previously (such as teamwork training) should leave behind an ongoing organizational structure that supports unit-based safety. For example, at UCSF, after more than 400 providers of all stripes participated in a crew resource management/teamwork training program, we launched a unit-based safety team on our medical ward that collected stories, organized interdisciplinary case conferences, and convened periodically to problem solve.[31] Their work was supported by e-CUSP, an electronic project management tool created for this purpose (Figure 22-1).[32,33]

Developing this kind of unit-based safety enterprise requires training, leadership, and some resources (a small amount of compensation for the unit-based champions, time for the group to meet, and—of course—food). It is also important to sort out the "cross-walk" between the unit-based efforts and the larger institutional safety program. On the one hand, the unit-based team must be free to discuss errors, develop educational materials, and problem solve without being encumbered by the organizational bureaucracy. On the other hand, the unit-based program cannot completely bypass the institutional incident reporting system, and it is vital that central leadership rapidly learns of major errors that should generate broader investigations (i.e., RCAs) or mandatory reports to external organizations.

DEALING WITH MAJOR ERRORS AND SENTINEL EVENTS

The RCA process is described in Chapter 14. The safety officer will often be charged with convening the RCA team, prepping senior leadership for the meetings, chairing the sessions, and converting the findings into meaningful action plans. Because many states and the Joint Commission now either

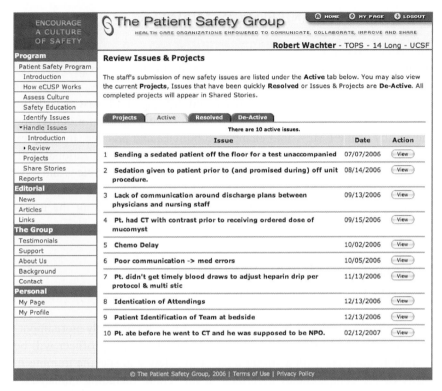

Figure 22-1 ■ Screenshot from e-CUSP, a project management tool for unit-based safety programs. (Reproduced with permission from UCSF implementation of e-CUSP, The Patient Safety Group.)

encourage or require that sentinel events (and the results of subsequent RCAs) be reported promptly, the safety officer plays a key role in managing this process, often collaborating with the compliance officer (in larger institutions), or the institutional risk manager if there are potential legal ramifications.

In addition, major errors often raise knotty questions regarding the role of the media (Chapter 19).[34,35] While certainly not every error needs to be shared with local reporters, particularly bad errors should be discussed with the institution's media relations department, if there is one, to consider the plusses and minuses of a proactive media strategy. This is a delicate balance, but organizations that have cultivated an open, honest, and mutually respectful relationship with their local media sometimes find that early disclosure of serious errors works better than waiting for reporters to discover them on their own.

The issue of disclosing errors to patients is discussed in Chapter 18.

FAILURE MODE AND EFFECTS ANALYSES

The safety officer may also be charged with spearheading efforts to proactively assess and mitigate safety risks. The Joint Commission now requires that every organization carry out at least one FMEA yearly. The process of and rationale behind FMEA is discussed in Chapter 14. Just as with the results of RCAs, the safety officer will often be responsible for converting the results of the FMEA into changes in policies and practice. In complex organizations, this requires tremendous diplomatic and organizational skill, because the changes often require approval by multiple committees and buy-in from a wide variety of stakeholders who may not have participated in the analysis and lack a full understanding of patient safety or the issues at hand.

QUALIFICATIONS AND TRAINING OF THE PATIENT SAFETY OFFICER

The personal qualities of the patient safety officer are probably more important than his or her training and pedigree. Ideally, a safety officer will be a credible clinician with a strong interest in safety and specific training in many of the competencies described in this book, including human factors, information technology, data management, and culture change. He or she will be a team player—needing to constantly assemble and motivate interdisciplinary teams to problem solve. The officer must work collaboratively not only with frontline providers and senior leadership but also with armies of individuals with overlapping job descriptions: the quality officer, risk manager, information technology officer, compliance officer, and more.[8] The larger the institution, the more likely that these functions will be managed by separate individuals. In smaller institutions, these hats (perhaps with the exception of the information technology leader) may all be worn by the same person.

There are now a number of excellent courses to teach individuals the skills needed to be patient safety officers and leaders. Two of the most popular are one run by the American Hospital Association–National Patient Safety Foundation (AHA–NPSF Patient Safety Leadership Fellowship) and another offered by the Institute for Healthcare Improvement (IHI Patient Safety Executive Development Program). Patient safety officers should also attend regional and national conferences on patient safety, and always be on the lookout for innovations and emerging best practices in the field.

Patient safety leaders also need to stay current on the literature, tools, and regulations in the field. The U.S. Agency for Healthcare Research and

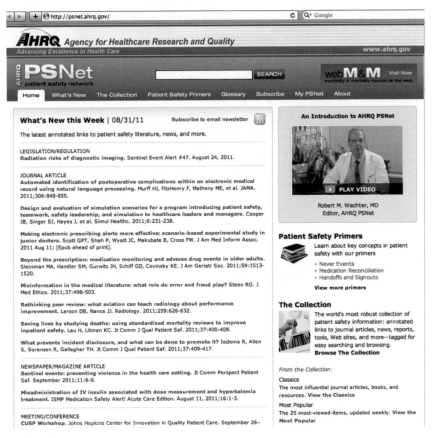

Figure 22-2 ▪ Screenshot from the homepage of AHRQ Patient Safety Network. (Available at http://psnet.ahrq.gov. Reproduced with permission.)

Quality (AHRQ) publishes *AHRQ Patient Safety Network* (http://psnet.ahrq. gov; Figure 22-2), a free Web site that posts 20 new resources each week in the field of patient safety, each with full annotations and rich links to related items (Figure 22-3). The site, which I edit, also hosts a searchable library of more than 10,000 safety resources, and offers a variety of other features, including advanced customizability ("My PSNet") and designated "Classics" in patient safety. It is an excellent resource for anyone interested in patient safety, and an indispensable one for the patient safety officer and his or her staff.

While AHRQ PSNet will deliver the week's most important safety resources to one's electronic doorstep, many people will want to also subscribe to key journals in the field, such as *BMJ Quality and Safety*, the *Joint Commission Journal of Quality and Patient Safety*, and the *Journal of Patient*

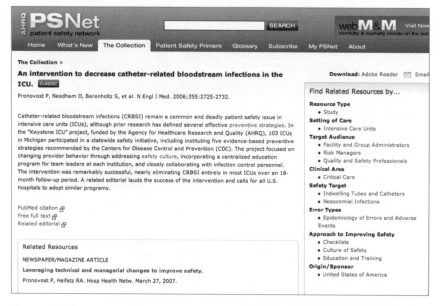

Figure 22-3 ▪ Screenshot from an individual resource annotation in AHRQ Patient Safety Network. (The resource is that of Pronovost P, Needham D, Berenholtz S, et al. An intervention to decrease catheter-related bloodstream infections in the ICU. *N Engl J Med* 2006;355:2725–2732. Reproduced with permission.)

Safety. In addition, several journals and textbooks focus on more specialized areas (informatics, device design, medication safety, cognitive errors, health policy) relevant to patient safety, and many clinical specialty journals (e.g., surgery, hospital medicine, critical care, nursing) now offer substantial safety content. Patient safety articles of interest to the broader healthcare community are often published in high-profile general journals such as the *New England Journal of Medicine*, *Annals of Internal Medicine*, *BMJ*, and *JAMA*. Finally, the patient safety officer should also be familiar with many of the key books and white papers in the field (Appendix I).

Increasingly, the patient safety officer needs to face outward as well as inward, cultivating positive relationships with state regulators, regional and national accreditors, and colleagues with similar roles at other institutions. Many patient safety officers work at hospitals that are part of larger health systems. This can make available additional resources and sources of learning—a real plus—but it also adds complexity, as solutions or policies developed for a system may need to be "localized" to meet the needs of an individual hospital or clinic. A similar problem with a slightly different twist arises when the patient safety officer's institution becomes part of a broader *patient safety organization* (PSO, Chapter 14).

THE ROLE OF THE PATIENT SAFETY COMMITTEE

Whether or not there is a designated patient safety officer, most institutions now have a patient safety committee, often a committee of the medical staff. This committee reviews adverse events and incident reports, helps to set and endorse safety-related policies, develops new safety initiatives, and disseminates information about patient safety to providers. It generally will be made up of a diverse group of clinicians (physicians, nurses, pharmacists) and hospital administrators; a few institutions include lay members.

Patient safety committees need to address certain challenges. One is how the committee's activities will relate to those of other overlapping committees, such as risk management and quality improvement. This issue parallels the one the safety officer faces in interacting with his or her peers in these departments. And, like the safety officer, the correct answer involves combining appropriate amounts of overlap (some personnel should be shared across committees, so that each can know what the other is doing) with a clear mandate to focus on certain exclusive areas. For example, while the involvement of the risk manager on the patient safety committee can be quite helpful (and, in certain states, required to shield the committee's deliberations from being legally discoverable), it is crucial that the committee's focus remain on improving safety rather than reducing the organization's legal exposure.[7]

A second issue is making sure that the committee reserves some time and energy to focus on issues that are not regulatory mandates and are not generated from specific cases of harm—also a parallel issue to the patient safety officer's prioritization challenges mentioned earlier. The committee that explicitly sets a goal of completing one to two group-generated projects per year is more likely to "think outside the box" than the group that spends all its time in reactive and compliance mode.

ENGAGING PHYSICIANS IN PATIENT SAFETY

Notwithstanding our emphasis on the role of teamwork and the vital contributions of all caregivers, the engagement of physicians is crucial in patient safety. In fact, the presence or absence of such engagement frequently predicts whether an organization's safety program is a smashing success or dismal failure.

Because so much of the accountability for patient safety (in the United States) is now being directed toward hospitals (Chapter 3, 14, and 20), cementing physician engagement tends to be comparatively (emphasis on "comparatively") easy in hospitals that either employ doctors (i.e., Veterans Affairs hospitals, many hospitals with hospitalists) or have physicians with strong links to the organization (i.e., Mayo and Cleveland Clinics, Kaiser Permanente, most academic health centers). In the thousands of hospitals in which physicians have weaker institutional links—members of the medical staff who use the hospital to provide care but receive no salary support and do not share in the organization's accountabilities—safety engagement tends to be more tenuous.

Taitz et al. conducted site visits and interviews at 10 high-performing teaching hospitals (mostly highly ranked academic medical centers) to highlight the best practices in engaging physicians in safety and quality.[36] Six themes emerging from this work are shown in Table 22-2, and major barriers to engagement are highlighted in Table 22-3. An important caveat is that these data come from medical centers that enjoy reasonably good physician–organizational alignment to begin with. The degree to which the results are applicable to community hospitals with lower baseline integration is unknown.

Table 22-2	SIX THEMES IN A FRAMEWORK FOR ENGAGING PHYSICIANS IN QUALITY AND SAFETY	
Theme	Selected Interviewee Quotes	% Endorsing Theme
1. Engaged leadership	"Leadership, that is, able to get physician buy-in to quality and safety, their commitment and belief in its value and the importance of making the final product better." "You need engaged leaders to have engaged physicians."	70
2. Physician compact	"The compact captures the focus on the patient. It also creates a common framework for why physicians are here, our relationship with the organizations, other physicians and our patients." "The compact is a living, breathing, dynamic reciprocal agreement that aligns expectations between the organization and our physicians."	15
3. Appropriate compensation	"Quality is not an add-on to busy physicians' schedules, otherwise you don't get full commitment."	50
4. Realignment of financial incentives		
Support financial incentives	"Have your professional values dominate and then align financial incentives around them." "Payment of incentives is important. Physicians are like everyone else, the monetary rewards are the power to drive behavior."	33
Oppose financial incentives	"Financial incentives are an insult to the professionalism of physicians." "We should rather reward value."	31

(continued)

Theme	Selected Interviewee Quotes	% Endorsing Theme
Table 22-2 SIX THEMES IN A FRAMEWORK FOR ENGAGING PHYSICIANS IN QUALITY AND SAFETY (*continued*)		
5a. Data and enablers	"Physicians are data connoisseurs—it is imperative to get accurate data." "There is no greater force than peer pressure in a structured format." "Physicians don't just need data, they also need enablers or processes to improve their performance."	66
5b. Data reporting Support internal transparency	"Need complete transparency internally to transform the culture of the organization." "Internal transparency is more a driver of change than external transparency."	95
Support external transparency	"We want to demystify the data and make it understandable to the public." "Data should be completely transparent so that patients know what we do well."	52
Oppose external transparency	"Be wary of publishing individual performance publically, external reporting should reflect system results." "Public reporting can be misleading."	26
6. Academic promotion*	"Tie academic promotion to outcomes and participation in quality-and-safety activities." "Quality-and-safety publications should be treated on a par with traditional research publications."	14

*Likely reflects study population: leaders at 10 teaching hospitals, mostly academic medical centers.
Reproduced with permission from Taitz JM, Lee TH, Sequist TD. A framework for engaging physicians in quality and safety. *BMJ Qual Saf* July 14, 2011 [Epub ahead of print].

BOARD ENGAGEMENT IN PATIENT SAFETY

Until recently, discussions about organizational leadership in safety tended to focus on the commitment and focus of the CEO and physician and nursing leaders. But in many healthcare organizations, the role of the board can be decisive.

Traditionally, hospital boards have delegated quality and safety to the medical staff, focusing instead on their fiduciary responsibilities. Why? Most board members are lay people (often prominent business and community

Table 22-3 **BARRIERS TO PHYSICIANS' ENGAGEMENT IN QUALITY AND SAFETY**

Barrier	% Reporting Barrier
Lack of time	45
Institutional culture	31
Physician desire for autonomy	17
Lack of medical school training	17
Lack of trust in data	15
Lack of information system support	12
Lack of quality improvement skills	12

Reproduced with permission from Taitz JM, Lee TH, Sequist TD. A framework for engaging physicians in quality and safety. *BMJ Qual Saf* July 14, 2011 [Epub ahead of print].

leaders) who felt that they did not—and perhaps could not—understand the clinical elements of quality and safety. Few board members or chairs were trained in quality and safety science,[37] and most boards lacked useful measures to help them judge the safety of their institutions.[38] A 2007–2008 survey of 722 board chairs found that fewer than half placed quality (and, by implication, safety) among the two most important priorities for evaluating their chief executive officers, and only slightly more than half considered quality to be one of their top two priorities for board oversight. Importantly, there was a strong association between the board chairs' stated priority for quality and the hospitals' actual quality performance (as assessed through publicly reported data [Figure 22-4]).[37]

The safety movement has catapulted boards into action. While some of this undoubtedly flows from boards' new appreciation of their ethical obligations to patients, the emergence of a powerful business case for safety (Table 3-5) is undoubtedly playing a part as well.[39] There is no question that an engaged board can help promote safety, particularly when the board spends more than one-quarter of its time on safety and quality issues, the board regularly reviews quality and safety data, incentives for senior executives are partly based on quality and safety, and there is active dialogue between the board and the medical staff.[40-42] The IHI's 5 Million Lives Campaign (Table 20-2) included a plank called "boards on board," highlighting activities to promote board engagement in patient safety (Table 22-4).[43]

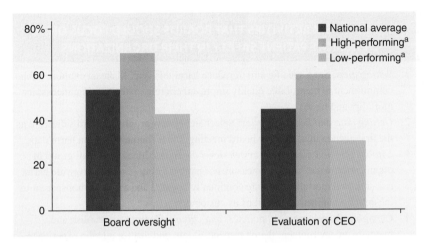

Figure 22-4 ▪ Percentage of hospital board chairs reporting that quality of care is one of the top two priorities for board oversight or evaluation of chief executive officer (CEO) performance. The superscript "a" denotes statistical significance (*P* < 0.001) for comparisons of the difference between the highest- and lowest-performing hospitals. Rates are adjusted for the number of beds, region, location (urban vs. rural), teaching status, and ownership. (Reproduced with permission from Jha AK, Epstein AM. Hospital governance and the quality of care. *Health Aff (Millwood)* 2010;29:182–187. © 2010 by Project HOPE—The People-to-People Health Foundation, Inc.)

As with other parts of the organization, board members should be given data (culled from the various data streams described in Table 22-1, but summarized into an easy-to-read, high-level "dashboard") that help illuminate the key patient safety issues and the organization's performance in addressing them. That said, it is also crucial that each board meeting include at least one story of an actual patient harmed or killed while receiving care in the system. It is the drama and poignancy of the individual case—a person with a name, face, and family who was seriously injured by an error—that provides the energy needed to inspire real action in safety. This energy can easily be sapped by a well-meaning recitation of bloodless statistics or the flashing of an endless series of PowerPoint graphs.

RESEARCH IN PATIENT SAFETY

Until a little more than a decade ago, there was scant research in patient safety. At the time, a simplistic understanding of errors (as individual failings rather than systems problems) led to little interest in empirical investigation. After

Table 22-4   **SIX ACTIVITIES THAT BOARDS SHOULD FOCUS ON TO PROMOTE PATIENT SAFETY IN THEIR ORGANIZATIONS**
1. *Setting aims*: Set a specific aim to reduce harm this year. Make an explicit, public commitment to measurable quality improvement (e.g., reduction in unnecessary mortality and harm).
2. *Getting data and hearing stories*: Select and review progress toward safer care as the first agenda item at every board meeting. Put a "human face" on harm data.
3. *Establishing and monitoring system-level measures*: Identify a small group of organization-wide "roll-up" measures of patient safety (e.g., facility-wide harm, risk-adjusted mortality) that are continually updated and are made transparent to the entire organization and all of its customers.
4. *Changing the environment, policies, and culture*: Commit to establish and maintain an environment that is respectful, fair, and just for all who experience pain and loss as a result of avoidable harm and adverse outcomes: the patients, their families, and the staff at the sharp end of error.
5. *Learning—starting with the board*: Develop your capability as a board. Learn about how "best in the world" boards work with executive and MD leaders to reduce harm. Set an expectation for similar levels of education and training for all staff.
6. *Establishing executive accountability*: Oversee the effective execution of a plan to achieve your aims to reduce harm, including executive team accountability for clear quality improvement targets.

Reproduced with permission from Get Boards on Board. *How to Guide*. Institute for Healthcare Improvement (IHI). Available at: http://www.ihi.org/knowledge/Pages/Tools/HowtoGuideGovernanceLeadership.aspx.

all, if an error was a screwup by an individual doctor or nurse, what exactly needed to be studied? This mindset led to little funding for patient safety research, few faculty who devoted their careers to it, and few journals interested in publishing the fruits of this research.

This has changed drastically over the past 10 to 12 years. As I mentioned earlier, *AHRQ Patient Safety Network* now hosts approximately 10,000 resources, including 3000 research studies. The AHRQ PSNet list of "Classic" articles (articles of "enduring importance") now numbers more than 400.[44] (Another more immediate and tactile example: the number of references in the book you are holding has more than doubled since the first edition, which was written only four years earlier.) AHRQ's annual funding for patient safety–oriented work is now approximately $100 million , and substantial additional funding comes from other federal agencies (such as the Centers for Disease Control and Prevention), foundations, and other worldwide organizations. Hundreds of faculty members have made patient safety research the focus of their professional careers, and many have been successful in garnering grants, publications, and promotion.

One of the exciting things about patient safety research is that it is inherently interdisciplinary and eclectic. Studies of medication errors, for example, often involve collaboration among physicians, nurses, pharmacists, and informatics experts. Studying errors at the person-machine interface may require engineers and human factors researchers. Studies of mistakes related to communication and poor teamwork may include psychologists and experts from other industries such as aviation.

Because patient safety involves real-world work processes, studies tend to be messier than controlled trials of new medications or laboratory studies of physiologic systems. It is very difficult to isolate the effect of one intervention (e.g., computerized provider order entry or Rapid Response Teams) from scores of other interventions occurring simultaneously.[45,46] It is nearly impossible to randomize hospital floors or institutions to one complex, expensive intervention or another, and institutions that embrace interventions often differ from those that don't in fundamental (and confounding) ways. Moreover, safety research cannot be standardized ("1 g of vancomycin IV" is approximately the same thing when administered in a big hospital in San Francisco and a small one in Peoria, but "teamwork training" is decidedly not). My colleagues and I have recently emphasized the importance of "context" in safety research, since the environmental and other contextual factors are often precisely what explains how a safety intervention that worked spectacularly in one setting failed miserably in another.[47,48]

All of this makes patient safety research harder than, say, drug trials. But young safety researchers should take heart, for safety research also has some unique advantages. Small studies that isolate the effect of a single intervention often lead to deeper understanding and give rise to larger research projects. For example, the simple matter of introducing "goal cards" to a clinical unit led to important improvements in communications and outcomes,[49,50] setting the stage for more ambitious teamwork and communication interventions (Chapter 9). A study that randomized ICU residents to longer versus shorter shifts found far fewer errors in the latter group[51] and informed the debate over resident duty hours (Chapter 16). Small studies that demonstrated the value of process changes in preventing central line–associated bloodstream infections[52–54] ultimately led to a multifaceted set of interventions that slashed the number of bloodstream infections in more than 100 ICUs (Chapter 10 and Figure 22-3).[55]

There is one more exciting aspect to patient safety research: in safety, unlike clinical medicine, the linkages to regulations, malpractice law, media scrutiny, and public pressure can lead to rapid dissemination of "safety practices." For example, laws, regulations, and accreditation requirements around nurse-to-patient ratios, medication reconciliation, and error disclosure all materialized after a relatively small number of studies demonstrated, or even hinted at, benefit. So too did a national, and even international, effort to use checklists to address error-prone systems of care. Because of this, well-designed and executed safety studies addressing important questions can rapidly lead to major changes in practice.

PATIENT SAFETY MEETS EVIDENCE–BASED MEDICINE

As research in safety has exploded, a fundamental question has arisen: what is the role of evidence in assessing patient safety practices? There are two schools of thought on this. One group points out that many safety practices have little downside, have substantial face validity, and are too complex to study effectively and efficiently. For these reasons, they argue, traditional standards of evidence-based medicine should be relaxed for practices like Rapid Response Teams and computerized provider order entry.[56,57] The other group (which I tend to find myself more comfortable with) holds that safety practices can be extremely expensive and disruptive, and they often have unforeseen consequences that only emerge over time. Because of this, the second group argues, most safety practices should be studied, if feasible, before widespread implementation.[46,58–60] In our 2001 AHRQ evidence report, *Making Health Care Safer*, my colleagues and I came down this way on this crucial question:

> In the end, we are left with our feet firmly planted in the middle of competing paradigms. One argues that an evidence-based, scientific approach has served health care well and should not be relaxed simply because a popular practice from a "safer" industry sounds attractive. The other counters that medicine's slavish devotion to the scientific and epidemiologic method has placed us in a patient safety straitjacket, unable to consider the value of practices developed in other fields because of our myopic traditions and "reality."
>
> We see the merits in both arguments. Health care clearly has much to learn from other industries. Just as physicians must learn the "basic sciences" of immunology and molecular biology, providers and leaders interested in making health care safer must learn the "basic sciences" of organizational theory and human factors engineering. Moreover, the "cases" presented on rounds should, in addition to classical clinical descriptions, also include the tragedy of the Challenger and the successes of Motorola. On the other hand, an unquestioning embrace of dozens of promising practices from other fields is likely to be wasteful, distracting, and potentially dangerous. We are drawn to a dictum from the Cold War era—"Trust, but verify."[61]

KEY POINTS

- Because of the intense focus on patient safety and increasing regulatory and accreditation requirements, many organizations have begun safety programs, hired patient safety officers, and formed patient safety committees.
- The challenges of measuring safety mean that the inputs to safety programs will come from multiple sources, including voluntary reporting, trigger tools, malpractice cases, patient and provider surveys, and structure, process, and outcome data relevant to patient safety.
- Safety officers and programs need to effectively collaborate with a variety of other personnel and programs: quality, risk management, information technology, and more.
- Effective safety programs blend elements of top-down management and bottom-up engagement and innovation. Boards and physicians must also be fully engaged for programs to be successful.
- Safety research is difficult to do, but its results can be highly influential, particularly when they lead to regulatory action or other broad-based mandates.
- There is debate regarding the degree to which traditional standards of evidence-based medicine should be relaxed for patient safety practices.

REFERENCES

1. In conversation with … Allan Frankel. *AHRQ WebM&M* (serial online); July 2006. Available at: http://webmm.ahrq.gov/perspective.aspx?perspective ID=26.
2. Whittington J. Key issues in developing a successful hospital safety program. *AHRQ WebM&M* (serial online); July 2006. Available at: http://webmm.ahrq.gov/perspective.aspx?perspectiveID=27.
3. Bagian JP, Lee C, Gosbee J, et al. Developing and deploying a patient safety program in a large health care delivery system: you can't fix what you don't know about. *Jt Comm J Qual Improv* 2001;27:522–532.
4. Hauck L, Jacob J. Implementing a patient safety program at a large national health system. *AHRQ WebM&M* (serial online); January 2008.
5. In conversation with … Steven J. Spear, DBA, MS. *AHRQ WebM&M* (serial online); August 2009. Available at: http://webmm.ahrq.gov/perspective.aspx?perspectiveID=77.
6. Kenney C. *Transforming Health Care: Virginia Mason Medical Center's Pursuit of the Perfect Patient Experience*. New York, NY: Productivity Press; 2011.

7. In conversation with …Geri Amori, PhD. *AHRQ WebM&M* (serial online); December 2010. Available at: http://webmm.ahrq.gov/perspective.aspx?perspectiveID=95.

8. Gandhi TK, Graydon-Baker E, Barnes JN, et al. Creating an integrated patient safety program. *Jt Comm J Qual Saf* 2003;29:383–390.

9. Shojania KG. The frustrating case of incident-reporting systems. *Qual Saf Health Care* 2008;17:400–402.

10. Cullen DJ, Bates DW, Small SD. Incident reporting system does not detect adverse drug events: a problem for quality improvement. *Jt Comm J Qual Improv* 1995;21: 541–548.

11. Pronovost PJ, Miller MR, Wachter RM. Tracking progress in patient safety: an elusive target. *JAMA* 2006;296:696–699.

12. Rowin EJ, Lucier D, Pauker SG. Does error and adverse event reporting by physicians and nurses differ. *Jt Comm J Qual Patient Saf* 2008;34:537–545.

13. In conversation with … Kaveh G. Shojania, MD. *AHRQ WebM&M* (serial online); September 2011. Available at: http://webmm.ahrq.gov/perspective.aspx?perspectiveId=107.

14. Levtzion-Korach O, Frankel A, Alcalai H, et al. Integrating incident data from five reporting systems to assess patient safety: making sense of the elephant. *Jt Comm J Qual Patient Saf* 2010;36:402–410.

15. Shojania KG. The elephant of patient safety: what you see depends on how you look. *Jt Comm J Qual Patient Saf* 2010;36:399–401, AP1–AP3.

16. Lipczak H, Knudsen JL, Nissen A. Safety hazards in cancer care: findings using three different methods. *BMJ Qual Saf* 2011;20:1052–1056.

17. Murff HJ, Forster AJ, Peterson JF, et al. Electronically screening discharge summaries for adverse medical events. *J Am Med Inform Assoc* 2003;10:339–350.

18. Classen DC, Resar R, Griffin F, et al. 'Global Trigger Tool' shows that adverse events in hospitals may be ten times greater than previously measured. *Health Aff (Millwood)* 2011;30:581–589.

19. Murff HJ, FitzHenry F, Matheny ME, et al. Automated identification of postoperative complications within an electronic medical record using natural language processing. *JAMA* 2011;306:848–855.

20. Waitman LR, Phillips IE, McCoy AB, et al. Adopting real-time surveillance dashboards as a component of an enterprise-wide medication safety strategy. *Jt Comm J Qual Patient Saf* 2011;37:326–332.

21. Colla JB, Bracken AC, Kinney LM, et al. Measuring patient safety climate: a review of surveys. *Qual Saf Health Care* 2005;14:364–366.

22. Agency for Healthcare Research and Quality. *Patient Safety Culture Surveys*. Rockville, MD: Agency for Healthcare Research and Quality; November 2010. Available at: http://www.ahrq.gov/qual/patientsafetyculture/.

23. Pronovost PJ, Sexton B. Assessing safety culture: guidelines and recommendations. *Qual Saf Health Care* 2005;14:231–233.

24. Huang DT, Clermont G, Sexton JB, et al. Perceptions of safety culture vary across the intensive care units of a single institution. *Crit Care Med* 2007;35:165–176.

25. In conversation with … J. Bryan Sexton. *AHRQ WebM&M* (serial online); December 2006. Available at: http://www.webmm.ahrq.gov/perspective.aspx?perspectiveID=34.

26. Peters TJ, Waterman RJ. *In Search of Excellence: Lessons from America's Best Run Companies*. New York, NY: Collins; 2004.

27. Frankel A, Graydon-Baker E, Neppl C, et al. Patient safety leadership walkrounds. *Jt Comm J Qual Improv* 2003;29:16–26.

28. Frankel A, Grillo SP, Baker EG, et al. Patient safety leadership walkrounds at Partners Healthcare: learning from implementation. *Jt Comm J Qual Patient Saf* 2005;31: 423–437.

29. Thomas EJ, Sexton JB, Neilands TB, et al. The effect of executive walk rounds on nurse safety climate attitudes: a randomized trial of clinical units. *BMC Health Serv Res* 2005;5:28.

30. Pronovost PJ. An interview with Peter Pronovost. *Jt Comm J Qual Saf* 2004;30: 659–664.

31. Sehgal NL, Fox M, Vidyarthi AR, et al.; TOPS Project. A multidisciplinary teamwork training program: the Triad for Optimal Patient Safety (TOPS) experience. *J Gen Intern Med*. 2008;23:2053–2057.

32. Pronovost P, Weast B, Rosenstein B. Implementing and validating a comprehensive unit-based safety program. *J Patient Saf* 2005;1:33–40.

33. Pronovost P, King J, Holzmueller CG, et al. A web-based tool for the Comprehensive Unit-based Safety Program (CUSP). *J Comm J Qual Patient Saf* 2006;32:119–129.

34. Conway JB, Weingart SN. Organizational change in the face of highly public errors—I. The Dana-Farber Cancer Institute experience. *AHRQ WebM&M* (serial online); May 2005. Available at: http://psnet.ahrq.gov/resource.aspx?resourceID=203.

35. Resnick D. The Jesica Santillan tragedy: lessons learned. *Hastings Center Report* 2003;33:15–20.

36. Taitz JM, Lee TH, Sequist TD. A framework for engaging physicians in quality and safety. *BMJ Qual Saf* July 14, 2011 [Epub ahead of print].

37. Jha AK, Epstein AM. Hospital governance and the quality of care. *Health Aff (Millwood)* 2010;29:182–187.

38. In conversation with ... Jim Reinertsen. *AHRQ WebM&M* (serial online); July 2007. Available at: http://webmm.ahrq.gov/perspective.aspx?perspective ID=45.

39. Weeks WB, Bagian JP. Making the business case for patient safety. *Jt Comm J Qual Saf* 2003;29:51–54.

40. Joshi MS, Hines SC. Getting the board on board: engaging hospital boards in quality and patient safety. *Jt Comm J Qual Patient Saf* 2006;32:179–187.

41. Lockee C, Kroom K, Zablocki E, et al. *Quality*. San Diego, CA: The Governance Institute; 2006.

42. Kroch E, Vaughn T, Koepke M, et al. Hospital boards and quality dashboards. *J Patient Saf* 2006;2:10–19.

43. McCannon CJ, Hackbarth AD, Griffin FA. Miles to go: an introduction to the 5 Million Lives Campaign. *Jt Comm J Qual Patient Saf* 2007;33:477–484.

44. Available at: http://psnet.ahrq.gov/classicBrowse.aspx.

45. Shojania KG, Duncan BW, McDonald KM, et al. Evidence-based review methodology. In: Shojania KG, Duncan BW, McDonald KM, et al., eds. *Making Health Care Safer: A Critical Analysis of Patient Safety Practices*. Evidence Report/Technology

Assessment No. 43, AHRQ Publication No. 01-E058. Rockville, MD: Agency for Healthcare Research and Quality; July 2001.

46. Shojania KG. Interpreting the patient safety literature. *AHRQ WebM&M* (serial online); June 2005. Available at: http://webmm.ahrq.gov/perspective.aspx?perspectiveID=5.

47. Shekelle PG, Pronovost PJ, Wachter RM, et al. Advancing the science of patient safety. *Ann Intern Med* 2011;154:693–696.

48. Taylor SL, Dy S, Foy R, et al. What context features might be important determinants of the effectiveness of patient safety practice interventions? *BMJ Qual Saf* 2011;20:611–617.

49. Pronovost P, Berenholz S, Dorman T, et al. Improving communication in the ICU using daily goals. *J Crit Care* 2003;18:71–75.

50. Narasimhan M, Eisen LA, Mahoney CD, et al. Improving nurse–physician communication and satisfaction in the intensive care unit with a daily goals worksheet. *Am J Crit Care* 2006;15:217–222.

51. Landrigan CP, Rothschild JM, Cronin JW, et al. Effect of reducing interns' work hours on serious medical errors in intensive care units. *N Engl J Med* 2004;351:1838–1848.

52. Raad II, Hohn DC, Gilbreath BJ, et al. Prevention of central venous catheter-related infections by using maximal sterile barrier precautions during insertion. *Infect Control Hosp Epidemiol* 1994;15(4 pt 1):231–238.

53. Chaiyakunapruk N, Veenstra DL, Lipsky BA, et al. Chlorhexidine compared with povidone–iodine solution for vascular catheter-site care: a meta-analysis. *Ann Intern Med* 2002;136:792–801.

54. Deshpande KS, Hatem C, Ulrich HL, et al. The incidence of infectious complications of central venous catheters at the subclavian, internal jugular, and femoral sites in an intensive care unit population. *Crit Care Med* 2005;33:13–20 [discussion 234–235].

55. Pronovost P, Needham D, Berenholtz S, et al. An intervention to decrease catheter-related bloodstream infections in the ICU. *N Engl J Med* 2006;355:2725–2732.

56. Leape LL, Berwick DM, Bates DW. What practices will most improve safety? Evidence-based medicine meets patient safety. *JAMA* 2002;288:501–507.

57. Berwick DM. The science of improvement. *JAMA* 2008;299:1182–1184.

58. Shojania KG, Duncan BW, McDonald KM, et al. Safe but sound: patient safety meets evidence-based medicine. *JAMA* 2002;288:508–513.

59. Wachter RM. Expected and unanticipated consequences of the quality and information technology revolutions. *JAMA* 2006;295:2780–2783.

60. Auerbach AD, Landefeld CS, Shojania KG. The tension between needing to improve care and knowing how to do it. *N Engl J Med* 2007;357:608–613.

61. Shojania KG, Duncan BW, McDonald KM, et al. Drawing on safety practices from outside healthcare. In: Shojania KG, Duncan BW, McDonald KM, et al., eds. *Making Health Care Safer: A Critical Analysis of Patient Safety Practices*. Evidence Report/Technology Assessment No. 43, AHRQ Publication No. 01-E058. Rockville, MD: Agency for Healthcare Research and Quality; July 2001.

ADDITIONAL READINGS

Bohmer RMJ. The four habits of high-value healthcare organizations. *N Engl J Med* 2011;365:2045–2047.

Burnett S, Benn J, Pinto A, Parand A, Iskander S, Vincent C. Organisational readiness: exploring the preconditions for success in organisation-wide patient safety improvement programmes. *Qual Saf Health Care* 2010;19:313–317.

Denham CR. Patient safety practices: leaders can turn barriers into accelerators. *J Patient Saf* 2005;1:41–55.

Denham CR. The new patient safety officer: a lifeline for patients, a life jacket for CEOs. *J Patient Saf* 2007;3:43–54.

Gandhi TK, Graydon-Baker E, Neppl Huber C, et al. Closing the loop: follow-up and feedback in a patient safety program. *Jt Comm J Qual Patient Saf* 2005;31:614–621.

Ginsburg LR, Chuang YT, Berta WB, et al. The relationship between organizational leadership for safety and learning from patient safety events. *Health Serv Res* 2010;45: 607–632.

Goeschel CA, Wachter RM, Pronovost PJ. Responsibility for quality improvement and patient safety: hospital board and medical staff leadership challenges. *Chest* 2010; 138:171–178.

The Joint Commission. *Leadership committed to safety. Sentinel event alert.* August 27, 2009;(43):1–3.

Keroack MA, Youngberg BJ, Cerese JL, et al. Organizational factors associated with high performance in quality and safety in academic medical centers. *Acad Med* 2007;82:1178–1186.

Parand A, Burnett S, Benn J, et al. The disparity of frontline clinical staff and managers' perceptions of a quality and patient safety initiative. *J Eval Clin Pract* 2011;17: 1184–1190.

Pronovost PJ. Learning accountability for patient outcomes. *JAMA* 2010;304:204–205.

Romig M, Goeschel C, Pronovost P, et al. Integrating CUSP and TRIP to improve patient safety. *Hosp Pract (Minneap)* 2010;38:114–121.

Spath PL, ed. *Error Reduction in Health Care: A Systems Approach to Improving Patient Safety.* 2nd ed. San Francisco, CA: Jossey-Bass; 2011.

Wachter RM. Patient safety at ten: unmistakable progress, troubling gaps. *Health Aff (Millwood)* 2010;29:165–173.

Youngberg BJ, ed. *Principles of Risk Management and Patient Safety.* Sudbury, MA: Jones Bartlett; 2011.

CONCLUSION

The fireworks that accompanied the publication of *To Err is Human* by the Institute of Medicine in late 1999 generated some magical thinking about how easy it would be to fix the problem of medical errors. A few computer systems here, some standard processes there (double checks, read backs), and maybe just a sprinkling of culture change—and poof, patients would be safer.

We now know how naive this point of view was. The problem of medical errors is remarkably complex, and the solutions will need to be as varied as the problems. Do we need better information technology? Yes. Improved teamwork? Yes. Stronger rules and regulations? Yes. Checklists, simulation, decision support, forcing functions? Yes, yes, yes, and yes.

Organizationally, we have come to understand that solutions must be *both* top down and bottom up. Resources need to be made available from senior leadership and boards—for teamwork training, computers, and appropriate staffing. Yet much of the action in patient safety happens at the frontline: will a nurse simply work around a hazardous situation, leaving it unaddressed, or take the time and trouble to report it and help fix it? Will residents enthusiastically participate in teamwork training programs and M&M conferences? Will the senior surgeon welcome—truly welcome—input from the intern or the nurse who sees something that might put a patient at risk?

The analogies from other industries are extraordinarily helpful, but they take us only so far. Computerizing the hospital is far more challenging than computerizing the supermarket. Changing an operating room's culture is many times more complex than creating an environment in a hermetically sealed cockpit that allows two people—with similar training, expertise, and social status—to feel comfortable raising their concerns. Giving a patient a dozen medications safely is much more difficult than avoiding defects as a car slides down an assembly line. And yet there is much we can learn from all these settings, and that learning has truly begun.

And what is the proper role of patients in all of this? It is clear that patients should be involved in their care, and that patient engagement can be an important part of a comprehensive safety strategy. Moreover, being open and honest about our errors with patients and their families is undeniably right, independent of pragmatic considerations regarding whether such disclosures change the risk of a malpractice suit.

But why should a patient have to check into a hospital or enter a clinic and be worried—quite appropriately—that he or she will be injured by the medical system? We should be proud of the progress we have made in the relatively short time since *To Err is Human* launched the modern patient safety movement. But we cannot rest until patients can approach the healthcare system with the trepidation and anxiety borne of their illness and its possible sequelae, while free of fear that they will be harmed or killed in the process of being helped. We still have much to do before we get there.

APPENDICES

SECTION

IV

APPENDICES

APPENDIX I. KEY BOOKS, REPORTS, SERIES, AND WEB SITES ON PATIENT SAFETY

Key Books and Reports on Medical Errors and Errors More Generally *

1. Agency for Healthcare Research and Quality. *Advances in Patient Safety: From Research to Implementation*. Rockville, MD: Agency for Healthcare Research and Quality; February 2005. AHRQ Publication Nos. 050021 (1–4).

2. Agency for Healthcare Research and Quality. *Advances in Patient Safety: New Directions and Alternative Approaches*. Rockville, MD: Agency for Healthcare Research and Quality; July 2008. AHRQ Publication Nos. 080034 (1–4).

3. Agency for Healthcare Research and Quality. *Advancing Patient Safety: A Decade of Evidence, Design, and Implementation*. Rockville, MD: Agency for Healthcare Research and Quality; November 2009. AHRQ Publication No. 09(10)-0084.

4. Antonsen S. *Safety Culture: Theory, Method and Improvement*. Burlington, VT: Ashgate; 2009.

5. Banja J. *Medical Errors and Medical Narcissism*. Sudbury, MA: Jones and Bartlett Publishers Inc; 2005.

6. Berwick DM. *Escape Fire: Designs for the Future of Health Care*. San Francisco, CA: Jossey-Bass; 2003.

7. Bogner MSE. *Human Error in Medicine*. Mahwah, NJ: Lawrence Erlbaum Associates; 1994.

8. Bosk CL. *Forgive and Remember: Managing Medical Failure*. 2nd ed. Chicago, IL: University of Chicago Press; 2003.

9. Bunting RF Jr, Schukman J, Wong WB. *A Comprehensive Guide to Managing Never Events and Hospital-Acquired Conditions*. Washington, DC: Atlantic Information Services Inc; 2009.

10. Casey SM. *Set Phasers on Stun: And Other True Tales of Design, Technology, and Human Error*. 2nd ed. Santa Barbara, CA: Aegean Publishing Company; 1998.

11. Cohen MR, ed. *Medication Errors*. 2nd ed. Washington, DC: American Pharmaceutical Association; 2006.

---

*Edited or written by Robert M. Wachter.

12. Columbia Accident Investigation Board. *Report of the Columbia Accident Investigation Board*; August 2003.

13. Conway J, Federico F, Stewart K, et al. *Respectful Management of Serious Clinical Adverse Events*. Cambridge, MA: Institute for Healthcare Improvement; 2010.

14. Cook RI, Woods DD, Miller C. *A Tale of Two Stories: Contrasting Views of Patient Safety*. National Patient Safety Foundation at the AMA: Annenberg Center for Health Sciences; 1998.

15. Dekker S. *Just Culture: Balancing Safety and Accountability*. Aldershot, England: Ashgate Publishing Limited; 2007.

16. Donaldson L. *An Organisation with a Memory: Report of an Expert Group on Learning from Adverse Events in the NHS Chaired by the Chief Medical Officer*. London: The Stationery Office; 2000.

17. Farley DO, Ridgely MS, Mendel P, et al. *Assessing Patient Safety Practices and Outcomes in the U.S. Health Care System*. Santa Monica, CA: RAND Corporation; 2009.

18. Frankel A, Leonard M, Simmonds T, et al., eds. *The Essential Guide for Patient Safety Officers*. Oakbrook Terrace, IL: Joint Commission on Accreditation of Healthcare Organizations and Institute for Healthcare Improvement; 2009.

19. Gawande A. *Complications: A Surgeon's Notes on an Imperfect Science*. New York, NY: Metropolitan Books; 2002.

20. Gawande A. *Better: A Surgeon's Notes on Performance*. New York, NY: Metropolitan Books; 2007.

21. Gawande A. *The Checklist Manifesto: How to Get Things Right*. New York, NY: Metropolitan Books; 2009.

22. Gibson R, Singh JP. *Wall of Silence: The Untold Story of the Medical Mistakes that Kill and Injure Millions of Americans*. Washington, DC: Lifeline; 2003.

23. Gosbee JW, Gosbee LL, eds. *Using Human Factors Engineering to Improve Patient Safety*. 2nd ed. Oakbrook Terrace, IL: Joint Commission Resources; 2010.

24. Griffin FA, Resar RK. *IHI Global Trigger Tool for Measuring Adverse Events*. 2nd ed. IHI Innovation Series White Paper. Cambridge, MA: Institute for Healthcare Improvement; 2009.

25. Groopman J. *How Doctors Think*. Boston, MA: Houghton Mifflin; 2007.

26. Helmreich RL, Merritt AC. *Culture at Work in Aviation and Medicine: National, Organizational, and Professional Influences*. Aldershot, Hampshire, UK: Ashgate; 1998.

27. Hughes RG, ed. *Patient Safety and Quality: An Evidence-Based Handbook for Nurses*. Rockville, MD: Agency for Healthcare Research and Quality; 2008. AHRQ Publication No. 08-0043.

28. Hurwitz B, Sheikh A, eds. *Health Care Errors and Patient Safety*. Hoboken, NJ: Wiley-Blackwell; 2009.

29. Jewell K, McGiffert L. *To Err is Human—To Delay is Deadly*. Austin, TX: Consumers Union; 2009.

30. Kahneman D, Slovic P, Tversky A. *Judgment Under Uncertainty: Heuristics and Biases*. Cambridge, England: Cambridge University Press; 1987.

31. Kahneman D. *Thinking Fast and Slow*. New York: Farrar, Strauss and Giroux; 2011.

32. King S. *Josie's Story*. New York, NY: Atlantic Monthly Press; 2009.

33. Krause TR, Hidley J. *Taking the Lead in Patient Safety: How Healthcare Leaders Influence Behavior and Create Culture*. Hoboken, NJ: Wiley; 2008.

34. Langley GJ, Moen R, Nolan KM, et al. *The Improvement Guide: A Practical Approach to Enhancing Organizational Performance*. 2nd ed. San Francisco, CA: Jossey-Bass; 2009.

35. Levinson DR. *Adverse Events in Hospitals: National Incidence Among Medicare Beneficiaries*. Washington, DC: US Department of Health and Human Services, Office of the Inspector General; November 2010. Report No. OEI-06-09-00090.

36. Lucian Leape Institute at the National Patient Safety Foundation. *Unmet Needs: Teaching Physicians to Provide Safe Patient Care*. Boston, MA: Lucian Leape Institute at the National Patient Safety Foundation; March 2010.

37. Marx D. *Whack-a-Mole: The Price We Pay for Expecting Perfection*. Plano, TX: By Your Side Studios; 2009.

38. Massachusetts Coalition for the Prevention of Medical Errors. *When Things Go Wrong: Responding to Adverse Events*. A Consensus Statement of the Harvard Hospitals. Burlington, VT: Massachusetts Coalition for the Prevention of Medical Errors; 2006.

39. Merry A, Smith AM. *Errors, Medicine, and the Law*. Cambridge, England: Cambridge University Press; 2001.

40. Millenson ML. *Demanding Medical Excellence. Doctors and Accountability in the Information Age*. Chicago, IL: University of Chicago Press; 1997.

41. Nance JJ. *Why Hospitals should Fly: The Ultimate Flight Plan to Patient Safety and Quality Care*. Boseman, MT: Second River Healthcare Press; 2008.

42. National Quality Forum. *Safe Practices for Better Healthcare—2009 Update*. Washington, DC: National Quality Forum; 2009.

43. Nemeth CP, ed. *Improving Healthcare Team Communication: Building on Lessons from Aviation and Aerospace*. Burlington, VT: Ashgate Publishing; 2008.

44. Norman DA. *The Design of Everyday Things*. New York, NY: Basic Books; 2002.

45. Paget MA. *Unity of Mistakes: A Phenomenological Interpretation of Medical Work*. Philadelphia, PA: Temple University Press; 1993.

46. Paget MA. In: DeVault ML, ed. *Reflections on Cancer and an Abbreviated Life*. Philadelphia, PA: Temple University Press; 1993.

47. Perrow C. *Normal Accidents: Living with High-Risk Technologies. With a New Afterword and a Postscript on the Y2K Problem*. Princeton, NJ: Princeton University Press; 1999.

48. Pronovost P, Vohr E. *Safe Patients, Smart Hospitals: How One Doctor's Checklist can Help Us Change Health Care from the Inside Out*. New York, NY: Hudson Street Press; 2010.

49. Reason JT. *Human Error*. New York, NY: Cambridge University Press; 1990.

50. Reason JT. *Managing the Risks of Organizational Accidents*. Aldershot, Hampshire, UK: Ashgate; 1997.

51. Reason J. *The Human Contribution: Unsafe Acts, Accidents and Heroic Recoveries*. Farnham Surrey, UK: Ashgate; 2008.

52. Reynard J, Reynolds J, Stevenson P. *Practical Patient Safety*. Oxford, UK: Oxford University Press; 2009.

53. Robins NS. *The Girl who Died Twice: Every Patient's Nightmare: The Libby Zion Case and the Hidden Hazards of Hospitals*. New York, NY: Delacorte Press; 1995.

54. Rogers EM. *Diffusion of Innovation*. 5th ed. New York, NY: Free Press; 2003.

55. Rosenthal MM, Sutcliffe KM, eds. *Medical Error. What do We Know? What do We Do?* San Francisco, CA: John Wiley & Sons; 2002.

56. Rozovsky FA, Woods JR Jr, eds. *The Handbook of Patient Safety Compliance: A Practical Guide for Health Care Organizations.* San Francisco, CA: Jossey-Bass; 2005.

57. Sagan SD. *The Limits of Safety: Organizations, Accidents and Nuclear Weapons.* Princeton, NJ: Princeton University Press; 1993.

58. Sanders L. *Every Patient Tells A Story: Medical Mysteries and the Art of Diagnosis.* New York, NY: Broadway Books; 2009.

59. Schuster PM, Nykolyn L. *Communication for Nurses: How to Prevent Harmful Events and Promote Patient Safety.* Philadelphia, PA: F.A. Davis Company; 2010.

60. Scobie S, Thomson R. *Building a Memory: Preventing Harm, Reducing Risks and Improving Patient Safety.* London, England: National Patient Safety Agency; 2005.

61. Sharpe VA, Faden AI. *Medical Harm: Historical, Conceptual, and Ethical Dimensions of Iatrogenic Illness.* New York, NY: Cambridge University Press; 1998.

62. *Shekelle PG, Pronovost PJ, Wachter RM, et al.; PSP Technical Expert Panel. *Assessing the Evidence for Context-Sensitive Effectiveness and Safety of Patient Safety Practices: Developing Criteria.* Rockville, MD: Agency for Healthcare Research and Quality; December 2010. AHRQ Publication No. 11-0006-EF.

63. *Shojania KG, Duncan BW, McDonald KM, Wachter RM, eds. *Making Health Care Safer: A Critical Analysis of Patient Safety Practices.* Evidence Report/Technology Assessment No. 43 from the Agency for Healthcare Research and Quality: AHRQ Publication No. 01-E058. Rockville, MD: Agency for Healthcare Research and Quality; July 2001. Available at: http://www.ahrq.gov/clinic/ptsafety/.

64. Spath P, ed. *Engaging Patients as Safety Partners.* Chicago, IL: AHA Press; 2008.

65. Spath PL. *Error Reduction in Health Care: A Systems Approach to Improving Patient Safety.* 2nd ed. San Francisco, CA: Jossey-Bass; 2011.

66. Stewart JB. *Blind Eye: How the Medical Establishment Let a Doctor Get Away with Murder.* New York, NY: Simon & Schuster; 1999.

67. Tenner E. *Why Things Bite Back: Technology and the Revenge of Unintended Consequences.* New York, NY: A.A. Knopf; 1996.

68. Truog RD, Browning DM, Johnson JA, et al. *Talking with Patients and Families about Medical Error: A Guide for Education and Practice.* Baltimore, MD: Johns Hopkins University Press; 2011.

69. Ulmer C, Wolman DM, Johns MME, eds. *Resident Duty Hours: Enhancing Sleep, Supervision, and Safety.* Committee on Optimizing Graduate Medical Trainee (Resident) Hours and Work Schedule to Improve Patient Safety, Institute of Medicine. Washington, DC: National Academies Press; 2008.

70. Vance JE. *A Guide to Patient Safety in the Medical Practice.* Chicago, IL: American Medical Association; 2008.

71. Vaughan D. *The Challenger Launch Decision: Risky Technology, Culture, and Deviance at NASA.* Chicago, IL: University of Chicago Press; 1997.

72. Vincent C. *Patient Safety.* 2nd ed. West Sussex, UK: Wiley-Blackwell; 2010.

73. *Wachter RM, Shojania KG. *Internal Bleeding: The Truth Behind America's Terrifying Epidemic of Medical Mistakes.* New York, NY: Rugged Land; 2004.

74. Weick KE. *Sensemaking in Organizations*. Thousand Oaks, CA: Sage Publications; 1995.

75. Weick KE, Sutcliffe KM. *Managing the Unexpected: Assuring High Performance in an Age of Complexity*. 2nd ed. San Francisco, CA: John Wiley & Sons; 2007.

76. Wiener EL, Kanki BG, Helmreich RL. *Cockpit Resource Management*. San Diego, CA: Academic Press; 1993.

77. Woods DD, Dekker S, Cook R, et al. *Behind Human Error*. 2nd ed. Burlington, VT: Ashgate; 2010.

78. Wu AW, ed. *The Value of Close Calls in Improving Patient Safety*. Oakbrook Terrace, IL: Joint Commission Resources; 2011.

79. Wu HW, Nishimi RY, Page-Lopez CM, et al. *Improving Patient Safety Through Informed Consent for Patients with Limited Health Literacy*. Washington, DC: National Quality Forum; 2005.

80. Youngberg BJ, ed. *Principles of Risk Management and Patient Safety*. Sudbury, MA: Jones Bartlett; 2011.

The Institute of Medicine (IOM) Reports on Medical Errors and Healthcare Quality (From its "Quality Chasm" Series)

1. Kohn L, Corrigan J, Donaldson M, eds. *To Err is Human: Building a Safer Health System*. Washington, DC: Committee on Quality of Health Care in America, Institute of Medicine: National Academy Press, 2000.

2. Committee on Quality of Health Care in America, IOM. *Crossing the Quality Chasm: A New Health System for the 21st Century*. Washington, DC: National Academy Press; 2001.

3. Page A, ed. *Keeping Patients Safe. Transforming the Work Environment of Nurses*. Committee on the Work Environment for Nurses and Patient Safety, Board on Health Care Services. Washington, DC: National Academy Press; 2004.

4. Aspden P, Corrigan JM, Wolcott J, et al. *Patient Safety: Achieving a New Standard for Care*. Washington, DC: National Academy Press; 2004.

5. Nielsen-Bohlman L, Panzer AM, Kindig DA. Institute of Medicine Committee on Health Literacy. *Health Literacy: A Prescription to End Confusion*. Washington, DC: National Academy Press; 2004.

6. Aspden P, Wolcott J, Bootman JL, et al., eds. *Preventing Medication Errors*. Committee on Identifying and Preventing Medication Errors. Washington, DC: National Academy Press; 2007.

Quality Grand Rounds Series, Annals of Internal Medicine*

1. *Wachter RM, Shojania KG, Saint S, et al. Learning from our mistakes: quality grand rounds, a new case-based series on medical errors and patient safety. *Ann Intern Med* 2002;136:850–852.

---

*Edited or written by Robert M. Wachter.

2. Chassin MR, Becher EC. The wrong patient. *Ann Intern Med* 2002;136:826–833.

3. Bates DW. Unexpected hypoglycemia in a critically ill patient. *Ann Intern Med* 2002;137:110–116.

4. Hofer TP, Hayward RA. Are bad outcomes from questionable clinical decisions preventable medical errors? A case of cascade iatrogenesis. *Ann Intern Med* 2002;137:327–333.

5. Gerberding JL. Hospital-onset infections: a patient safety issue. *Ann Intern Med* 2002;137:665–670.

6. Cleary PD. A hospitalization from hell: a patient's perspective on quality. *Ann Intern Med* 2003;138:33–39.

7. Lynn J, Goldstein NE. Advance care planning for fatal chronic illness: avoiding commonplace errors and unwarranted suffering. *Ann Intern Med* 2003;138:812–818.

8. Brennan TA, Mello MM. Patient safety and medical malpractice: a case study. *Ann Intern Med* 2003;139:267–273.

9. Goldman L, Kirtane AJ. Triage of patients with acute chest pain and possible cardiac ischemia: the elusive search for diagnostic perfection. *Ann Intern Med* 2003;139: 987–995.

10. Pronovost PJ, Wu AW, Sexton JB. Acute decompensation after removing a central line: practical approaches to increasing safety in the intensive care unit. *Ann Intern Med* 2004;140:1025–1033.

11. Redelmeier DA. Improving patient care. The cognitive psychology of missed diagnoses. *Ann Intern Med* 2005;142:115–120.

12. Gandhi TK. Fumbled hand-offs: one dropped ball after another. *Ann Intern Med* 2005;142:352–358.

13. McDonald CJ. Computerization can create safety hazards: a bar-coding near miss. *Ann Intern Med* 2006;144:510–516.

14. Shojania KG, Fletcher KE, Saint S. Graduate medical education and patient safety: a busy—and occasionally hazardous—intersection. *Ann Intern Med* 2006;145:592–598.

15. *Wachter RM, Shojania KG, Markowitz AJ, et al. Quality grand rounds: the case for patient safety. *Ann Intern Med* 2006;148:629–630.

Selected Theme Issues on Medical Errors

Focus on computerized provider order systems. *J Am Med Inform Assoc* 2007;14:25–75. Available at: http://www.jamia.org/content/vol14/issue1/.

Profiles in patient safety. Case-based series of articles. *Acad Emerg Med*. Available at: http://www.aemj.org/cgi/content/full/9/4/324.

Theme issue on medical error. *BMJ* 2000;320:7237. Available at: http://bmj.com/content/vol320/issue7237/.

Theme issue on medical error. *Eff Clin Pract* 2000. Available at: http://www.acponline.org/journals/ecp/pastiss/nd00.htm.

Theme issue: contributions from ergonomics and human factors. *Qual Saf Health Care* 2010;19(suppl 3):i1–i79.

Theme issue: diagnostic error in medicine. Berner ES, Graber ML, eds. *Adv Health Sci Educ Theory Pract* 2009;14(suppl 1):1–112.

Theme issue: human factors and ergonomics in patient safety. Carayon P, Buckle P, eds. *App Ergon* 2010:41:643–718.

Theme issue: knowledge for improvement. *BMJ Qual Saf* 2011;20(suppl 1):1–105.

Theme issue: medical malpractice and errors. *Health Aff (Millwood)* 2010;29:1564–1619.

Theme issue: new approaches to researching patient safety. Iedema R, ed. *Soc Sci Med* 2009;69:1701–1783.

Theme issue: nurses transforming care. *Am J Nurs* 2009;109(suppl 11):3–80, C3.

Theme issue: quality and safety in medicine. Nash DB, Goldfarb NI, Patow C, eds. *Acad Med* 2009;84:1641–1846.

Theme issue: safety by design. *Qual Saf Health Care* December 2006;15(suppl 1):i1–i90.

Theme issue: safety. Simmons D, ed. *Crit Care Nurs Clin North Am* 2010;22:161–290.

Theme issue: special issue on health information technology. *J Gen Intern Med* 2008;23:353–507.

Theme issue: still crossing the quality chasm. *Health Aff (Millwood)* 2011;30:554–800.

Selected Websites on Medical Errors

Agency for Healthcare Research and Quality (AHRQ). *Patient Safety & Medical Errors.* Available at: http://ahrq.gov/qual/errorsix.htm.

*AHRQ Patient Safety Network (PSNet). Available at: http://www.psnet.ahrq.gov.

*AHRQ WebM&M: Morbidity and Mortality Rounds on the Web. Available at: http://www.webmm.ahrq.gov/.

AHRQ Patient Safety Organizations. Available at: http://www.pso.ahrq.gov/index.html.

AHRQ Health Care Innovations Exchange. Available at: http://www.innovations.ahrq.gov/.

American College of Surgeons. National Surgical Quality Improvement Program (NSQIP). Available at: http://www.acsnsqip.org/.

American Hospital Association Patient Safety Center. Available at: http://www.ahaqualitycenter.org/ahaqualitycenter/dimQualityServlet?keywordId=3.

Association for Professionals in Infection Control and Epidemiology. PreventInfection.org. Available at: http://www.preventinfection.org//AM/Template.cfm?Section=Home4.

FDA Patient Safety News. Available at: http://www.fda.gov/cdrh/psn.

Institute for Healthcare Improvement (IHI). Available at: http://www.ihi.org.

Institute for Safe Medication Practices. Available at: http://www.ismp.org/.

Joint Commission. Available at: http://www.jointcommission.org.

Joint Commission Center for Transforming Healthcare. Available at: http://www.centerfortransforminghealthcare.org/.

Joint Commission National Patient Safety Goals: Available at: http://www.jointcommission.org/standards_information/npsgs.aspx.

Leapfrog Group for Patient Safety. Available at: http://www.leapfroggroup.org/.

*Edited or written by Robert M. Wachter.

National Patient Safety Agency (United Kingdom). Available at: http://www.npsa.nhs.uk/.

National Patient Safety Agency (United Kingdom). *Safer Healthcare*. Available at: http://www.saferhealthcare.org.uk/ihi.

National Patient Safety Foundation. Available at: http://www.npsf.org/.

National Quality Forum. Available at: http://www.qualityforum.org.

US Department of Health and Human Services. *Partnership for Patients*. Available at: http://www.healthcare.gov/center/programs/partnership/index.html.

World Health Organization (WHO) Patient Safety. Available at: http://www.who.int/patientsafety/en/.

WHO Patient Safety Human Factors Web Site. Available at: http://www.who.int/patientsafety/research/methods_measures/human_factors/en/.

APPENDIX II. THE AHRQ PATIENT SAFETY NETWORK (AHRQ PSNET) GLOSSARY OF SELECTED TERMS IN PATIENT SAFETY

Active error (or active failure)—The terms *active* and *latent* as applied to errors were coined by James Reason. Active errors occur at the point of contact between a human and some aspect of a larger system (e.g., a human–machine interface). They are generally readily apparent (e.g., pushing an incorrect button, ignoring a warning light) and almost always involve someone at the frontline. Active failures are sometimes referred to as errors at the sharp end, figuratively referring to a scalpel. In other words, errors at the sharp end are noticed first because they are committed by the person closest to the patient. This person may literally be holding a scalpel (e.g., an orthopedist operating on the wrong leg) or figuratively be administering any kind of therapy (e.g., a nurse programming an intravenous pump) or performing any aspect of care. Latent errors (or latent conditions), in contrast, refer to less apparent failures of organization or design that contributed to the occurrence of errors or allowed them to cause harm to patients. To complete the metaphor, latent errors are those at the other end of the scalpel—the blunt end—referring to the many layers of the healthcare system that affect the person "holding" the scalpel.

Adverse drug event (ADE)—An adverse event (i.e., injury resulting from medical care) involving medication use.

Examples:

- Anaphylaxis to penicillin
- Major hemorrhage from heparin
- Aminoglycoside-induced renal failure
- Agranulocytosis from chloramphenicol

As with the more general term adverse event, the occurrence of an ADE does not necessarily indicate an error or poor quality of care. ADEs that involve an element of error (of either omission or commission) are often referred to as *preventable* ADEs. Medication errors that reached the patient but by good fortune did not cause any harm are often called *potential* ADEs. For instance, a serious allergic reaction to penicillin in a patient with no prior such history is an ADE, but so is the same reaction in a patient who has a known allergy history but receives penicillin due to a prescribing oversight. The former occurrence would count as an adverse drug reaction or nonpreventable ADE, while the latter would represent a preventable ADE. If a patient with a documented serious penicillin allergy received a penicillin-like antibiotic but happened not to react to it, this event would be characterized as a potential ADE.

An *ameliorable* ADE is one in which the patient experienced harm from a medication that, while not completely preventable, could have been mitigated. For instance, a patient taking a cholesterol-lowering agent (statin) may develop muscle pains and eventually progress to a more serious condition called rhabdomyolysis. Failure to periodically check a blood test that assesses muscle damage or failure to recognize this possible diagnosis in a patient taking statins who subsequently develops rhabdomyolysis would make this event an ameliorable ADE: harm from medical care that could have been lessened with earlier, appropriate management. Again, the initial development of some problem was not preventable, but the eventual harm that occurred need not have been so severe, hence the term ameliorable ADE.

Adverse event—Any injury caused by medical care.

Examples:

- Pneumothorax from central venous catheter placement
- Anaphylaxis to penicillin
- Postoperative wound infection
- Hospital-acquired delirium (or "sundowning") in elderly patients

Identifying something as an adverse event does not imply "error," "negligence," or poor quality care. It simply indicates that an undesirable clinical outcome resulted from some aspect of diagnosis or therapy, not an underlying disease process. Thus, pneumothorax from central venous catheter placement counts as an adverse event regardless of insertion technique. Similarly, a postoperative wound infection counts as an adverse event even if the operation proceeded with optimal adherence to sterile procedures, the patient received appropriate antibiotic prophylaxis in the perioperative setting, and so on. (See also "iatrogenic").

Anchoring error (or bias)—Refers to the common cognitive trap of allowing first impressions to exert undue influence on the diagnostic process.

Clinicians often latch on to features of a patient's presentation that suggest a specific diagnosis. Often, this initial diagnostic impression will prove correct, hence the use of the phrase *anchoring heuristic* in some contexts, as it can be a useful rule of thumb to "always trust your first impressions." However, in some cases, subsequent developments in the patient's course will prove inconsistent with the first impression. Anchoring bias refers to the tendency to hold on to the initial diagnosis, even in the face of disconfirming evidence.

Authority gradient—Refers to the balance of decision-making power or the steepness of command hierarchy in a given situation. Members of a crew or organization with a domineering, overbearing, or dictatorial team leader experience a steep authority gradient. Expressing concerns, questioning, or even simply clarifying instructions would require considerable determination on the part of team members who perceive their input as devalued or frankly unwelcome. Most teams require some degree of authority gradient; otherwise roles are blurred and decisions cannot be made in a timely fashion. However, effective team leaders consciously establish a command hierarchy appropriate to the training and experience of team members.

Authority gradients may occur even when the notion of a team is less well defined. For instance, a pharmacist calling a physician to clarify an order may encounter a steep authority gradient, based on the tone of the physician's voice or a lack of openness to input from the pharmacist. A confident, experienced pharmacist may nonetheless continue to raise legitimate concerns about an order, but other pharmacists might not.

Availability bias (or heuristic)—Refers to the tendency to assume, when judging probabilities or predicting outcomes, that the first possibility that comes to mind (i.e., the most cognitively "available" possibility) is also the most likely possibility. For instance, suppose a patient presents with intermittent episodes of very high blood pressure. Because episodic hypertension resembles textbook descriptions of pheochromocytoma, a memorable but uncommon endocrinologic tumor, this diagnosis may immediately come to mind. A clinician who infers from this immediate association that pheochromocytoma is the most likely diagnosis would be exhibiting availability bias. In addition to resemblance to classic descriptions of disease, personal experience can also trigger availability bias, as when the diagnosis underlying a recent patient's presentation immediately comes to mind when any subsequent patient presents with similar symptoms. Particularly memorable cases may similarly exert undue influence in shaping diagnostic impressions.

Bayesian approach—Probabilistic reasoning in which test results (not just laboratory investigations but also history, physical exam, or any aspect for the diagnostic process) are combined with prior beliefs about the probability of a particular disease. One way of recognizing the need for a Bayesian approach is to recognize the difference between the performance of a test in a population and that in an individual. At the population level, we can say that a test has a sensitivity and specificity of, say, 90%—that is, 90% of patients with the condition of interest have a positive result and 90% of patients without the condition have a negative result. In practice, however, a clinician needs to attempt to predict whether an individual patient with a positive or negative result does or does not have the condition of interest. This prediction requires combining the observed test result not just with the known sensitivity and specificity but also with the chance the patient could have had the disease in the first place (based on demographic factors, findings on exam, or general clinical gestalt).

Benchmark—A benchmark in healthcare refers to an attribute or achievement that serves as a standard for other providers or institutions to emulate. Benchmarks differ from other standard of care goals, in that they derive from empiric data—specifically, performance or outcomes data. For example, a statewide survey might produce risk-adjusted 30-day rates for death or other major adverse outcomes. After adjusting for relevant clinical factors, the top 10% of hospitals can be identified in terms of particular outcome measures. These institutions would then provide benchmark data on these outcomes. For instance, one might benchmark "door-to-balloon" time at 90 minutes, based on the observation that the top-performing hospitals all had door-to-balloon times in this range. In regard to infection control, benchmarks would typically be derived from national or regional data on the rates of relevant nosocomial infections. The lowest 10% of these rates might be regarded as benchmarks for other institutions to emulate.

Blunt end—The blunt end refers to the many layers of the healthcare system not in direct contact with patients, but which influence the personnel and equipment at the sharp end who do contact patients. The blunt end thus consists of those who set policy, manage healthcare institutions, and design medical devices, and other people and forces, which, though removed in time and space from direct patient care, nonetheless affect how care is delivered. Thus, an error programming an intravenous pump would represent a problem at the sharp end, while the institution's decision to use multiple different types of infusion pumps, making programming errors more likely, would represent a problem at the blunt end. The terminology of "sharp" and "blunt" ends corresponds roughly to active failures and latent conditions.

Checklist—Algorithmic listing of actions to be performed in a given clinical setting (e.g., advanced cardiac life support [ACLS] protocols for treating cardiac arrest) to ensure that, no mater how often performed by a given practitioner, no step will be forgotten. An analogy is often made to flight preparation in aviation, as pilots and air traffic controllers follow pretakeoff checklists regardless of how many times they have carried out the tasks involved.

Clinical decision support system (CDSS)—Any system designed to improve clinical decision making related to diagnostic or therapeutic processes of care. Typically a decision support system responds to "triggers" or "flags"—specific diagnoses, laboratory results, medication choices, or complex combinations of such parameters—and provides information or recommendations directly relevant to a specific patient encounter.

CDSSs address activities ranging from the selection of drugs (e.g., the optimal antibiotic choice given specific microbiologic data) or diagnostic tests to detailed support for optimal drug dosing and support for resolving diagnostic dilemmas. Structured antibiotic order forms represent a common example of paper-based CDSSs. Although such systems are still commonly encountered, many people equate CDSSs with computerized systems in which software algorithms generate patient-specific recommendations by matching characteristics, such as age, renal function, or allergy history, with rules in a computerized knowledge base.

The distinction between decision support and simple reminders can be unclear, but usually reminder systems are included as decision support if they involve patient-specific information. For instance, a generic reminder (e.g., "Did you obtain an allergy history?") would not be considered decision support, but a warning (e.g., "This patient is allergic to codeine.") that appears at the time of entering an order for codeine would be.

Close call—An event or situation that did not produce patient injury, but only because of chance. This good fortune might reflect robustness of the patient (e.g., a patient with penicillin allergy receives penicillin, but has no reaction) or a fortuitous, timely intervention (e.g., a nurse happens to realize that a physician wrote an order in the wrong chart). Such events have also been termed near miss incidents.

Competency—Having the necessary knowledge or technical skill to perform a given procedure within the bounds of success and failure rates deemed compatible with acceptable care. The medical education literature often refers to core competencies, which include not just technical skills with respect to procedures or medical knowledge but also competencies with respect to communicating with patients, collaborating with other members of the healthcare team, and acting as a manager or agent for change in the health system.

Complexity science (or complexity theory)—Provides an approach to understanding the behavior of systems that exhibit nonlinear dynamics, or the ways in which some adaptive systems produce novel behavior not expected from the properties of their individual components. Such behaviors emerge as a result of interactions between agents at a local level in the complex system and between the system and its environment.

Complexity theory differs importantly from systems thinking in its emphasis on the interaction between local systems and their environment (such as the larger system in which a given hospital or clinic operates). It is often tempting to ignore the larger environment as unchangeable and therefore outside the scope of quality improvement or patient safety activities. According to complexity theory, however, behavior within a hospital or clinic (e.g., noncompliance with a national practice guideline) can often be understood only by identifying interactions between local attributes and environmental factors.

Computerized provider order entry or computerized physician order entry (CPOE)—Refers to a computer-based system of ordering medications and often other tests. Physicians (or other providers) directly enter orders into a computer system that can have varying levels of sophistication. Basic CPOE ensures standardized, legible, complete orders, and thus primarily reduces errors caused by poor handwriting and ambiguous abbreviations.

Almost all CPOE systems offer some additional capabilities, which fall under the general rubric of CDSS. Typical CDSS features involve suggested default values for drug doses, routes of administration, or frequency. More sophisticated CDSSs can perform drug allergy checks (e.g., the user orders ceftriaxone and a warning flashes that the patient has a documented penicillin allergy), drug-laboratory value checks (e.g., initiating an order for gentamicin prompts the system to alert you to the patient's last creatinine), drug–drug interaction checks, and so on. At the highest level of sophistication, CDSS prevents not only errors of commission (e.g., ordering a drug in excessive doses or in the setting of a serious allergy) but also errors of omission. For example, an alert may appear such as, "You have ordered heparin; would you like to order a partial thromboplastin time (PTT) in 6 hours?" Or, even more sophisticated: "The admitting diagnosis is hip fracture; would you like to order heparin for deep vein thrombosis (DVT) prophylaxis?" See also "Clinical decision support system."

Confirmation bias—Refers to the tendency to focus on evidence that supports a working hypothesis, such as a diagnosis in clinical medicine, rather than to look for evidence that refutes it or provides greater support to an alternative diagnosis. Suppose that a 65-year-old man with a past history of angina presents to the emergency department with acute onset of shortness of breath. The physician immediately considers the possibility of cardiac ischemia, so asks the patient if he has experienced any chest pain. The patient replies affirmatively. Because the physician perceives this answer as confirming his working diagnosis, he does not ask if the chest pain was pleuritic in nature, which would decrease the likelihood of an acute coronary syndrome and increase the likelihood of pulmonary embolism (a reasonable alternative diagnosis for acute shortness of breath accompanied by chest pain). The physician then orders an ECG and cardiac troponin. The ECG shows nonspecific ST changes and the troponin returns slightly elevated.

Of course, ordering an ECG and testing cardiac enzymes is appropriate in the work-up of acute shortness of breath, especially when it is accompanied by chest pain and in a patient with known angina. The problem is that these tests may be misleading, since positive results are consistent not only with acute coronary syndrome but also with pulmonary embolism. To avoid confirmation bias in this case, the physician might have obtained an arterial blood glass or a D-dimer level. Abnormal results for either of these tests would be relatively unlikely to occur in a patient with an acute coronary syndrome (unless complicated by pulmonary edema), but likely to occur with pulmonary embolism. These results could be followed up by more direct testing for pulmonary embolism (e.g., with a helical CT scan of the chest), while normal results would allow the clinician to proceed with greater confidence down the road of investigating and managing cardiac ischemia.

This vignette was presented as if information were sought in sequence. In many cases, especially in acute care medicine, clinicians have the results of numerous tests in hand when they first meet a patient. The results of these tests often do not all suggest the same diagnosis. The appeal of accentuating confirmatory test results and ignoring nonconfirmatory ones is that it minimizes cognitive dissonance.

A related cognitive trap that may accompany confirmation bias and compound the possibility of error is "anchoring bias"—the tendency to stick with one's first impressions, even in the face of significant disconfirming evidence.

Crew resource management (CRM)—Also called crisis resource management in some contexts (e.g., anesthesia), encompasses a range of approaches to training groups to function as teams, rather than as collections of individuals. Originally developed in aviation, CRM emphasizes the role of human factors—the effects of fatigue, expected or predictable perceptual errors (such as misreading monitors or mishearing instructions), as well as the impact of different management styles and organizational cultures in high-stress, high-risk environments. CRM training develops communication skills, fosters a more cohesive environment among team members, and creates an atmosphere in which junior personnel will feel free to speak up when they think that something is amiss. Some CRM programs emphasize education on the settings in which errors occur and the aspects of team decision making conducive to "trapping" errors before they cause harm. Other programs may provide more hands-on training involving simulated crisis scenarios followed by debriefing sessions in which participants assess their own and others' behavior.

Critical incidents—A term made famous by a classic human factors study by Jeffrey Cooper of "anesthetic mishaps," though the term had first been coined in the 1950s. Cooper and colleagues brought the technique of critical incident analysis to a wide audience in healthcare but followed the definition of the originator of the technique. They defined critical incidents as occurrences that are "significant or pivotal, in either a desirable or an unde-sirable way," though Cooper and colleagues (and most others since) chose to focus on incidents that had potentially undesirable consequences. This con-cept is best understood in the context of the type of investigation that follows, which is very much in the style of root cause analysis. Thus, *significant* or *pivotal* means that there was significant potential for harm (or actual harm), but also that the event has the potential to reveal important hazards in the organization. In many ways, it embodies the expression in quality improve-ment circles that "every defect is a treasure." In other words, these incidents, whether near misses or disasters in which significant harm occurred, provide valuable opportunities to learn about individual and organizational factors that can be remedied to prevent similar incidents in the future.

Decision support—Refers to any system for advising or providing guid-ance about a particular clinical decision at the point of care. For example, a copy of an algorithm for antibiotic selection in patients with community-acquired pneumonia would count as clinical decision support if made available at the point of care. Increasingly, decision support occurs via a computerized clinical information or order entry system. Computerized decision support includes any software employing a knowledge base designed to assist clini-cians in decision making at the point of care.

Typically a decision support system responds to "triggers" or "flags"—specific diagnoses, laboratory results, medication choices, or complex com-binations of such parameters—and provides information or recommendations directly relevant to a specific patient encounter. For instance, ordering an aminoglycoside for a patient with creatinine above a certain value might trig-ger a message suggesting a dose adjustment based on the patient's decreased renal function.

Error—An act of commission (doing something wrong) or omission (failing to do the right thing) that leads to an undesirable outcome or signifi-cant potential for such an outcome. For instance, ordering a medication for a patient with a documented allergy to that medication would be an act of commission. Failing to prescribe a proven medication with major benefits for an eligible patient (e.g., low-dose unfractionated heparin as venous throm-boembolism prophylaxis for a patient after hip replacement surgery) would represent an error of omission.

Errors of omission are more difficult to recognize than errors of com-mission but likely represent a larger problem. In other words, there are likely many more instances in which the provision of additional diagnostic, ther-apeutic, or preventive modalities would have improved care than there are instances in which the care provided quite literally should not have been pro-vided. In many ways, this point echoes the generally agreed-upon view in the healthcare quality literature that underuse far exceeds overuse, even though the latter historically received greater attention. (See definition for "Under-use, overuse, and misuse"). In addition to commission versus omission, three other dichotomies commonly appear in the literature on errors: active failures versus latent conditions, errors at the sharp end versus errors at the blunt end, and slips versus mistakes.

Error chain—Error chain generally refers to the series of events that led to a disastrous outcome, typically uncovered by a root cause analysis. Sometimes the chain metaphor carries the added sense of inexorability, as many of the causes are tightly coupled, such that one problem begets the next. A more specific meaning of error chain, especially when used in the phrase "break the error chain," relates to the common themes or categories of causes that emerge from root cause analyses. These categories go by different names in different settings, but they generally include (1) failure to follow standard operating procedures, (2) poor leadership, (3) breakdowns in communication or teamwork, (4) overlooking or ignoring individual fallibility, and (5) losing track of objectives. Used in this way, "break the error chain" is shorthand for an approach in which team members continually address these links as a crisis or routine situation unfolds. The checklists that are included in teamwork training programs have categories corresponding to these common links in the error chain (e.g., establish a team leader, assign roles and responsibilities, and monitor your teammates).

Face validity—The extent to which a technical concept, instrument, or study result is plausible, usually because its findings are consistent with prior assumptions and expectations.

Failure mode and effects analysis (FMEA)—A common process used to prospectively identify error risk within a particular process. FMEA begins with a complete process mapping that identifies all the steps that must occur for a given process to occur (e.g., programming an infusion pump or preparing an intravenous medication in the pharmacy). With the process mapped out, the FMEA then continues by identifying the ways in which each step can go wrong (i.e., the "failure modes" for each step), the probability that each error will be detected (i.e., so that it can be corrected before causing harm), and the consequences or impact of the error not being detected. The estimates of the likelihood of a particular process failure, the chance of detecting such failure, and its impact are combined numerically to produce a *criticality index*.

This criticality index provides a rough quantitative estimate of the magnitude of hazard posed by each step in a high-risk process. Assigning a criticality index to each step allows prioritization of targets for improvement. For instance, an FMEA analysis of the medication-dispensing process on a general hospital ward might break down all steps from receipt of orders in the central pharmacy to filling automated dispensing machines by pharmacy technicians. Each step in this process would be assigned a probability of failure and an impact score, so that all steps could be ranked according to the product of these two numbers. Steps ranked at the top (i.e., those with the highest criticality indices) would be prioritized for error proofing.

FMEA makes sense as a general approach and it (or similar prospective error-proofing techniques) has been used in other high-risk industries. However, the reliability of the technique is not clear. Different teams charged with analyzing the same process may identify different steps in the process, assign different risks to the steps, and consequently prioritize different targets for improvement.

Failure to rescue—Failure to rescue is shorthand for failure to rescue (i.e., prevent a clinically important deterioration, such as death or permanent disability) from a complication of an underlying illness (e.g., cardiac arrest in a patient with acute myocardial infarction) or a complication of medical care (e.g., major hemorrhage after thrombolysis for acute myocardial infarction). Failure to rescue thus provides a measure of the degree to which providers responded to adverse occurrences (e.g., hospital-acquired infections, cardiac arrest or shock) that developed on their watch. It may reflect the quality of monitoring, the effectiveness of actions taken once early complications are recognized, or both.

The technical motivation for using failure to rescue to evaluate the quality of care stems from the concern that some institutions might document adverse occurrences more assiduously than others. Therefore, using lower rates of in-hospital complications by themselves may simply reward hospitals with poor documentation. However, if the medical record indicates that a complication has occurred, the response to that complication should provide an indicator of the quality of care that is less susceptible to charting bias.

Forcing function—An aspect of a design that prevents a target action from being performed or allows its performance only if another specific action is performed first. For example, automobiles are now designed so that the driver cannot shift into reverse without first putting his or her foot on the brake pedal. Forcing functions need not involve device design. For instance, one of the first forcing functions identified in healthcare was the removal of concentrated potassium from general hospital wards. This action is intended to prevent the inadvertent preparation of intravenous solutions with concentrated potassium, an error that has produced small but consistent numbers of deaths for many years.

"Five Rights"—The "Five Rights"—administering the Right Medication, in the Right Dose, at the Right Time, by the Right Route, to the Right Patient—are the cornerstone of traditional nursing teaching about safe medication practice.

While the Five Rights represent goals of safe medication administration, they contain no procedural detail, and thus may inadvertently perpetuate the traditional focus on individual performance rather than system improvement. Procedures for ensuring each of the Five Rights must take into account human factor and systems design issues (such as workload, ambient distractions, poor lighting, problems with wristbands, ineffective double-check protocols, etc.) that can threaten or undermine even the most conscientious efforts to comply with the Five Rights. In the end, the Five Rights remain an important goal for safe medication practice, but one that may give the illusion of safety if not supported by strong policies and procedures, a system organized around modern principles of patient safety, and a robust safety culture.

Handoffs and handovers—Refer to the process when one healthcare professional updates another on the status of one or more patients for the purpose of taking over their care. Typical examples involve a physician who has been on call overnight telling an incoming physician about patients she has admitted so he can continue with their ongoing management, know what immediate issues to watch out for, and so on. Nurses similarly conduct a handover at the end of their shift, updating their colleagues about the status of the patients under their care and tasks that need to be performed. When the outgoing nurses return for their next duty period, they will in turn receive new updates during the change of shift handover.

Handovers in care have always carried risks: a professional who spent hours assessing and managing a patient, on completion of her work, provides a brief summary of the salient features of the case to an incoming professional who typically has other unfamiliar patients he must get to know. The summary may leave out key details due to oversight, exacerbated by an unstructured process and being rushed to finish work. Even structured, fairly thorough summaries during handovers may fail to capture nuances that could subsequently prove relevant.

Despite these long-recognized problems, handovers received relatively little attention until recent years, when they became more frequent. For instance, with reductions in duty hours for physician trainees, more handovers must occur in any given 24-hour period. And, with shorter lengths of stay in hospitals and other occupancy issues, patients more often move from one ward to another or from one institution to another (e.g., from an acute care hospital to a rehabilitation facility or skilled nursing facility).

Due to the increasing recognition of hazards associated with these transitions in care, the term "handovers" is often used to refer to the information transfer that occurs from one clinical setting to another (e.g., from hospital to nursing home), not just from one professional to another.

Health literacy—Individuals' ability to find, process, and comprehend the basic health information necessary to act on medical instructions and make decisions about their health. Numerous studies have documented the degree to which patients frequently do not understand basic information or instructions related to general aspects of their medical care, their medications, and procedures they will undergo. The limited ability to comprehend medical instructions or information in some cases reflects obvious language barriers (e.g., reviewing medication instructions in English with a patient who speaks very little English), but the scope of the problem reflects broader issues related to levels of education, cross-cultural differences, and overuse of technical terminology by clinicians.

Heuristic—Loosely defined or informal rules often arrived at through experience or trial and error that influence assessments and decisions (e.g., gastrointestinal complaints that wake patients up at night are unlikely to be benign in nature). Heuristics provide cognitive shortcuts in the face of complex situations, and thus serve an important purpose. Unfortunately, they can also turn out to be wrong, with frequently used heuristics often forming the basis for the many cognitive biases, such as anchoring bias, availability bias, confirmation bias, and others, that have received attention in the literature on diagnostic errors and medical decision making.

The Health Insurance Portability and Accountability Act (HIPAA)—HIPAA, passed by the U.S. Congress in 1996, was intended to increase privacy and security of patient information during electronic transmission or communication of "protected health information" (PHI) among providers or between providers and payers or other entities.

PHI includes all medical records and other individually identifiable health information. "Individually identifiable information" includes data explicitly linked to a patient, as well as health information with data items that carry a reasonable potential for allowing individual identification.

HIPAA also requires providers to offer patients certain rights with respect to their information, including the right to access and copy their records and the right to request amendments to the information contained in their records.

Administrative protections specified by HIPAA to promote the above regulations and rights include requirements for a Privacy Officer and staff training regarding the protection of patients' information.

High reliability organizations (HROs)—HROs refer to organizations or systems that operate in hazardous conditions but have fewer than their fair share of adverse events. Commonly discussed examples include air traffic control systems, nuclear power plants, and naval aircraft carriers. It is worth noting that, in the safety literature, organizations labeled as HROs are ones that operate with nearly failure-free performance records, not simply better than average ones. This shift in meaning is understandable given that the failure rates in these other industries are much lower than rates of errors and adverse events in healthcare. This comparison glosses over the difference in significance of a "failure" in the nuclear power industry compared with one in healthcare. The point remains, however, that some organizations achieve consistently safe and effective performance records despite unpredictable operating environments or intrinsically hazardous endeavors. Detailed case studies of specific HROs have identified some common features, which have been offered as models for other organizations to achieve substantial improvements in their safety records. These features include:

- Preoccupation with failure—the acknowledgment of the high-risk, error-prone nature of an organization's activities and the determination to achieve consistently safe operations.
- Commitment to resilience—the development of capacities to detect unexpected threats and contain them before they cause harm, or bounce back when they do.
- Sensitivity to operations—an attentiveness to the issues facing workers at the frontline. This feature comes into play when conducting analyses of specific events (e.g., frontline workers play a crucial role in root cause analysis by bringing up unrecognized latent threats in current operating procedures), but also in connection with organizational decision making.
- Decentralized decision making—management units at the frontline are given some autonomy in identifying and responding to threats, rather than adopting a rigid top-down approach.
- A culture of safety, in which individuals feel comfortable drawing attention to potential hazards or actual failures without fear of censure from management.

Hindsight bias—In a very general sense, hindsight bias relates to the common expression, "hindsight is 20/20." This expression captures the tendency for people to regard past events as expected or obvious, even when, in real time, the events perplexed those involved. More formally, one might say that after learning the outcome of a series of events—whether the outcome of the World Series or the steps leading to a war—people tend to exaggerate the extent to which they had foreseen the likelihood of its occurrence.

In the context of safety analysis, hindsight bias refers to the tendency to judge the events leading up to an accident as errors because the bad outcome is known. The more severe the outcome, the more likely that decisions leading up to this outcome will be judged as errors. Judging the antecedent decisions as errors implies that the outcome was preventable. In legal circles, one might use the phrase "but for," as in "but for these errors in judgment, this terrible outcome would not have occurred." Such judgments return us to the concept of "hindsight is 20/20." Those reviewing events after the fact see the outcome as more foreseeable and therefore more preventable than they would have appreciated in real time.

Human factors (or human factors engineering)—Refers to the study of human abilities and characteristics as they affect the design and smooth operation of equipment, systems, and jobs. The field concerns itself with considerations of the strengths and weaknesses of human physical and mental abilities and how these affect the systems design. Human factors analysis does not require designing or redesigning existing objects. For instance, the now generally accepted recommendation that hospitals standardize equipment such as ventilators, programmable IV pumps, and defibrillators (i.e., each hospital picks a single type, so that different floors do not have different defibrillators) is an example of a very basic application of a heuristic from human factors that equipment be standardized within a system wherever possible.

Iatrogenic—An adverse effect of medical care, rather than of the underlying disease (literally "brought forth by healer," from Greek *iatros*, for healer, and *gennan*, to bring forth); equivalent to adverse event.

Incident reporting—Refers to the identification of occurrences that could have led, or did lead, to an undesirable outcome. Reports usually come from personnel directly involved in the incident or events leading up to it (e.g., the nurse, pharmacist, or physician caring for a patient when a medication error occurred) rather than, say, floor managers. From the perspective of those collecting the data, incident reporting counts as a *passive* form of surveillance, relying on those involved in target incidents to provide the desired information. Compared with medical record review and direct observation (*active* methods), incident reporting captures only a fraction of incidents, but has the advantages of relatively low cost and the involvement of frontline personnel in the process of identifying important problems for the organization.

Informed consent—Refers to the process whereby a physician informs a patient about the risks and benefits of a proposed therapy or test. Informed consent aims to provide sufficient information about the proposed course and any reasonable alternatives that the patient can exercise autonomy in deciding whether to proceed.

Legislation governing the requirements of, and conditions under which, consent must be obtained varies by jurisdiction. Most general guidelines require patients to be informed of the nature of their condition, the proposed procedure, the purpose of the procedure, the risks and benefits of the proposed treatments, the probability of the anticipated risks and benefits, alternatives to the treatment and their associated risks and benefits, and the risks and benefits of not receiving the treatment or procedure.

Although the goals of informed consent are irrefutable, consent is often obtained in a haphazard, pro forma fashion, with patients having little true understanding of procedures to which they have consented. Evidence suggests that asking patients to restate the essence of the informed consent improves the quality of these discussions and makes it more likely that the consent is truly informed.

Just culture—The phrase "Just Culture" was popularized in the patient safety lexicon by David Marx, who outlined principles for achieving a culture in which frontline personnel feel comfortable disclosing errors—including their own—while maintaining professional accountability.

Traditionally, healthcare's culture has held individuals accountable for all errors or mishaps that befall patients under their care. By contrast, a Just Culture recognizes that individual practitioners should not be held accountable for system failings over which they have no control. It also recognizes many individual or "active" errors are the result of predictable interactions between human operators and the systems in which they work. However, in contrast to a culture that touts "no blame" as its governing principle, a Just Culture does not tolerate conscious disregard of clear risks to patients or gross misconduct (e.g., falsifying a record, performing professional duties while intoxicated).

In summary, a Just Culture recognizes that competent professionals make mistakes and acknowledges that even competent professionals will develop unhealthy norms (shortcuts, "routine rule violations"), but has zero tolerance for reckless behavior.

Latent error (or latent condition)—The terms *active* and *latent* as applied to errors were coined by James Reason. Latent errors (or latent conditions) refer to less apparent failures of organization or design that contributed to the occurrence of errors or allowed them to cause harm to patients. For instance, whereas the active failure in a particular adverse event may have been a mistake in programming an intravenous pump, a latent error might be that the institution uses multiple different types of infusion pumps, making programming errors more likely. Thus, latent errors are quite literally "accidents waiting to happen." Latent errors are sometimes referred to as errors at the blunt end, referring to the many layers of the healthcare system that affect the person "holding" the scalpel. Active failures, in contrast, are sometimes referred to as errors at the sharp end, or the personnel and parts of the healthcare system in direct contact with patients.

Learning curve—The acquisition of any new skill is associated with the potential for lower-than-expected success rates or higher-than-expected complication rates. This phenomenon is often known as a learning curve. In some cases, this learning curve can be quantified in terms of the number of procedures that must be performed before an operator can replicate the outcomes of more experienced operators or centers. While learning curves are almost inevitable when new procedures emerge or new providers are in training, minimizing their impact is a patient safety imperative. One option is to perform initial operations or procedures under the supervision of more experienced operators. Surgical and procedural simulators may play an increasingly important role in decreasing the impact of learning curves on patients, by allowing acquisition of relevant skills in laboratory settings.

Magnet hospital status—Refers to a designation by the Magnet Hospital Recognition Program administered by the American Nurses Credentialing Center. The program has its genesis in a 1983 study conducted by the American Academy of Nursing that sought to identify hospitals that retained nurses for longer than average periods of time. The study identified institutional characteristics correlated with high retention rates, an important finding in light of a major nursing shortage at the time. These findings provided the basis for the concept of magnet hospital and led 10 years later to the formal Magnet Program.

Without taking anything away from the particular hospitals that have achieved magnet status, the program has its critics. Regardless of the particulars of the Magnet Recognition Program and the lack of persuasive evidence linking magnet status to quality, to many the term magnet hospital connotes a hospital that delivers superior patient care and, partly on this basis, attracts and retains high-quality nurses.

Medical Emergency Team—See "Rapid Response Team."

Medication reconciliation—Patients admitted to a hospital commonly receive new medications or have changes made to their existing medications. As a result, the new medication regimen prescribed at the time of discharge may inadvertently omit needed medications that patients have been receiving for some time. Alternatively, new medications may unintentionally duplicate existing medications. Such unintended inconsistencies in medication regimens may occur at any point of transition in care (e.g., transfer from an intensive care unit [ICU] to a general ward), not just hospital admission or discharge. Medication reconciliation refers to the process of avoiding such inadvertent inconsistencies across transitions in care by reviewing the patient's complete medication regimen at the time of admission, transfer, and discharge and comparing it with the regimen being considered for the new setting of care.

Mental model—Mental models are psychological representations of real, hypothetical, or imaginary situations. Scottish psychologist Kenneth Craik (1943) first proposed mental models as the basis for anticipating events and explaining events (i.e., for reasoning). Though easiest to conceptualize in terms of mental pictures of objects (e.g., a DNA double helix or the inside of an internal combustion engine), mental models can also include "scripts" or processes and other properties beyond images. Mental models create differing expectations, which suggest different courses of action. For instance, when you walk into a fast-food restaurant, you are invoking a different mental model than when you enter a fancy restaurant. Based on this model, you automatically go to place your order at the counter, rather than sitting at a booth and expecting a waiter to take your order.

Metacognition—Metacognition refers to thinking about thinking—that is, reflecting on the thought processes that led to a particular diagnosis or decision to consider whether biases or cognitive short cuts may have had a detrimental effect. In some ways, metacognition amounts to playing devil's advocate with oneself when it comes to working diagnoses and important therapeutic decisions. However, the devil is often in the details—one must become familiar with the variety of specific biases that commonly affect medical reasoning. For instance, when discharging a patient with atypical chest pain from the emergency department, you might step back and consider how much the discharge diagnosis of musculoskeletal pain reflects the sign-out as a "soft rule out" you received from a colleague on the night shift. Or, you might mull over the degree to which your reaction to and assessment of a particular patient stemmed from his having been labeled a "frequent flyer." Another cognitive bias is that clinicians tend to assign more importance to pieces of information that required personal effort to obtain.

Mistakes—In some contexts, errors are dichotomized as slips or mistakes, based on the cognitive psychology of task-oriented behavior. Mistakes reflect failures during attentional behaviors—behavior that requires conscious thought, analysis, and planning, as in active problem solving. Rather than lapses in concentration (as with slips), mistakes typically involve insufficient knowledge, failure to correctly interpret available information, or application of the wrong cognitive heuristic or rule. Thus, choosing the wrong diagnostic test or ordering a suboptimal medication for a given condition represents a mistake. Mistakes often reflect lack of experience or insufficient training. Reducing the likelihood of mistakes typically requires more training, supervision, or occasionally disciplinary action (in the case of negligence).

Unfortunately, healthcare has typically responded to all errors as if they were mistakes, with remedial education and/or added layers of supervision. In point of fact, most errors are actually slips, which are failures of schematic behavior that occur due to fatigue, stress, or emotional distractions, and are prevented through sharply different mechanisms.

Near miss—See "close call."

"Never Events" list—Nickname for a list launched and managed by the National Quality Forum, initially intended to be "things that should never happen in healthcare." The list, whose real name is the "Serious Reportable Events" list, has expanded over time to include adverse events that are unambiguous, serious, and to a reasonable degree preventable (Appendix VI). While most are rare, never events may be devastating to patients and indicate serious underlying organizational safety problems.

Normal accident theory—Though less often cited than high reliability theory in the healthcare literature, normal accident theory has played a prominent role in the study of complex organizations. In contrast to the optimism of high reliability theory, normal accident theory suggests that, at least in some settings, major accidents become inevitable and, thus, in a sense, "normal."

Safety expert Charles Perrow proposed two factors that create an environment in which a major accident becomes increasingly likely over time: complexity and tight coupling. The degree of complexity envisioned by Perrow occurs when no single operator can immediately foresee the consequences of a given action in the system. Tight coupling occurs when processes are intrinsically time dependent—once a process has been set in motion, it must be completed within a certain period of time. Importantly, normal accident theory contends that accidents become inevitable in complex, tightly coupled systems regardless of steps taken to increase safety. In fact, these steps sometimes increase the risk for future accidents through unintended collateral effects and general increases in system complexity.

Even if one does not believe the central contention of normal accident theory—that the potential for catastrophe emerges as an intrinsic property of certain complex systems—analyses informed by this theory's perspective have offered some fascinating insights into possible failure modes for high-risk organizations, including hospitals.

Normalization of deviance—The term "normalization of deviance" was coined by Diane Vaughan in her book *The Challenger Launch Decision*, in which she analyzes the interactions between various cultural forces within NASA that contributed to the Challenger disaster. Vaughn used this expression to describe the gradual shift in what is regarded as normal after repeated exposures to "deviant behavior" (behavior straying from correct [or safe] operating procedure). Corners get cut, safety checks bypassed, and alarms ignored or turned off, and these behaviors become *normal*—not just common but also stripped of their significance as warnings of impending danger. In their 2002 *Annals of Internal Medicine* discussion of a catastrophic error in healthcare, Chassin and Becher coined the phrase "a culture of low expectations." When a system routinely produces errors (paperwork in the wrong chart, major miscommunications between different members of a given healthcare team, patients in the dark about important aspects of the care), providers in the system become inured to malfunction. In such a system, what should be regarded as a major warning of impending danger is ignored as a *normal* operating procedure.

Patient safety—Fundamentally, patient safety refers to freedom from accidental or preventable injuries produced by medical care. Thus, practices or interventions that improve patient safety are those that reduce the occurrence of preventable adverse events.

Pay for performance ("P4P")—Refers to the general strategy of promoting quality improvement by rewarding providers (meaning individual clinicians or, more commonly, clinics or hospitals) who meet certain performance expectations with respect to healthcare quality or efficiency.

Performance can be defined in terms of patient outcomes but is more commonly defined in terms of processes of care (e.g., the percentage of eligible diabetics referred for annual retinal examinations, the percentage of children who received immunizations appropriate for their age, patients admitted to the hospital with pneumonia who receive antibiotics within six hours). P4P initiatives reflect the efforts of purchasers of healthcare—from the federal government to private insurers—to use their purchasing power to encourage providers to develop whatever specific quality improvement initiatives are required to achieve the specified targets. Thus, rather than committing to a specific quality improvement strategy, such as a new information system or a disease management program, which may have variable success in different institutions, P4P creates a climate in which provider groups will be strongly incentivized to find whatever solutions will work for them.

Plan–do–study–act—Commonly referred to as PDSA, refers to the cycle of activities advocated for achieving process or system improvement. The cycle was first proposed by Walter Shewhart, one of the pioneers of statistical process control (see "run charts") and popularized by his student, quality expert W. Edwards Deming. The PDSA cycle represents one of the cornerstones of continuous quality improvement (CQI). The components of the cycle are briefly described as follows:

- Plan: Analyze the problem you intend to improve and devise a plan to correct the problem.
- Do: Carry out the plan (preferably as a pilot project to avoid major investments of time or money in unsuccessful efforts).
- Study: Did the planned action succeed in solving the problem? If not, what went wrong? If partial success was achieved, how could the plan be refined?
- Act: Adopt the change piloted above as is, abandon it as a complete failure, or modify it and run through the cycle again.

Regardless of which action is taken, the PDSA cycle continues, with either the same problem or a new one.

Potential ADE—A potential ADE is a medication error or other drug-related mishap that reached the patient but happened not to produce harm (e.g., a penicillin-allergic patient receives penicillin but happens not to have an adverse reaction). In some studies, potential ADEs refer to errors or other problems that, if not intercepted, would be expected to cause harm. Thus, in some studies, if a physician ordered penicillin for a patient with a documented serious penicillin allergy, the order would be characterized as a potential ADE, on the grounds that administration of the drug would carry a substantial risk of harm to the patient.

Production pressure—Represents the pressure to put quantity of output—for a product or a service—ahead of safety. This pressure is seen in its starkest form in the line speed of factory assembly lines, famously demonstrated by Charlie Chaplin in *Modern Times*, as he is carried away on a conveyor belt and into the giant gears of the factory by the rapidly moving assembly line.

In healthcare, production pressure refers to delivery of services—the pressure to run hospitals at 100% capacity, with each bed filled with the sickest possible patients who are discharged at the first sign that they are stable, or the pressure to leave no operating room unused and to keep moving through the schedule for each room as fast as possible. In a survey of anesthesiologists, half of respondents stated that they had witnessed at least one case in which production pressure resulted in what they regarded as unsafe care. Examples included elective surgery in patients without adequate preoperative evaluation and proceeding with surgery despite significant contraindications.

Production pressure produces an organizational culture in which frontline personnel (and often managers) are reluctant to suggest any course of action that compromises productivity, even temporarily. For instance, in the survey of anesthesiologists, respondents reported pressure by surgeons to avoid delaying cases through additional patient evaluation or canceling cases, even when patients had clear contraindications to surgery.

Rapid Response Team (RRT)—The concept of RRTs (also known as Medical Emergency Teams) is that of a Code Blue team with more liberal calling criteria. Instead of just frank respiratory or cardiac arrest, RRTs respond to a wide range of worrisome, acute changes in patients' clinical status, such as low blood pressure, difficulty breathing, or altered mental status. In addition to less stringent calling criteria, RRTs (now sometimes called "Rapid Response Systems," to highlight the importance of the activation criteria as well as the response) de-emphasize the traditional hierarchy in patient care in that anyone can initiate the call. Nurses, junior medical staff, or others involved in the care of patients (and, in some hospitals, patients or family members) can call for the assistance of the RRT whenever they are worried about a patient's condition, without having to wait for more senior personnel to assess the patient and approve the decision to call for help.

Read-backs—When information is conveyed verbally, miscommunication may occur in a variety of ways, especially when transmission may not occur clearly (e.g., by telephone or radio, or if communication occurs under stress). For names and numbers, the problem often is confusing the sound of one letter or number with another. To address this possibility, the military, civil aviation, and many high-risk industries use protocols for mandatory read-backs, in which the listener repeats the key information, so that the transmitter can confirm its correctness.

Because mistaken substitution or reversal of alphanumeric information is such a potential hazard, read-back protocols typically include the use of phonetic alphabets, such as the NATO system ("Alpha–Bravo–Charlie–Delta–Echo … X-ray–Yankee–Zulu") now familiar to many. In healthcare, traditionally, read-back has been mandatory only in the context of checking to ensure accurate identification of recipients of blood transfusions. However, there are many other circumstances in which healthcare teams could benefit from following such protocols, for example, when communicating key lab results or patient orders over the phone, and even when exchanging information in person (e.g., handoffs).

Red rules—Rules that must be followed to the letter. In the language of nonhealthcare industries, red rules "stop the line." In other words, any deviation from a red rule will bring work to a halt until compliance is achieved. Red rules, in addition to relating to important and risky processes, must also be simple and easy to remember.

An example of a red rule in healthcare might be the following: "No hospitalized patient can undergo a test of any kind, receive a medication or blood product, or undergo a procedure if they are not wearing an identification bracelet." The implication of designating this a red rule is that the moment a patient is identified as not meeting this condition, all activity must cease in order to verify the patient's identity and supply an identification band.

Healthcare organizations already have numerous rules and policies that call for strict adherence. The reason that some organizations are using red rules is that, unlike many standard rules, red rules will always be supported by the entire organization. In other words, when someone at the frontline calls for work to cease on the basis of a red rule, top management must always support this decision. Thus, when properly implemented, red rules should foster a culture of safety, as frontline workers will know that they can stop the line when they notice potential hazards, even when doing so may result in considerable inconvenience or be time consuming and costly, for their immediate supervisors or the organization as a whole.

Root cause analysis—A structured process for identifying the causal or contributing factors underlying adverse events or other critical incidents. The key advantage of RCA over traditional clinical case reviews is that it follows a predefined protocol for identifying specific contributing factors in various causal categories (e.g., personnel, training, equipment, protocols, scheduling) rather than attributing the incident to the first error one finds or to preconceived notions investigators might have about the case.

Rule of thumb—See "Heuristic."

Run charts—A type of statistical process control or quality control graph in which some observation (e.g., manufacturing defects or adverse outcomes) is plotted over time to see if there are "runs" of points above or below a center line, usually representing the average or median. In addition to the number of runs, the length of the runs conveys important information. For run charts with more than 20 useful observations, a run of 8 or more dots would count as a "shift" in the process of interest, suggesting some nonrandom variation. Other key tests applied to run charts include tests for "trends" (sequences of successive increases or decreases in the observation of interest) and "zigzags" (alternation in the direction—up or down—of the lines joining pairs of dots). If a nonrandom change for the better, or shift, occurs, it suggests that an intervention has succeeded. The expression "moving the dots" refers to this type of shift.

Safety culture—Safety culture refers to a commitment to safety that permeates all levels of an organization, from frontline personnel to executive management. More specifically, "safety culture" calls up a number of features identified in studies of high reliability organizations, organizations outside of healthcare with exemplary performance with respect to safety, including:

- Acknowledgment of the high-risk, error-prone nature of an organization's activities
- A blame-free environment where individuals are able to report errors or close calls without fear of reprimand or punishment
- An expectation of collaboration across ranks to seek solutions to vulnerabilities
- A willingness on the part of the organization to direct resources to addressing safety concerns

Sentinel event—An adverse event in which death or serious harm to a patient has occurred; usually used to refer to events that are not at all expected or acceptable—for example, an operation on the wrong patient or body part. The choice of the word *sentinel* reflects the egregiousness of the injury (e.g., amputation of the wrong leg) and the likelihood that investigation of such events will reveal serious problems in current policies or procedures.

Sensemaking—A term from organizational theory that refers to the processes by which an organization takes in information to make sense of its environment, to generate knowledge, and to make decisions. It is the organizational equivalent of what individuals do when they process information, interpret events in their environments, and make decisions based on these activities. More technically, organizational sensemaking constructs the shared meanings that define the organization's purpose and frame the perception of problems or opportunities that the organization needs to work on.

Sharp end—The sharp end refers to the personnel or parts of the health-care system in direct contact with patients. Personnel operating at the sharp end may literally be holding a scalpel (e.g., an orthopedist who operates on the wrong leg) or figuratively be administering any kind of therapy (e.g., a nurse programming an intravenous pump) or performing any aspect of care. To complete the metaphor, the blunt end refers to the many layers of the healthcare system that affect the scalpels, pills, and medical devices, or the personnel wielding, administering, and operating them. Thus, an error in programming an intravenous pump would represent a problem at the sharp end, while the institution's decision to use multiple types of infusion pumps (making programming errors more likely) would represent a problem at the blunt end. The terminology of "sharp" and "blunt" ends corresponds roughly to active failures and latent conditions.

Situational awareness—Situational awareness refers to the degree to which one's perception of a situation matches reality. In the context of crisis management, where the phrase is most often used, situational awareness includes awareness of fatigue and stress among team members (including oneself), environmental threats to safety, appropriate immediate goals, and the deteriorating status of the crisis (or patient). Failure to maintain situational awareness can result in various problems that compound the crisis. For instance, during a resuscitation, an individual or entire team may focus on a particular task, such as a difficult central line insertion or a particular medication to administer. Fixation on this problem can result in loss of situational awareness to the point that steps are not taken to address immediately life-threatening problems such as respiratory failure or a pulseless rhythm. In this context, maintaining situational awareness might be seen as equivalent to keeping the big picture in mind. Alternatively, in assigning tasks in a crisis, the leader may ignore signals from a team member, which may result in escalating anxiety for the team member, failure to perform the assigned task, or further patient deterioration.

Slips (or lapses)—Errors can be dichotomized as slips or mistakes, based on the cognitive psychology of task-oriented behavior. Slips refer to failures of schematic behaviors, or lapses in concentration (e.g., overlooking a step in a routine task due to a lapse in memory, an experienced surgeon nicking an adjacent organ during an operation due to a momentary lapse in concentration).

Slips occur in the face of competing sensory or emotional distractions, fatigue, and stress. Reducing the risk of slips requires attention to the designs of protocols, devices, and work environments—using checklists so key steps will not be omitted, reducing fatigue among personnel (or shifting high-risk work away from personnel who have been working extended hours), removing unnecessary variation in the design of key devices, eliminating distractions (e.g., phones and pagers) from areas where work requires intense concentration, and other redesign strategies. Slips can be contrasted with mistakes, which are failures that occur in attentional behavior such as active problem solving.

Standard of care—What the average, prudent clinician would be expected to do under certain circumstances. The standard of care may vary by community (e.g., due to resource constraints). When the term is used in the clinical setting, the standard of care is generally felt not to vary by specialty or level of training. In other words, the standard of care for a condition may well be defined in terms of the standard expected of a specialist, in which case a generalist (or trainee) would be expected to deliver the same care or make a timely referral to the appropriate specialist (or supervisor, in the case of a trainee). Standard of care is also a term of art in malpractice law, and its definition varies from jurisdiction to jurisdiction. When used in this legal sense, often the standard of care is specific to a given specialty; it is often defined as the care expected of a reasonable practitioner with similar training practicing in the same location under the same circumstances.

Structure–process–outcome triad ("Donabedian Triad")—Most definitions of quality emphasize favorable patient outcomes as the gold standard for assessing quality. In practice, however, one would like to detect quality problems without waiting for poor outcomes to develop in such sufficient numbers that deviations from expected rates of morbidity and mortality can be detected. Donabedian first proposed that quality could be measured using aspects of care with proven relationships to desirable patient outcomes. For instance, if proven diagnostic and therapeutic strategies are monitored, quality problems can be detected long before demonstrable poor outcomes occur.

Aspects of care with proven connections to patient outcomes fall into two general categories: process and structure. Processes encompass all that is done to patients in terms of diagnosis, treatment, monitoring, and counseling. Cardiovascular care provides classic examples of the use of process measures to assess quality. Given the known benefits of aspirin and beta-blockers for patients with myocardial infarction, the quality of care for patients with myocardial infarction can be measured in terms of the rates at which eligible patients receive these proven therapies. The percentage of eligible women who undergo mammography at appropriate intervals would provide a process-based measure for quality of preventive care for women.

Structure refers to the setting in which care occurs and the capacity of that setting to produce quality. Traditional examples of structural measures related to quality include credentials, patient volume, and academic affiliation. More recent structural measures include the adoption of organizational models for inpatient care (e.g., closed ICUs and dedicated stroke units) and possibly the presence of sophisticated clinical information systems. Cardiovascular care provides another classic example of structural measures of quality. Numerous studies have shown that institutions that perform more cardiac surgeries and invasive cardiology procedures achieve better outcomes than institutions that see fewer patients. Given these data, patient volume represents a structural measure of quality of care for patients undergoing cardiac procedures.

Swiss cheese model—James Reason developed the "Swiss cheese model" (Figure 2-1) to illustrate how analyses of major accidents and catastrophic systems failures tend to reveal multiple, smaller failures leading up to the actual hazard.

In the model, each slice of cheese represents a safety barrier or precaution relevant to a particular hazard. For example, if the hazard were wrong-site surgery, slices of the cheese might include conventions for identifying sidedness on radiology tests, a protocol for signing the correct site when the surgeon and patient first meet, and a second protocol for reviewing the medical record and checking the previously marked site in the operating room. Many more layers exist. The point is that no single barrier is foolproof. They each have "holes," hence the Swiss cheese. For some serious events (e.g., operating on the wrong site or wrong person), even though the holes will align infrequently, even rare cases of harm (errors making it "through the cheese") will be unacceptable.

While the model may convey the impression that the slices of cheese and the location of their respective holes are independent, this may not be the case. For instance, in an emergency situation, all three of the surgical identification safety checks mentioned above may fail or be bypassed. The surgeon may meet the patient for the first time in the operating room. A hurried x-ray technologist might mislabel a film (or simply hang it backwards and a hurried surgeon not notice), "signing the site" may not take place at all (e.g., if the patient is unconscious), or, if it takes place, be rushed and offer no real protection. In the technical parlance of accident analysis, the different barriers may have a common failure mode, in which several protections are lost at once (i.e., the holes in several layers of the cheese line up).

In healthcare, such failure modes, in which slices of the cheese line up more often than one would expect if the location of their holes were independent of each other (and certainly more often than wings fall off airplanes), occur distressingly commonly. In fact, many of the systems problems discussed by Reason and others—poorly designed work schedules, lack of teamwork, and variations in the design of important equipment between and even within institutions—are sufficiently common that many of the slices of cheese already have their holes aligned. In such cases, one slice of cheese may be all that is left between the patient and significant hazard.

Systems approach—Medicine has traditionally treated quality problems and errors as failings on the part of individual providers, perhaps reflecting inadequate knowledge or skill levels. The systems approach, by contrast, takes the view that most errors reflect predictable human failings in the context of poorly designed systems (e.g., expected lapses in human vigilance in the face of long work hours or predictable mistakes on the part of relatively inexperienced personnel faced with cognitively complex situations). Rather than focusing corrective efforts on reprimanding individuals or pursuing remedial education, the systems approach seeks to identify situations or factors likely to give rise to human error and implement systems changes that will reduce their occurrence or minimize their impact on patients. This view holds that efforts to catch human errors before they occur or block them from causing harm will ultimately be more fruitful than ones that seek to somehow create flawless providers.

This systems focus includes paying attention to human factors engineering (or ergonomics), including the design of protocols, schedules, and other factors that are routinely addressed in other high-risk industries but have traditionally been ignored in medicine.

"Time outs"—Refer to planned periods of quiet and/or interdisciplinary discussion focused on ensuring that key procedural details have been addressed. For instance, protocols for ensuring correct site surgery often recommend a time out to confirm the identification of the patient, the surgical procedure, site, and other key aspects, often stating them aloud for double-checking by other team members. In addition to avoiding major misidentification errors involving the patient or surgical site, such a time out ensures that all team members share the same "game plan," so to speak. Taking the time to focus on listening and communicating the plans as a team can rectify miscommunications and misunderstandings before a procedure gets underway.

Triggers—Refer to signals for detecting likely adverse events. Triggers alert providers involved in patient safety activities to probable adverse events so they can review the medical record to determine if an actual or potential adverse event has occurred. For instance, if a hospitalized patient received naloxone (a drug used to reverse the effects of narcotics), the patient probably received an excessive dose of morphine or some other opiate. In the emergency department, the use of naloxone would more likely represent treatment of a self-inflicted opiate overdose, so the trigger would have little value in that setting. But, among patients already admitted to hospital, a pharmacy could use the administration of naloxone as a "trigger" to investigate possible ADEs.

In cases in which the trigger correctly identified an adverse event, causative factors can be identified and, over time, interventions developed to reduce the frequency of particularly common causes of adverse events. The traditional use of triggers has been to efficiently identify adverse events after the fact. However, using triggers in real time has tremendous potential as a patient safety tool. In a study of real-time triggers in a single community hospital, for example, more than 1000 triggers were generated in 6 months, and approximately 25% led to physician action and would not have been recognized without the trigger.

As with any alert or alarm system, the threshold for generating triggers has to balance true and false positives. The system will lose its value if too many triggers prove to be false alarms. This concern is less relevant when triggers are used as chart review tools. In such cases, the tolerance of false alarms depends only on the availability of sufficient resources for medical record review. Reviewing four false alarms for every true adverse event might be quite reasonable in the context of an institutional safety program, but frontline providers would balk at (and eventually ignore) a trigger system that generated four false alarms for every true one.

Underuse, overuse, and misuse—For process of care, quality problems can arise in one of the three ways: underuse, overuse, and misuse.

Underuse refers to the failure to provide a healthcare service when it would have produced a favorable outcome for a patient. Standard examples include failures to provide appropriate preventive services to eligible patients (e.g., Pap smears, flu shots for elderly patients, screening for hypertension) and proven medications for chronic illnesses (steroid inhalers for asthmatics; aspirin, beta-blockers, and lipid-lowering agents for patients who have suffered a recent myocardial infarction).

Overuse refers to providing a process of care in circumstances where the potential for harm exceeds the potential for benefit. Prescribing an antibiotic for a viral infection such as a cold, for which antibiotics are ineffective, constitutes overuse. The potential for harm includes adverse reactions to the antibiotics and increases in antibiotic resistance among bacteria in the community. Overuse can also apply to diagnostic tests and surgical procedures.

Misuse occurs when an appropriate process of care has been selected but a preventable complication occurs and the patient does not receive the full potential benefit of the service. Avoidable complications of surgery or medication use are misuse problems. A patient who suffers a rash after receiving penicillin for strep throat, despite having a known allergy to that antibiotic, is an example of misuse. A patient who develops a pneumothorax after an inexperienced operator attempted to insert a subclavian line would represent another example of misuse.

Workaround—From the perspective of frontline personnel trying to accomplish their work, the design of equipment or the policies governing work tasks can seem counterproductive. When frontline personnel adopt consistent patterns of bypassing safety features of medical equipment, these patterns and actions are referred to as workarounds. Although workarounds "fix the problem," the system remains unaltered and thus continues to present potential safety hazards for future patients.

From a definitional point of view, it does not matter if frontline users are justified in working around a given policy or equipment design feature. What does matter is that the motivation for a workaround lies in getting work done, not laziness or whim. Thus, the appropriate response by managers to the existence of a workaround should not consist of reflexively reminding staff about the policy and restating the importance of following it. Rather, workarounds should trigger assessment of workflow and the various competing demands for the time of frontline personnel. In busy clinical areas where efficiency is paramount, managers can expect workarounds to arise whenever policies create added tasks for frontline personnel, especially when the extra work is perceived to be out of proportion to the importance of the safety goal.

Reproduced with permission from Shojania KG, Wachter RM, Hartman E. *The AHRQ WebM&M Glossary*. Available at: http://webmm.ahrq.gov/glossary.aspx.

APPENDIX III. SELECTED MILESTONES IN THE FIELD OF PATIENT SAFETY

Year	Event
Fourth century BC	Hippocrates writes, "I will never do harm to anyone," which is later translated (and changed) into "Primum non nocere," or "first do no harm."
1857	Ignaz Semmelweiss publishes his findings, demonstrating that hand disinfection leads to fewer infections (puerperal fever).
1863	Florence Nightingale, in *Notes on Hospitals*, writes, "It may seem a strange principle to enunciate as the very first requirement in a Hospital that it should do the sick no harm."
1911	Ernest Codman, a Boston surgeon, establishes his "End Result" hospital—with a goal of following and learning from patient outcomes, include errors in treatment.
1917	The first specialty board (ophthalmology) is formed. Ultimately, 24 boards are founded to certify physicians in the United States.
1918	The American College of Surgeons begins the first program of hospital inspection and certification. In 1951, the program becomes the Joint Commission on Accreditation of Healthcare Organizations (JCAHO), now the Joint Commission.
1959	Robert Moser, an Army physician, publishes *Diseases of Medical Progress*, arguing that iatrogenic disease is common and preventable.
1964	Elihu Schimmel, a Yale physician, publishes one of the first studies of iatrogenic illness, finding that 20% of patients admitted to a university hospital experienced an "untoward episode."

(continued)

Year	Event
1977	Ivan Illich publishes *Limits of Medicine. Medical Nemesis: the Expropriation of Health*, arguing that healthcare is actually a threat to health.
1985	The Anesthesia Patient Safety Foundation (APSF) is founded, a year after Jeffrey Cooper's seminal paper analyzing failures in anesthesia machines. Twelve years later, the National Patient Safety Foundation is founded, modeled on the APSF.
1990	James Reason publishes *Human Error* (and, 7 years later, *Managing the Risks of Organisational Accidents*), describing his new theory of error as systems failure. His work will go undiscovered by healthcare until Leape's 1994 *JAMA* article.
1991	Publication of Harvard Medical Practice studies (from which the IOM later derives its 44,000–98,000 deaths/year estimate).
1994	Lucian Leape publishes *Error in Medicine* in *JAMA*, the first mainstream article in the healthcare literature arguing for a systems approach to safety.
1999	The release of the IOM report, *To Err is Human*, creates a media sensation and begins the modern patient safety movement.
2000	Following the IOM report, the UK's National Health Service releases another major report, *An Organisation with a Memory*.
2001	The IOM releases its *Quality Chasm* report.
2001	The Agency for Healthcare Research and Quality (AHRQ) receives $50 million from Congress to begin an aggressive patient safety research and improvement program.
2002	The Joint Commission releases its first National Patient Safety Goals.
2002	The National Quality Forum launches its list of Serious Reportable Events (the "Never Events" list), which later becomes the scaffolding for public reporting and "no pay" programs.
2003	The Accreditation Council on Graduate Medical Education (ACGME) institutes duty-hour regulations, limiting residents to 80 hours/week.
2004	The U.S. government creates the Office of the National Coordinator for Healthcare IT (ONCHIT), the first federal initiative to computerize healthcare.
2005–2006	The Institute for Healthcare Improvement launches its 100,000 Lives Campaign, followed a year later by its 5 Million Lives Campaign.
2005	The U.S. Congress passes the Patient Safety Act, paving the way for the creation of patient safety organizations beginning in 2009.
2006	Pronovost and colleagues report the results of the Keystone project, which slashed the rate of central line–associated bloodstream infections in Michigan intensive care units, and highlights the role of checklists in patient safety.

(continued)

Year	Event
2008	Medicare launches its "no pay for errors" initiative.
2010	Patient safety leader Don Berwick becomes director of the U.S. Centers for Medicare & Medicaid Services (CMS). A year later, he announces a "Partnership for Patients," with nearly $1 billion in support of patient safety and quality activities.
2011	The U.S. government begins distributing incentive payments to hospitals and doctors for implementing healthcare information technology (HIT) systems that meet certain "meaningful use" criteria.
2011	ACGME further tightens its residency duty-hour and supervision requirements.

Adapted from various sources, particularly Vincent C. *Patient Safety*. London: Elsevier; 2006; Sharpe VA, Faden AI. *Medical Harm: Historical, Conceptual, and Ethical Dimensions of Iatrogenic Illness*. New York, NY: Cambridge University Press; 1998; and author's own analysis.

APPENDIX IV. THE JOINT COMMISSION'S NATIONAL PATIENT SAFETY GOALS (HOSPITAL VERSION, 2011)

NPSG.01.01.01
Use at least two patient identifiers when providing care, treatment, and services.

NPSG.01.03.01
Eliminate transfusion errors related to patient misidentification.

NPSG.02.03.01
Report critical results of tests and diagnostic procedures on a timely basis.

NPSG.03.04.01
Label all medications, medication containers, and other solutions on and off the sterile field in perioperative and other procedural settings. *Note*: Medication containers include syringes, medicine cups, and basins.

NPSG.03.05.01
Reduce the likelihood of patient harm associated with the use of anticoagulant therapy.

NPSG.03.06.01
Maintain and communicate accurate patient medication information.

NPSG.07.01.01
Comply with either the current Centers for Disease Control and Prevention (CDC) hand hygiene guidelines or the current World Health Organization (WHO) hand hygiene guidelines.

NPSG.07.03.01

Implement evidence-based practices to prevent healthcare-associated infections due to multidrug-resistant organisms in acute care hospitals. *Note*: This requirement applies to, but is not limited to, epidemiologically important organisms such as methicillin-resistant *Staphylococcus aureus* (MRSA), *Clostridium difficile* (CDI), vancomycin-resistant enterococci (VRE), and multidrug-resistant gram-negative bacteria.

NPSG.07.04.01

Implement evidence-based practices to prevent central line–associated blood-stream infections. *Note*: This requirement covers short- and long-term central venous catheters and peripherally inserted central catheter (PICC) lines.

NPSG.07.05.01

Implement evidence-based practices for preventing surgical site infections.

NPSG.07.06.01

Implement evidence-based practices to prevent indwelling catheter-associated urinary tract infections (CAUTI).

NPSG.15.01.01

Identify patients at risk for suicide. *Note*: This requirement applies only to psychiatric hospitals and patients being treated for emotional or behavioral disorders in general hospitals.

UP.01.01.01

Conduct a preprocedure verification process.

UP.01.02.01

Mark the procedure site.

UP.01.03.01

A time out is performed before the procedure.

Reproduced with permission from http://www.jointcommission.org/assets/1/6/NPSG_EPs_Scoring_HAP_20110706.pdf.

Skipped numbers represent retired Goals (the numbers are not replaced).

NPSG, National Patient Safety Goal; UP, Universal Protocol.

APPENDIX V. AGENCY FOR HEALTHCARE RESEARCH AND QUALITY'S (AHRQ) PATIENT SAFETY INDICATORS (PSIs)

Hospital-level PSIs (n = 18)

- Death in low-mortality diagnosis-related groups
- Pressure ulcer
- Death among surgical inpatients with treatable serious complications
- Foreign body left in during procedure

- Iatrogenic pneumothorax
- Central venous catheter-related bloodstream infections
- Postoperative hip fracture
- Postoperative hemorrhage or hematoma
- Postoperative physiologic and metabolic derangements
- Postoperative respiratory failure
- Postoperative pulmonary embolism or deep vein thrombosis
- Postoperative sepsis
- Postoperative wound dehiscence
- Accidental puncture or laceration
- Transfusion reaction
- Birth trauma—injury to neonate
- Obstetric trauma—vaginal delivery with instrument
- Obstetric trauma—vaginal delivery without instrument

Area-level indicators (e.g., county, state) (n = 7)

- Foreign body left in during procedure
- Iatrogenic pneumothorax
- Central venous catheter-related bloodstream infection
- Accidental puncture or laceration
- Postoperative hemorrhage or hematoma
- Postoperative wound dehiscence
- Transfusion reaction

Reprinted from *Patient Safety Indicators. A Tool to Help Assess Quality and Safety of Care to Adults in the Hospital* [brochure]. AHRQ Publication No. 10-M043-4. Rockville, MD: Agency for Healthcare Research and Quality; July 2010. Available at: http://www.qualityindicators.ahrq.gov/modules/psi_resources.aspx.

APPENDIX VI. THE NATIONAL QUALITY FORUM'S LIST OF SERIOUS REPORTABLE EVENTS, 2011

1. **Surgical or invasive procedure events (*n* = 5)**
   - Surgery or other invasive procedure performed on the wrong site
   - Surgery or other invasive procedure performed on the wrong patient
   - Wrong surgical or other invasive procedure performed on a patient
   - Unintended retention of a foreign object in a patient after surgery or other invasive procedure
   - Intraoperative or immediately postoperative/postprocedure death in an ASA Class 1 patient

2. **Product or device events (*n* = 3)**
   - Patient death or serious injury associated with the use of contaminated drugs, devices, or biologics provided by the healthcare setting

- Patient death or serious injury associated with the use or function of a device in patient care, in which the device is used for functions other than as intended
- Patient death or serious injury associated with intravascular air embolism that occurs while being cared for in a healthcare setting

3. **Patient protection events (*n* = 3)**
   - Discharge or release of a patient/resident of any age, who is unable to make decisions, to other than an authorized person
   - Patient death or serious injury associated with patient elopement (disappearance)
   - Patient suicide, attempted suicide, or self-harm that results in serious injury, while being cared for in a healthcare setting

4. **Care management events (*n* = 9)**
   - Patient death or serious injury associated with a medication error (e.g., errors involving the wrong drug, wrong dose, wrong patient, wrong time, wrong rate, wrong preparation, or wrong route of administration)
   - Patient death or serious injury associated with unsafe administration of blood products
   - Maternal death or serious injury associated with labor or delivery in a low-risk pregnancy while being cared for in a healthcare setting
   - Death or serious injury of a neonate associated with labor or delivery in a low-risk pregnancy (*new in 2011*)
   - Patient death or serious injury associated with a fall while being cared for in a healthcare setting
   - Any Stage 3, Stage 4, and unstageable pressure ulcers acquired after admission/presentation to a healthcare setting
   - Artificial insemination with the wrong donor sperm or wrong egg
   - Patient death or serious injury resulting from the irretrievable loss of an irreplaceable biological specimen (*new in 2011*)
   - Patient death or serious injury resulting from failure to follow up or communicate laboratory, pathology, or radiology test results (*new in 2011*)

5. **Environmental events (*n* = 4)**
   - Patient or staff death or serious injury associated with an electric shock in the course of a patient care process in a healthcare setting
   - Any incident in which systems designated for oxygen or other gas to be delivered to a patient contain no gas, the wrong gas, or are contaminated by toxic substances

- Patient or staff death or serious injury associated with a burn incurred from any source in the course of a patient care process in a health-care setting
- Patient death or serious injury associated with the use of physical restraints or bedrails while being cared for in a healthcare setting

6. **Radiologic events ($n = 1$)**
   - Death or serious injury of a patient or staff associated with the introduction of a metallic object into the MRI area (*new in 2011*)

7. **Potential criminal events ($n = 4$)**
   - Any instance of care ordered by or provided by someone impersonating a physician, nurse, pharmacist, or other licensed healthcare provider
   - Abduction of a patient/resident of any age
   - Sexual abuse/assault on a patient or staff member within or on the grounds of a healthcare setting
   - Death or serious injury of a patient or staff member resulting from a physical assault (i.e., battery) that occurs within or on the grounds of a healthcare setting

Reproduced with permission from The National Quality Forum. Available at: http://www.qualityforum.org/projects/hacs_and_sres.aspx. This list is still commonly known as the "Never Events" list.

APPENDIX VII. THE NATIONAL QUALITY FORUM'S LIST OF "SAFE PRACTICES FOR BETTER HEALTHCARE—2010 UPDATE"

Safe Practice	Practice Statement
1. Leadership structures and systems	Leadership structures and systems must be established to ensure that there is organization-wide awareness of patient safety performance gaps, leaders are directly accountable for those gaps and there is adequate investment in performance improvement abilities, and actions are taken to ensure safe care of every patient served.
2. Culture measurement, feedback, and intervention	Healthcare organizations must measure their culture, provide feedback to the leadership and staff, and undertake interventions that will reduce patient safety risk.
3. Teamwork training and skill building	Healthcare organizations must establish a proactive, systematic, organization-wide approach to developing team-based care through teamwork training, skill building, and team-led performance improvement interventions that reduce preventable harm to patients.

(continued)

Safe Practice	Practice Statement
4. Identification and mitigation of risks and hazards	Healthcare organizations must systematically identify and mitigate patient safety risks and hazards with an integrated approach in order to continuously drive down preventable patient harm.
5. Informed consent	Ask every patient or legal surrogate to "teach back," in his or her own words, key information about the proposed treatments or procedures for which he or she is being asked to provide informed consent.
6. Life-sustaining treatment	Ensure that written documentation of the patient's preferences for life-sustaining treatment is prominently displayed in his or her chart.
7. Disclosure	Following serious unanticipated outcomes, including those that are clearly caused by systems failures, the patient and, as appropriate, the family, should receive timely, transparent, and clear communication concerning what is known about the event.
8. Care of the caregiver	Following serious unintentional harm due to systems failures and/or errors that resulted from human performance failures, the involved caregivers should receive timely and systematic care—and the opportunity to fully participate in event investigation and risk identification and mitigation activities that will prevent future events.
9. Nursing workforce	Implement critical components of a well-designed nursing workforce, including (a) an adequate nursing plan, (b) senior nurse administrative leaders as part of the hospital's senior management team, (c) governance board engagement in nurse staffing decisions, and (d) budget to support nursing education and skill building.
10. Direct caregivers	Ensure that non-nursing direct care staffing levels are adequate, that staff are competent, and that they have had adequate orientation, training, and education.
11. Intensive care unit care	All patients in general ICUs should be managed by physicians who have specific training and certification in critical care medicine.
12. Patient care information	Ensure that care information is transmitted and appropriately documented in a timely manner and in a clearly understandable form to patients and to all relevant caregivers.
13. Order read-back and abbreviations	Incorporate a safe, effective communication strategy, structure, and systems to include (a) record and "read-backs" for verbal orders and critical test results; (b) use of a standard "do not use" abbreviation list.
14. Labeling of diagnostic studies	Implement standardized policies, processes, and systems to ensure accurate labeling of radiographs, lab specimens, and other studies to ensure accuracy.
15. Discharge systems	A "discharge plan" must be prepared for each patient at the time of hospital discharge, and a concise discharge summary must be relayed to the caregiver accepting responsibility for postdischarge care in a timely manner. Organizations should confirm receipt of this communication.

(continued)

Safe Practice	Practice Statement
16. Safe adoption of computerized provider order entry	Implement a CPOE system built on the requisite foundation of reengineered evidence-based care, an assurance of healthcare organization staff and independent practitioner readiness, and an integrated information technology infrastructure.
17. Medication reconciliation	The healthcare organization must develop, reconcile, and communicate an accurate patient medication list throughout the continuum of care.
18. Pharmacist leadership structures and systems	Pharmacy leaders should have an active role on the administrative leadership team that reflects their authority and accountability for medication management systems performance across the organization.
19. Hand hygiene	Comply with current Centers for Disease Control and Prevention (CDC) Hand Hygiene guidelines.
20. Influenza prevention	Comply with current CDC guidelines regarding influenza vaccination and prevention/control.
21. Central line–associated bloodstream infection prevention	Take actions to prevent central line–associated bloodstream infections by implementing evidence-based intervention practices.
22. Surgical site infection prevention	Take actions to prevent surgical site infections by implementing evidence-based intervention practices.
23. Care of the ventilated patient	Take actions to prevent complications associated with ventilated patients: ventilator-associated pneumonia, venous thromboembolism, peptic ulcer disease, dental complications, and pressure ulcers.
24. Multidrug-resistant organism prevention	Implement a systematic multidrug-resistant organization prevention program.
25. Catheter-associated urinary tract infection prevention	Take actions to prevent catheter-associated urinary tract infections by implementing evidence-based intervention practices.
26. Wrong-site, wrong-procedure, wrong-person surgery prevention	Implement the Universal Protocol for preventing wrong-site, wrong-procedure, wrong-person surgery for all procedures.
27. Pressure ulcer prevention	Take actions to prevent pressure ulcers by implementing evidence-based intervention practices.
28. Venous thromboembolism prevention	Evaluate each patient on admission and regularly thereafter for the risk of developing venous thromboembolism. Utilize clinically appropriate evidence-based prophylaxis methods.

(continued)

Safe Practice	Practice Statement
29. Anticoagulation practice	Organizations should implement practices to prevent harm due to anticoagulant therapy.
30. Contrast media–induced renal failure prevention	Utilize validated protocols to evaluate patients who are at risk for contrast media–induced renal failure and gadolinium-associated nephrogenic systemic fibrosis.
31. Organ donation	Hospital policies that are consistent with applicable law and regulations should be in place and should address patient and family preferences for organ donations.
32. Glycemic control	Take actions to improve glycemic control by implementing evidence-based intervention practices that prevent hypoglycemia and optimize the care of patients with hyperglycemia and diabetes.
33. Fall prevention	Take actions to prevent patient falls and to reduce fall-related injuries by implementing evidence-based intervention practices.
34. Pediatric imaging	When CT imaging studies are undertaken on children, "child-size" techniques should be used to reduce unnecessary exposure to ionizing radiation.

Adapted with permission from National Quality Forum. *Safe Practice for Better Healthcare—2010 Update. A Consensus Report.* Available at www.qualityforum.org.

APPENDIX VIII. MEDICARE'S "NO PAY FOR ERRORS" LIST*

- Stage III and IV pressure ulcers
- Fall or trauma resulting in serious injury
- Vascular catheter-associated infection
- Catheter-associated urinary tract infection
- Foreign object retained after surgery
- Certain surgical site infections
- Air embolism
- Blood incompatibility
- Certain manifestations of poor blood sugar control
- Certain deep vein thromboses or pulmonary embolisms

Source: Centers for Medicare & Medicaid Services.

---

*The policy works this way: if under the old payment system an item on this list would have increased the reimbursement for a given hospitalization under Medicare's system of diagnosis-related groups (DRGs), the hospital no longer receives that additional reimbursement under this policy. However, if there are any other so-called "complicating conditions," the hospital still does receive the higher reimbursement, markedly muting the financial impact of the policy. List is current as of January 2012.

APPENDIX IX. THINGS PATIENTS AND FAMILIES CAN DO, AND QUESTIONS THEY CAN ASK, TO IMPROVE THEIR CHANCES OF REMAINING SAFE IN THE HOSPITAL

What to Do or Check	Discussion or Recommendation
Make friends with your nurses, phlebotomists, and other hospital personnel. Make sure they address you by name at least once each shift.	
Before you are given a medication, ask what it is and what it's for.	
Before you are given a medication, a transfusion, an x-ray, or a procedure, make sure the nurse confirms your name by both asking you and checking your wristband.	Some hospitals may supplement this through the use of bar coding, for example, checking that the bar code on your wristband and the bar code on a medication bottle match.
Before being taken off the floor for a procedure, ask what it is and be sure you understand where you are going and why.	
Be sure your family members' contact information is available to the hospital or nursing home personnel.	It is not a bad idea to place a card with your family members' contact information by your bedside (in addition to being sure that this information is in the chart).
Before being transferred from floor to floor in a hospital (such as from the ICU to the general medical or surgical floor) or from one institution to another, check to be sure all catheters and other paraphernalia that should be removed have been.	Sometimes (particularly when there are no checklists), caregivers will forget to remove an IV line or urinary catheter before a transfer, which creates an unnecessary risk of infections. Believe it or not, doctors (one out of three in one study) will often forget whether their patient even has a urinary catheter in place. Don't be reluctant to ask your doctors or nurses whether you still need your catheters after the urgent need for them has passed.
Ask your caregivers whether they have washed (or cleaned) their hands.	Increasingly, you won't see them wash their hands, because they will be rubbing their hands with an antiseptic hand gel placed in a dispenser outside your room. I'd also want to know the hospital's overall hand hygiene rate, which should be above 80%.

(continued)

What to Do or Check	Discussion or Recommendation
What is the hospital's rate of central line–associated bloodstream infections?	Most hospitals with strong safety and infection prevention programs have driven this rate down to less than 1.5 per 1000 catheter-days. Similar benchmark rates for adverse events such as falls are likely to emerge in the next few years.
If you have an advance directive (and you should), keep a copy with you, make sure your family has one, give one to your nurse or doctor to place on your chart, and be certain it is transferred from site to site with you.	
Does the hospital have CPOE, an electronic medical record, and bar coding? If not, when do they plan to have them?	It would be great if they had them and they were up and running. If they have CPOE, ask what percent of physicians' orders are written on the computerized system (if it is less than half, then the doctors are still kicking the tires and the system is not really implemented). If CPOE and bar coding are not in place, it should be budgeted to be in place in the next few years. If not, I'd worry.
Is there a functioning, preferably computerized, incident reporting system, on which hospital personnel can report errors and near misses?	The computerized systems make reporting, and dissemination of the information, much easier. So it would be good to hear, "yes we do." Unfortunately, there is no guarantee that the hospital is using the reports productively to improve safety.
How many incident reports are logged each month?	Although it might seem counterintuitive, this is probably a case of the more the better. If a midsized hospital (approximately 300 beds) doesn't receive a few hundred reports a month, then it may be that workers aren't sharing errors and near misses because either they are worried about blame or they are convinced that it isn't worth reporting because reports enter a black hole.
What is done with these reports?	You'd like to know that they go to the relevant managers in the area (the catheterization lab, the OR), who are expected to respond to them. Also, there should be an uber manager who watches for trends (e.g., an uptick in patient falls, bed ulcers, or medication administration errors).
How many detailed root cause analyses have been done in the past year?	Like the incident reports, you might think that "zero" would be a great answer because it would mean there were no major errors. But you can be sure that there were. So I'd expect that the average hospital will have done at least 20 full-blown RCAs in the past year.

(continued)

What to Do or Check	Discussion or Recommendation
Is there a Patient Safety Officer who is compensated for this role? What are his or her qualifications?	Some small hospitals will not have a paid Patient Safety Officer, but all midsized and large hospitals should have one. This guarantees that it is someone's job to be concerned about safety. It should be a respected physician, nurse, or pharmacist with additional training in human factors, systems engineering, quality improvement, and similar areas.
Is there an active Patient Safety Committee that meets at least monthly?	The answer must be yes.
Are there trained intensivists in the critical care units (ICUs) and hospitalists on the medical wards?	There is strong evidence that the on-site presence of intensivists, at least during the day, is associated with better ICU outcomes. For small hospitals without intensivists, linking the ICU electronically to trained intensivists who remotely monitor the patients also may improve outcomes. The evidence supporting the value of hospitalists caring for general medical and surgical patients is not quite as strong, but two studies did show lower death rates. I believe that the on-site presence of physicians who specialize in overseeing and coordinating patients' hospital care is likely to improve safety.
Which physicians are "in house" overnight?	I'd like to know that there is at least one senior attending physician in the building overnight to deal with acute issues, even if there are also residents.
Are the physicians who will care for you board certified in their specialty?	All else being equal, board certification indicates that your physician has demonstrated a certain level of knowledge and competence, and is keeping up in his or her field.
What is the nurse-to-patient ratio, and what percentage of the nurses are registered nurses (RNs)?	Ratios of more than 6–7:1 on the medical and surgical wards are associated with higher rates of errors (it should be much lower, such as 2:1, in the ICUs). Error rates also seem to be higher when more than about 30% of total nursing care is delivered by non-RNs (i.e., licensed practical nurses or nurses' aides).
Are there clinical pharmacists on the hospital wards who can help you understand and organize your medications?	There is good evidence that the involvement of clinical pharmacists, particularly in the discharge process, improves safety.
What is the hospital's system to prevent readmissions?	Good hospitals now have organized programs to do this, including robust discharge counseling, some type of postdischarge follow-up (phone call or visit), a prompt discharge summary, and a well-organized and rapid visit to the follow-up provider.

(continued)

What to Do or Check	Discussion or Recommendation
Does the hospital run simulator or other specific teamwork training?	Ideally, the hospital would require simulator training for people working in high-risk areas such as the OR, ER, and on Code Blue teams. In addition, specific teamwork training (CRM) is helpful, and a hospital that has an organized simulator and CRM program is probably ahead of the patient safety curve.
What does the hospital do to prevent handoff errors?	I would want to know that, at very least, there are read-backs of verbal orders and checklists before patients move from one unit to another (such as the ICU to the floor or from the floor to a nursing home).
What patient safety initiatives has the hospital undertaken in the past year?	They should have several that they can describe proudly, preferably with measurable results they can cite.

Reproduced and updated with permission from Wachter RM, Shojania KG. *Internal Bleeding: The Truth Behind America's Terrifying Epidemic of Medical Mistakes*. New York, NY: Rugged Land; 2004.

Index

telephone, 126
telephonic interpretation services in care
of hospitalized patients, 374
therapeutic benefit, 7
thoracentesis, 88, 89
Ticket to Ride system, 139
time out, 80
"time outs," 447
Torrence, Scott (pseudonym), 341, 342
tort law and malpractice system, 322–327
dealing with judgment calls, 323
defensive medicine, 326
expert witnesses role in, 324
fault and compensation, 322, 324
injured patients' cases, 326–327
liability of caregivers, 323
medical error interpretation, 326
physicians facing malpractice claim,
324–326
rule violations, 323–324
trainee autonomy and supervising
physicians, 304–305
trainee-related transition, 292
training issues
autonomy *vs.* oversight, 304–307
demands of medical practice
and, 303
training programs, patient safety
education in, 315–316
transitions coach, 140
transitions, patient-related, 125–144
basic concepts, 126, 127
information, 128
preventing readmissions, 140–144
Trans World Airlines (TWA), 239
triggers, 447–448
trigger tools, use of, 9
Trowbridge, R. L., 101
TWA (Trans World Airlines), 239

U

UCSF Crew Resource Management, 268
UCSF Medical Center, 133
attending presence at, 305
root cause analysis process, 245–247
ultrasound, bedside, 89
underuse, 448
unit-based safety enterprise, 392–393

University of California, San Francisco,
See UCSF
University of Michigan Health System's
disclosure-with-offer program,
328–329
unstructured data, 209–210
urinary catheters, urinary tract infection
by, 169, 171, *See also* catheter-
associated urinary tract infection
urologic simulator, 313
usability testing, 114–118
U.S. healthcare system, transparency
in, 364
U.S. nursing shortage, 282
U.S. population growth, 373
U.S. Veterans Affairs (VA) hospitals, *See*
Veterans Affairs hospitals

V

value, 46–47
value-based purchasing program, 36
Van Zanten, Jacob, 150, 151
VAP. *See* Ventilator-associated pneumonia
Vasquez, Ramon, 55, 57
Vaughan, Diana, 273
Venn diagram, patient safety, 5
venous thromboembolism
clinical diagnosis of, 180
prevention strategies, 180
ACCP guidelines, 180
evidence-based prophylaxis,
180–181
national programs, 181
reimbursement strategy, 181
risk in hospitalized patient, 179–180
ventilator-associated pneumonia
incidence of, 166
prevention strategies, 165–167
Verghese, Abraham, 210, 211
Veterans Affairs Medical Centers
computer system, 207, 209
MRSA prevention efforts, 171, 172
policy of disclosure, apology, and
reasonable settlement, 327–328
surgical outcomes of VA healthcare
system, 264–265
teamwork training, 83
VA healthcare system, 135, 209